NAVIGATING THE ADULT SPINE

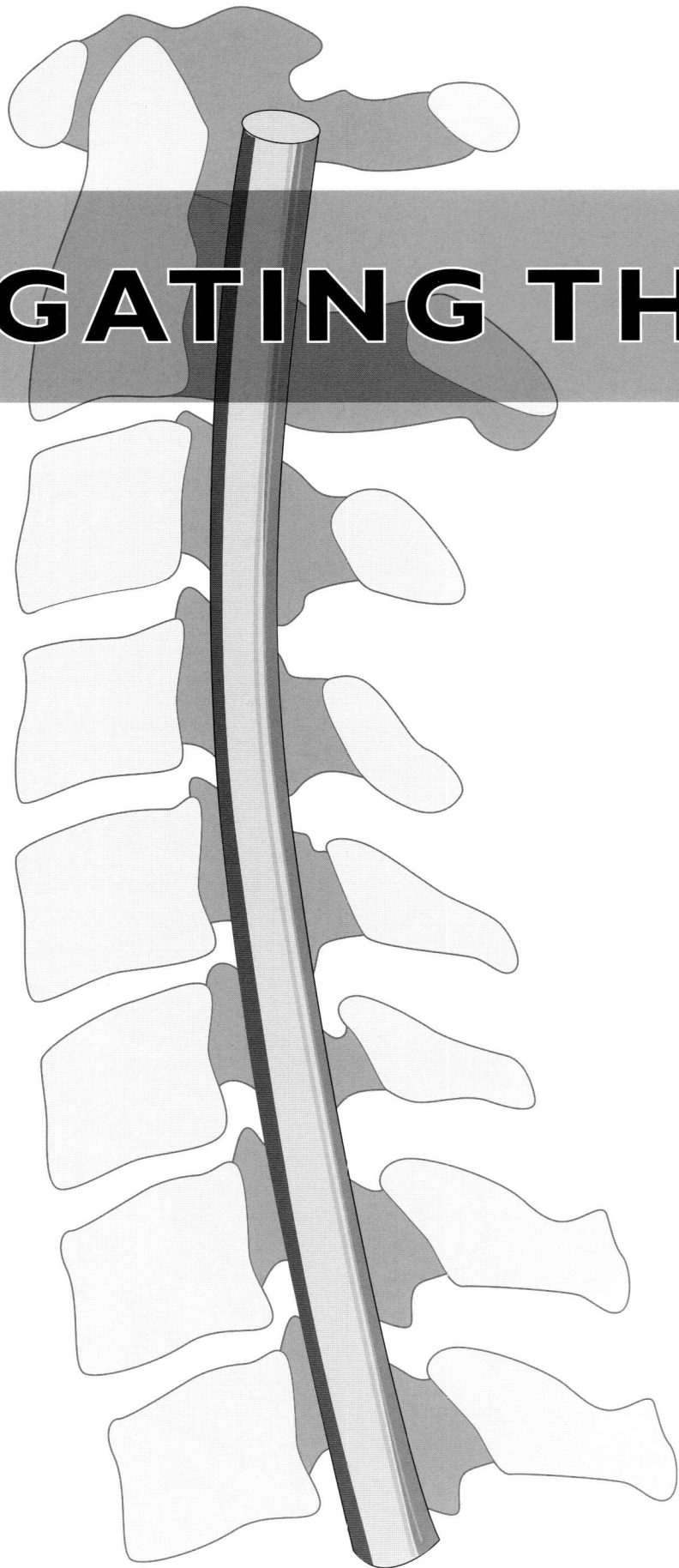

NAVIGATING THE

ADULT SPINE
BRIDGING CLINICAL PRACTICE AND NEURORADIOLOGY

Avital Fast, MD
Professor and Chairman
Department of Rehabilitation Medicine
Albert Einstein College of Medicine
Montefiore Medical Center
Bronx, NY

Dorith Goldsher, MD
Director, MRI Institute and Neuroradiology
Department of Medical Imaging
Rambam Health Care Campus
  and
Senior Lecturer in Medical Imaging
The Ruth and Bruce Rappaport Faculty of Medicine
Technion—Israel Institute of Technology
Haifa, Israel

Illustrations by Oliver Funk

Demos

DEMOS MEDICAL PUBLISHING, LLC
386 Park Avenue South
New York, New York 10016

Visit our website at www.demosmedpub.com

LIBRARY OF CONGRESS CATALOGING-IN-PUBLICATION DATA
Fast, Avital, 1947–
Navigating the adult spine : bridging clinical practice and neuroradiology /
Avital Fast, Dorith Goldsher ; illustrations by Oliver Funk.
p. ; cm.
Includes bibliographical references and index.
ISBN-13: 978-1-888799-98-9 (hardcover)
ISBN-10: 1-888799-98-6 (hardcover)
1. Spine—Diseases—Treatment. 2. Clinical medicine. 3. Spine—
Abnormalities. I. Goldsher, Dorith. II. Title.
[DNLM: 1. Spinal Diseases—diagnosis. 2. Spinal Cord Diseases
—diagnosis. 3. Spinal Cord Diseases—therapy. 4. Spinal Diseases
—therapy. WE 725 F251n 2007]
RD768.F37 2007
616.7'3—dc22
2006020444

Designed by Steven Pisano

MANUFACTURED IN THE UNITED STATES OF AMERICA

06 07 08 09 10   5 4 3 2 1

This book is dedicated to our families in gratitude for their unwavering support.

CONTENTS

PREFACE

Physicians from wide-ranging disciplines such as physiatry, gerontology, neurology, internal medicine, orthopedics, and neurosurgery frequently encounter patients complaining of spinal pain. Although most patients with neck or back pain do not require a major workup, and their symptoms remit or resolve within a few weeks, some suffer from serious ailments that may compromise their quality of life or result in permanent disability or death. For patients with spinal disorders such as malignancy or infection, timely diagnosis is critical and may improve the patient's chances of recovery.

Diagnostic tools such as computed tomography (CT) and magnetic resonance imaging (MRI) provide important information that enhance the physician's ability to understand the origin of the patient's complaints and make the most appropriate therapeutic choices, be they conservative or surgical. Frequently, however, X-rays, CT scans, and MRI examinations are ordered and the reports provided from the radiologist are read without the referring physician personally viewing the actual images. On many occasions, only the radiologist's conclusions are read, while the full radiological report is ignored. Though this approach may be expeditious, it does not assure the best possible care. Ignoring the actual films may deprive the physician of key information and lead to wrong therapeutic decisions. Furthermore, in many instances the radiologist who interprets the films is provided with scant clinical information or receives none at all. All he or she can do is report what is seen without being able to correlate the neuroradiological material with the patient's clinical history and physical examination. As a result, the referring physician is frequently provided with a "menu" of neuroradiological abnormalities affecting various spinal levels, many of which, or sometimes most of which, bear no clinical relevance.

Careful clinical correlation between the patient's history, physical examination, and imaging studies may help both the radiologist and the referring physician identify the structures and processes responsible for the patient's symptoms.

Our book is designed to serve as an introductory guide for those physicians who strive to enhance their clinical skills and ability to provide excellent care to patients suffering from axial pain due to spinal diseases. The clinical presentation of various diseases is presented along with basic critical imaging studies. It is hoped that after reading this book physicians will become familiar with the clinical history, the salient physical findings, and the correlating imaging studies of spinal disorders.

CONTRIBUTORS

Yizhar Floman, MD
Professor Emeritus of Orthopedic Surgery
Hebrew University Hadassah Medical School
Chief, Israel Spine Center
Assuta Hospital
Tel Aviv, Israel

Julian Sosner, MD, FAAPMR, FIPP
Associate Professor of Clinical Physical Medicine and
    Rehabilitation and Pain Medicine
New York Medical College
Valhalla, New York
    and
Chairman and Residency Program Director
Department of Rehabilitation Medicine
St. Vincent Catholic Medical Centers of New York,
    Manhattan Division
New York, New York

NAVIGATING THE ADULT SPINE

ANATOMY OF THE SPINE

The spinal column consists of vertebrae, intervertebral discs, ligaments, and muscles.

VERTEBRAE

There are seven cervical, twelve thoracic, five lumbar, and five sacral vertebrae. The coccyx consists of up to five fused segments. Vertebral shape and size vary in different regions of the spine. Figures 1-1A, 1-1B, and 1-1C demonstrate typical cervical, thoracic, and lumbar vertebrae, respectively, as seen from the front, in a lateral view, and from above. It can be clearly seen that the lower vertebrae, which carry a heavier load, have larger and stronger vertebral bodies.

The pedicles connect the vertebral bodies to the posterior elements—laminae and spinous processes. Their contours can be clearly seen in plain films in the AP views. The superior and inferior articular facets are also clearly seen (Figures 1-2A, 1-2B, and 1-2C).

The orientation of the facet joints, which is different in the cervical, thoracic, and lumbar regions, has a great impact on spinal stability and mobility. In the cervical region the superior articular facets face cranially and posteriorly, thus providing some stability in forward motion while allowing significant mobility. The thoracic facets are oriented in the coronal plane, thus preventing forward motion, whereas the lumbar facets are oriented mostly in the sagittal plane, preventing axial rotation and lateral movement of one vertebra in relation to neighboring vertebrae while allowing flexion and extension. The transverse processes can be identified in plain films. A progressive increase in the space between the articular facets is noted in the caudal end of the spinal column. This allows for the development of lumbar lordosis. The transverse processes of the upper six cervical vertebrae contain an additional foramen, the foramen transversarium, in order to accommodate the vertebral arteries. The transverse process of the seventh cervical vertebra does not have a foramen transversarium (Figure 1-3).

The spinal canal occupies the space between the posterior wall of the vertebral bodies and the discs, and the anterior aspect of the laminae and

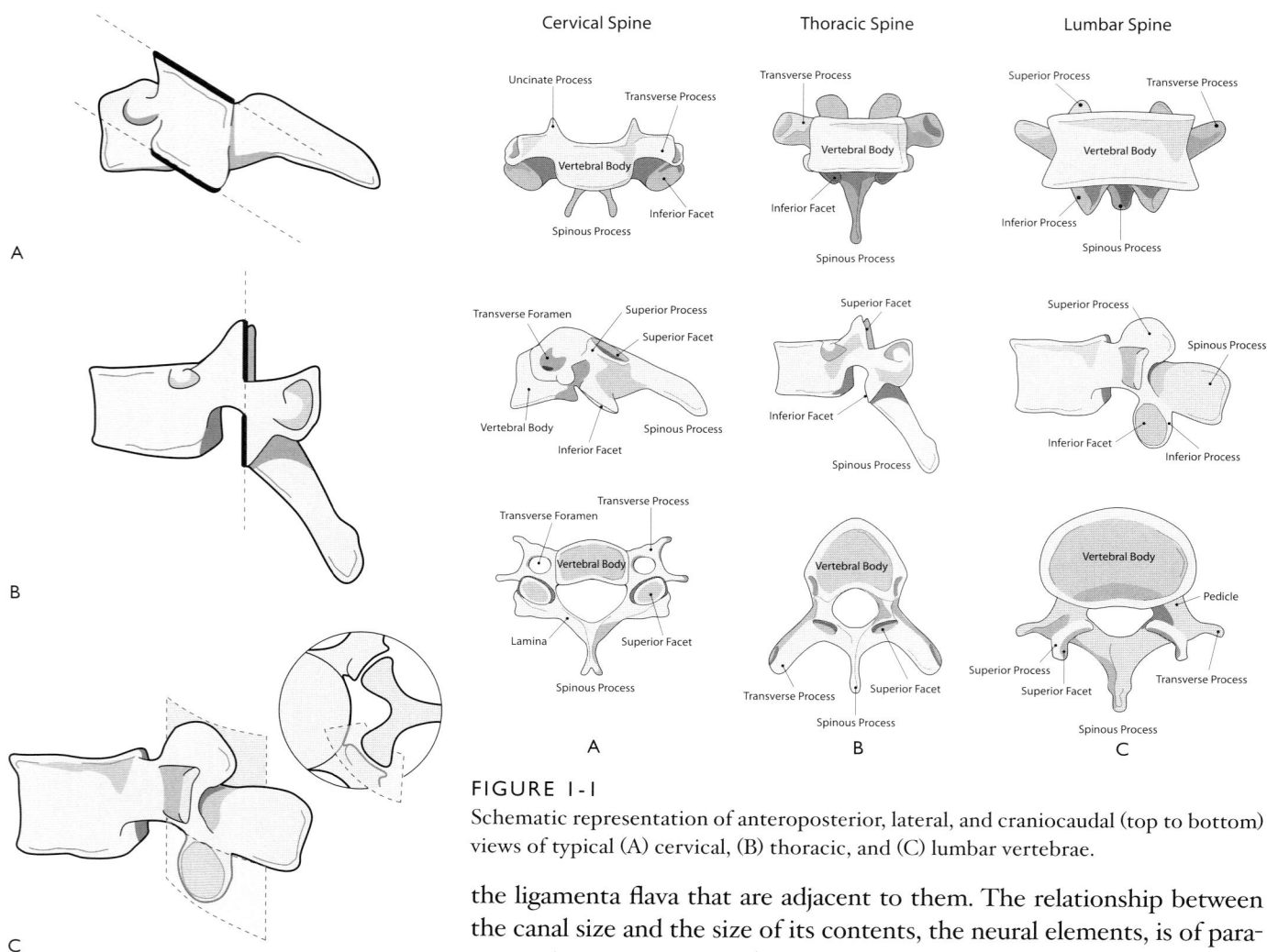

A

B

C

FIGURE 1-2
Schematic representation of the orientation of articular facets of a typical (A) cervical, (B) dorsal, or (C) lumbar vertebra.

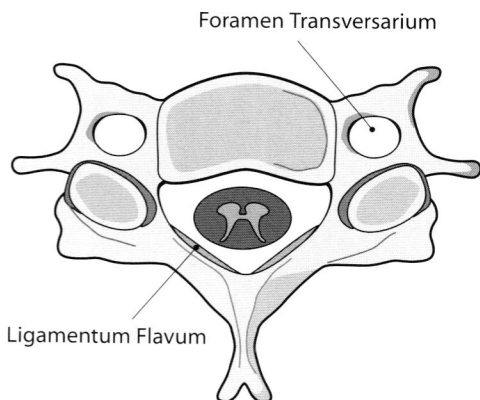

FIGURE 1-3
Schematic representation of transverse process of a typical cervical vertebra. Note the foramen transversarium.

Cervical Spine   Thoracic Spine   Lumbar Spine

A   B   C

FIGURE 1-1
Schematic representation of anteroposterior, lateral, and craniocaudal (top to bottom) views of typical (A) cervical, (B) thoracic, and (C) lumbar vertebrae.

the ligamenta flava that are adjacent to them. The relationship between the canal size and the size of its contents, the neural elements, is of paramount importance. In tight spots such as the thoracic spine region, the spinal cord fills most of the available space. Here, even a moderate-sized space-occupying lesion, such as a herniated disc or tumor, may lead to progressive, severe neurological compromise due to cord compression. In the lumbar region, however, where the canal is wider, lesions of the same size may remain asymptomatic for a long time because there is ample space left for the nerve roots to move away from the offending structure.

Spinal Canal and Neural Elements

The spinal canal contains the spinal cord and the nerve roots. The spinal cord, which is the continuation of the brain stem, extends from the foramen magnum to the L1-L2 level. The lower tip of the spinal cord—the conus medullaris—is a cone-shaped structure pointing downward that contains the centers for micturition and defecation. Because it is shorter than the spinal column, its lower segments do not correspond with the vertebrae at the same level. Below the L1-L2 level the spinal canal contains the lumbar and sacral nerve roots, which exit through their respective foraminae. As they course down toward their exit points they form the cauda equina.

There are eight cervical nerves. The first through the seventh cervical nerves exit above their respective vertebrae. The eighth cervical nerve exits the spine between C7 and the first thoracic vertebra (Figure 1-4). As a result, all the nerves below C8 (thoracic, lumbar, sacral) exit the spine below their respective vertebrae (e.g., T7 nerve root exits under T7 vertebral body).

The nerves exit the spine through the intervertebral foraminae. The anterior "wall" of the foramen is formed by the posterolateral region of the vertebral bodies and discs. The "ceiling" and "floor" are formed by the pedicles, and the posterior "wall" is formed by the facet joints. The dorsal root ganglia are located within the intervertebral foraminae (Figure 1-5).

The Cervical Spine

The first two cervical vertebrae, C1 and C2, are known as the atlas and the axis, respectively. C1 and C2 are anatomically very different from the rest of the cervical vertebrae. The first cervical vertebra, the atlas, does not have a vertebral body per se; it has been incorporated into the dens. It consists of a ring. The anterior arch of this ring is rather short and stays in close proximity to the dens. The posterior arch of the atlas is much longer in order to accommodate the spinal cord (Figures 1-6A, 1-6B, and 1-6C).

The superior articular facets of C1 articulate with the occipital condyles, and the inferior articular facets articulate with C2. There is no intervertebral disc between the C1 and C2 vertebrae. The second cervical vertebra, the axis, carries the odontoid process upon which the atlas rotates. The odontoid process "articulates" with the posterior aspect of the anterior ring of the atlas and remains close to it in all positions, including flexion. It is kept in this position by the transverse ligament. The atlanto-axial complex can be well visualized in plain films in lateral and open mouth views (Figures 1-7A and 1-7B). Finer details of this region can be obtained with CT and/or MRI scans.

The C3 through C7 vertebrae have a quadrangular shape with sagittal diameter shorter than the coronal one. They bear a ridge on their superior posterolateral aspect—the uncinate process. These ridges add lateral stability to the mobile cervical spine and protect the exiting nerve roots from lateral disc herniations (Figure 1-8).

The "articulations" between the uncinate processes and the vertebral bodies above them, the joints of Luschka, are not true synovial joints.

The cervical nerve roots exit the spine between the uncinate processes and the facet joints. Uncinate process degeneration is a common cause of nerve root compression and may result in cervical radiculopathy. The cervical intervertebral foraminae are not well demonstrated on plain lateral films. In order to better visualize them, an oblique view should be obtained. Normally the foraminae look like inverted tear drops. The nerve roots are located in the upper one-third of the foramen and are surrounded by fatty tissue. The foraminae may be well demonstrated on oblique plain films and axial CT and MR images (Figures 1-9A and 1-9B).

The diameter of the cervical spinal canal can be roughly estimated on lateral views of the cervical spine. The anterior border of the canal can be easily identified: it is the posterior border of the vertebral bodies. The

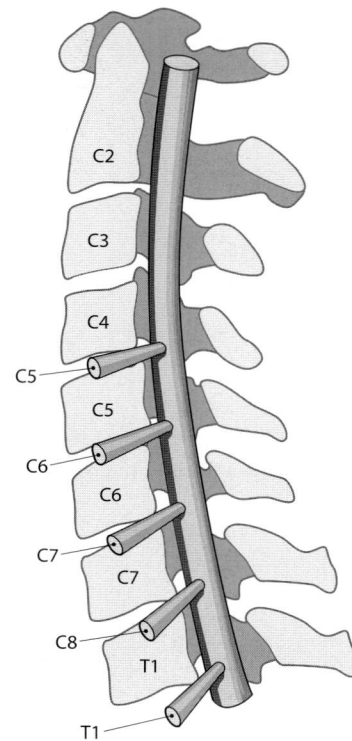

FIGURE 1-4
Schematic representation of exit points of cervical nerve roots along the cervical spine. Note that C8 nerve root exits the spine between C7 and T1 vertebral bodies.

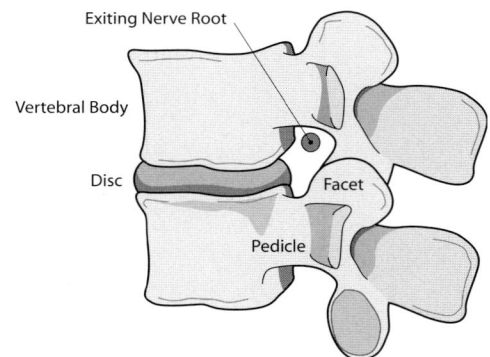

FIGURE 1-5
Schematic representation of location of the nerve root within the upper third of the intervertebral foramen.

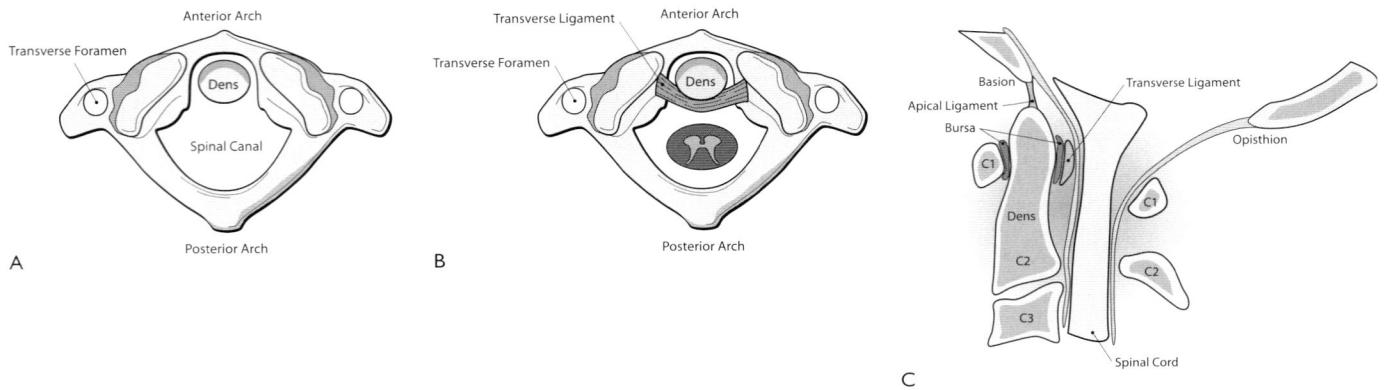

FIGURE 1-6
Schematic representation of axial view of the first cervical vertebra, or axis (A). The transverse ligament is tightly bound around the dens and keeps it close to the anterior arch of the atlas and away from the cord, as seen in (B) axial view and (C) sagittal view.

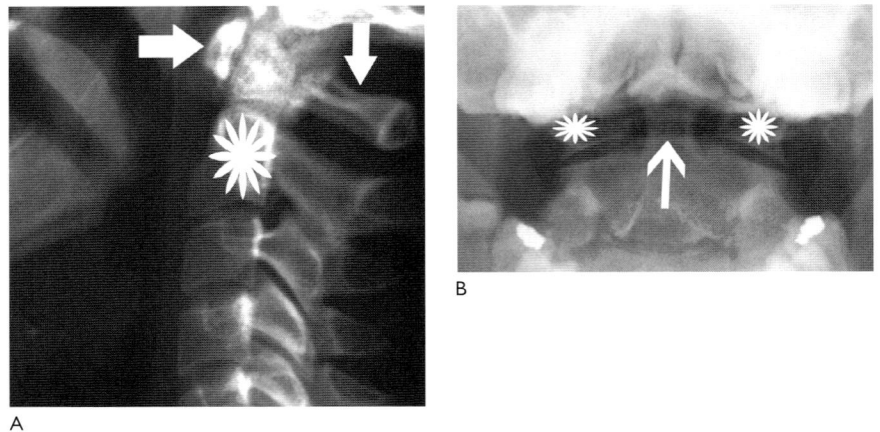

FIGURE 1-7
Plain films of the atlanto-axial complex. (A) Lateral view showing the second vertebral body (star), the anterior arch of C1 (horizontal arrow), and the posterior arch (vertical arrow). Note the odontoid process between them. (B) Open mouth view. Stars indicate the lateral masses of C1 in the coronal plane. The arrow points toward the odontoid process.

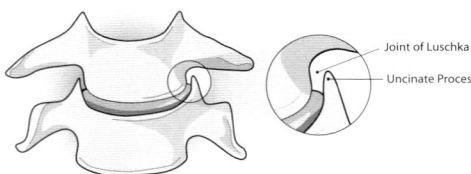

FIGURE 1-8
Schematic representation of the joints of Luschka in the coronal plane.

posterior spinal canal border is formed at the spot where the laminae meet to form the spinous process—the spinolaminar line (Figure 1-10).

The Thoracic Spine

There are twelve thoracic vertebrae. The lower thoracic vertebrae are larger than the upper thoracic vertebrae and resemble the lumbar vertebrae. The thoracic spine has less mobility than the cervical or the lumbar spine. Its stability is enhanced mostly through the rib attachments and their connection to the sternum and also by the coronally oriented facet joins. As a result of its limited mobility the thoracic spine does not tend to degenerate as much as the cervical and lumbar regions. In the anteroposterior (AP) view, the thoracic pedicles appear as vertically oriented dense calcific oval rings that are perpendicular to the vertebral bodies (Figure 1-11). The distance between the pedicles should be evaluated. Increased interpedicular distance may suggest the presence of an expanding intraspinal lesion. All the pedicles should be visible in

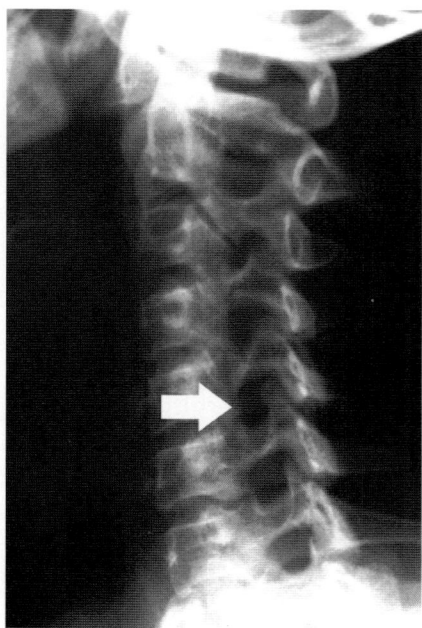

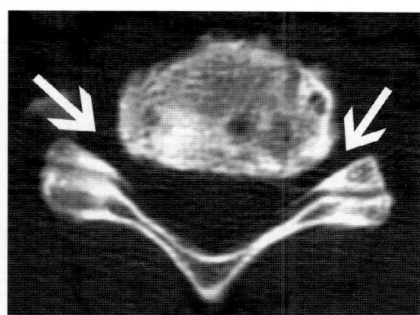

A

FIGURE 1-9

Plain film of an oblique view of the cervical spine (A) and axial CT cut (B) demonstrating the intervertebral foraminae (arrows).

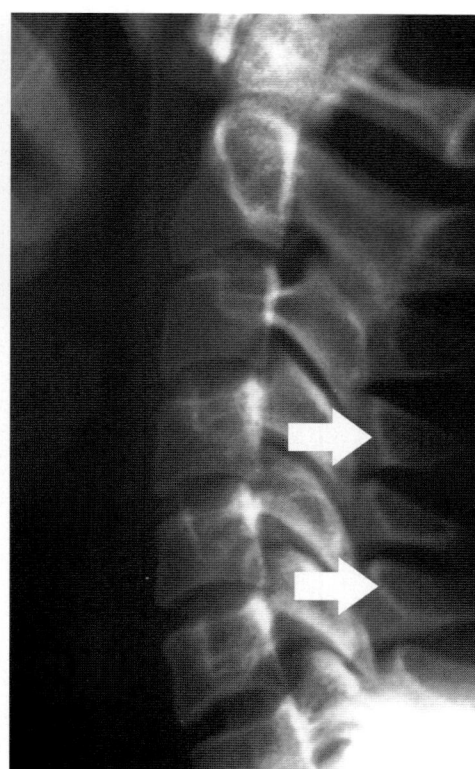

FIGURE 1-10

The spino-laminar line is demonstrated on lateral plain films (arrows).

the AP view. An absent pedicle may be the first clue to the presence of a bone-destroying lesion and should be diligently worked up.

Whenever an attempt is made to number the thoracic vertebrae, as is frequently done when pathology is found, one should start from the top and count from C2 downward, as the C2 vertebra can be easily identified. When films do not include the cervical spine, the last rib-carrying vertebral body should be identified. This should be considered as T12, and then the rest can be numbered cranially. The thoracic and lumbar intervertebral foraminae can be well identified on lateral spinal views because they are parallel to the vertical axis of the vertebral bodies (Figure 1-12).

The Lumbar Spine

There are five lumbar vertebrae. These vertebrae are the largest in the body as they bear the heaviest load. Their shape can be best assessed in the lateral view. The AP view allows good visualization of the pedicles, transverse processes, and psoas shadows (Figure 1-13). Oblique views clearly show the "Scottie dogs" (Figures 1-14 and 1-15). The "nose" represents the transverse process, the "front leg" the inferior articular process, the "ear" the superior articular process, the "body" the lamina, and the "eye" the pedicle. Special attention should be devoted to the "dog's neck," which is the pars interarticularis. A break in this region exists in up to 6% of the population and is called spondylolysis. Should the break occur bilaterally, it may compromise the stability of the spine and lead to vertebral slippage called spondylolisthesis. The upper lumbar facet joints are oriented mostly in the sagittal plane, whereas the lower facets are oriented more coronally (Figure 1-1A).

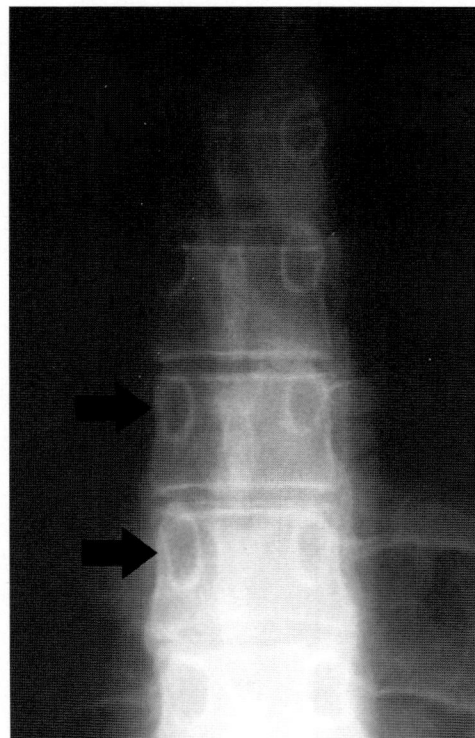

FIGURE 1-11

AP view of the dorsal spine in a plain film demonstrating the pedicles (arrow).

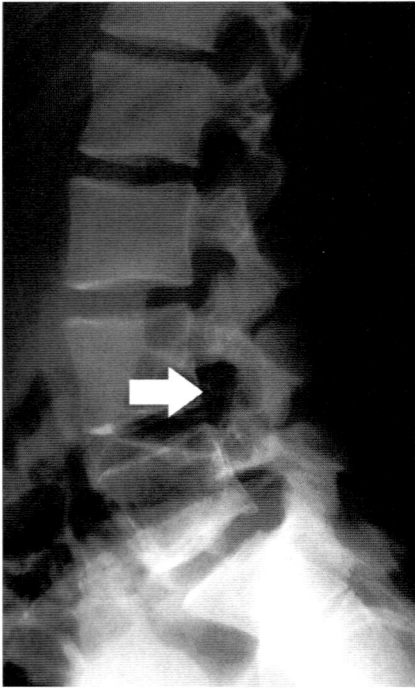

FIGURE 1-12
Plain film of the lumbar spine showing the intervertebral foramina on a lateral view (arrow).

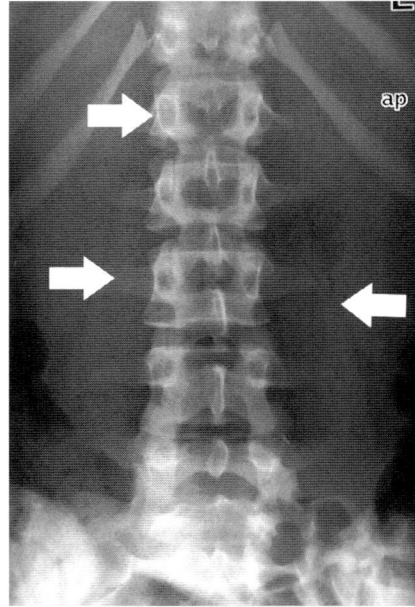

FIGURE 1-13
AP view of the lumbar spine indicating the pedicle (upper arrow), transverse process (lower arrow same side), and the fat stripe bordering the psoas shadow (contralateral arrow).

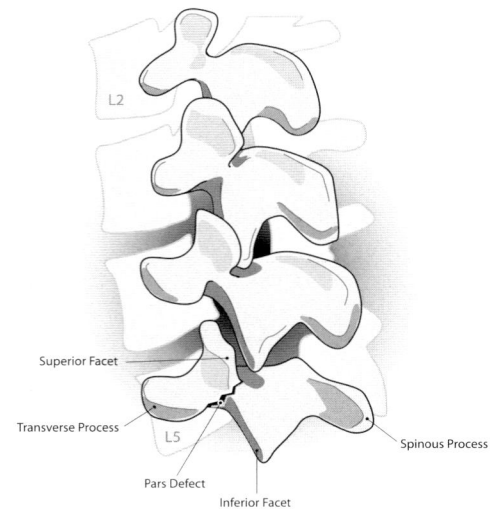

FIGURE 1-14
Schematic representation of the Scottie dogs as they appear in the oblique view.

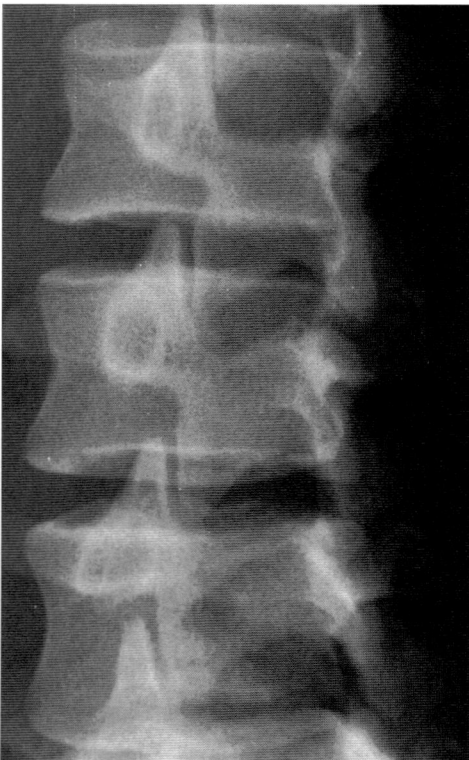

FIGURE 1-15
Plain X-ray (oblique view) demonstrating the Scottie dogs.

The Sacrum and Coccyx

The five sacral vertebrae and the articular processes of the last four sacral vertebrae are fused together to form the sacrum. The superior processes of the first sacral vertebra articulate with the inferior processes of the L5 vertebra. There are four pairs of anterior and posterior sacral foraminae. The sacral spinal canal is triangular in shape and is relatively large, providing ample space for the cauda equina. The anterior rami of the S2 through S5 roots conduct the parasympathetic fibers that are responsible for the bladder and rectum.

The sacrum joins the iliac bones at the sacroiliac joints. These are remarkably stable joints that may become completely fused with aging. The stability of the sacroiliac joints is maintained by massive, dense ligaments. The coccyx is shaped like a bird's beak. It consists of four or five fused vertebral bodies. The first two coccygeal vertebrae carry rudimentary transverse processes. The sacrococcygeal joint is a symphysis joint and has some mobility. Minimal or no motion exists in the rest of the coccygeal segments. The sacrococcygeal ligaments enhance stability and fix the coccyx to the sacrum.

INTERVERTEBRAL DISCS

The intervertebral discs are large fibrocartilaginous structures that connect the vertebral bodies while allowing significant mobility. These excellent load-bearing shock absorbers maintain the distance between the vertebrae, thus preserving foraminal patency. They also resist shear stress. The discs consist of two major parts: the nucleus pulposus and the annulus fibrosus. The nucleus pulposus consists of ground substance containing cells, collagen (mostly type II), and proteoglycans that have a high water-retaining capacity. Normally the nucleus consists of up to 90% water. With aging, the water-retaining capacity of the discs decreases, and the discs tend to lose height.

The annulus fibrosus surrounds the nucleus as a multilayered crisscrossing set of rings and attaches to the vertebral bodies. The periphery of the annulus consists of dense collagen with low water retention capacity. The inner annulus is less dense and lacks the organization of the outer annulus.

Adult discs have no blood supply and are, metabolically, tenuously maintained. Their nutrition is provided by diffusion from end plate blood vessels.

Healthy normal discs are not visible on plain X-rays. They appear simply as the space available between the vertebral bodies (Figure 1-16). The intervertebral discs can be visualized on CT or MRI studies. The contours of the discs can be easily determined on axial cuts when the cuts are parallel to the discs. The easiest way to determine whether an axial slice goes through the disc is by identifying the facet joints in the same cut. Their presence in the slice confirms that the cut is through the disc, as they occupy the same level (Figure 1-17).

LIGAMENTS

Several important ligaments contribute to and enhance spinal stability: the anterior and posterior longitudinal ligaments, the ligamenta flava, and the interspinous and supraspinous ligaments.

The anterior longitudinal ligament (ALL) is more extensive than the posterior longitudinal ligament (PLL). It extends from C1 to the sacrum and attaches to the anterior aspect of the vertebral bodies, mostly at the cranial and caudal portions of the vertebral bodies, and to the anterior aspect of the intervertebral discs. The PLL extends from the axis to the sacrum, is located within the spinal canal, and is attached to the posterior wall of the vertebral bodies as well as to the discs. In the lumbar region the PLL narrows and decreases in thickness.

The ligamenta flava are located just anterior to the laminae and are attached to them. They tend to get thicker and stronger in the low thoracic and lumbar regions. Spinal degeneration exposes the ligamenta flava to added stress, which causes them to hypertrophy and thicken. This may contribute to canal narrowing, known as spinal stenosis (Figure 1-18).

The interspinous ligaments are located between the spinous processes and are attached to them, whereas the supraspinous ligaments attach to the tip of the spinous processes and extend from C7 to the sacrum. The ligaments are not visible in plain films. The best radiological modality that allows visualization of the ligaments is MRI. As the ligaments have a very low water content they will appear hypointense on T1 and T2 weighted

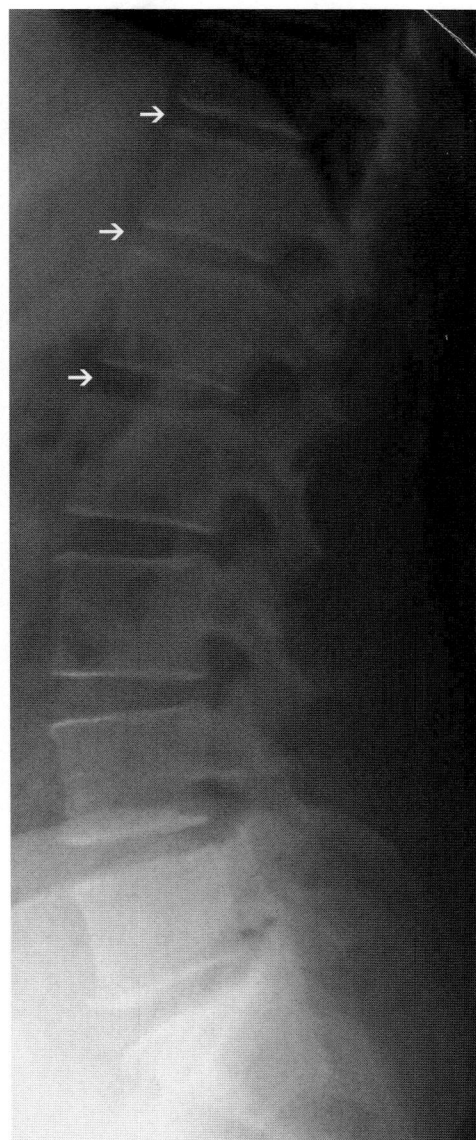

FIGURE 1-16
Lateral plain film demonstrating the spaces between the vertebral bodies that represent the intervertebral discs.

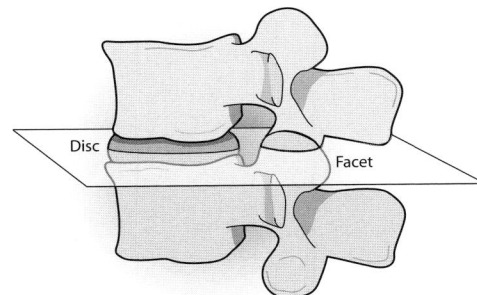

FIGURE 1-17
Schematic representation of the lumbar spine demonstrating the axial plane through the disc and the facet joints.

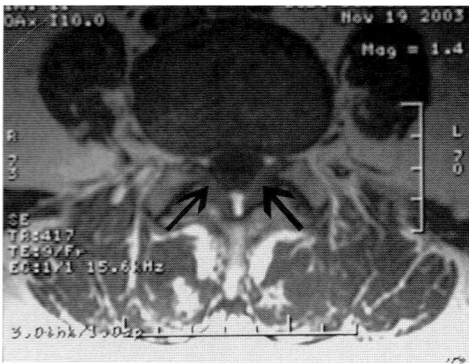

FIGURE 1-18
Axial MRI (T1-weighted image) showing thickened ligamenta flava (arrows).

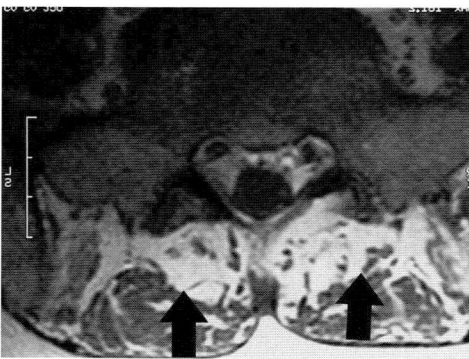

FIGURE 1-19
Axial MR image (T1WI) showing fairly massive fatty infiltration of the paraspinal / retrovertebral muscles (arrows).

images. The anterior and posterior longitudinal ligaments can be easily identified on sagittal cuts, whereas the ligamenta flava, especially when thickened, can be well demonstrated on both sagittal and axial cuts.

MUSCLES

Spinal stability is further enhanced by muscles that are attached to the transverse and spinous processes. The most extensive muscles belong to the extensor group. Some of these muscles are unisegmental and extend over a short distance, and thus have little leverage, whereas others cross over several vertebral bodies and have a much greater mechanical advantage. These muscles tend to undergo fatty degeneration and atrophy in people with a sedentary lifestyle, in aging individuals, and in patients with chronic back pain (Figure 1-19).

Bibliography

Boden SD, Riew KD, Yamaguchi K, Branch TP, Schellinger D, Wiesel S: Orientation of the lumbar facet joints: Association with degenerative disc disease. J Bone Joint Surg Am 78: 403–411, 1996.

Bogduk H: The lumbar disc and low back pain. Neurosurg Clin N Am 2: 791–806, 1991.

Bogduk N: The anatomic basis for spinal pain syndromes. J Manipulative Physiol Ther 18: 603–605, 1995.

Bogduk N: The anatomy and pathophysiology of neck pain. Phys Med Rehabil Clin N Am 14: 455–472, 2003.

Bogduk N, Cole AJ, Herring SA, eds.: Anatomy and biomechanics, pp. 9–26 in Low back pain handbook: A guide for the practicing clinician, 2nd edition. Hanley & Belfus, 2003.

Cavanaugh JM, Cuneyt Ozaktay A, Toshihiko Yamashita H, King AI: Lumbar facet pain: Biomechanics, neuroanatomy and neurophysiology. J Biomech 29: 1117–1129, 1996.

Ebraheim NA, Xu R, Darwich M, Yeasting RA: Anatomic relations between the lumbar pedicle and the adjacent neural structures. Spine 22: 2338–2341, 1997.

Hasue M, Kikuchi S, Sakuyama Y, Ito T: Anatomic study of the interrelation between lumbosacral nerve roots and their surrounding tissues. Spine 8: 50–58, 1983.

Lawson TL, Foley WD, Carrera GF, Berland LL: The sacroiliac joints: anatomic, plain roentgenographic, and computed tomographic analysis. J Comput Assist Tomogr 6: 307– 314, 1982.

Macintosh JE, Bogduk N: 1987 Volvo award in basic science: The morphology of the lumbar erector spinae. Spine 12: 658–668, 1987.

Macnab I, McCulloch J: Anatomy, pp. 1–21 in Backache, 2nd edition. Williams and Wilkins, 1990.

Mercer SR, Bogduk N: Joints of the cervical vertebral column. J Orthop Sports Phys Ther 31: 174–182, 2001.

Mikhael MA, Ciric I, Tarkington JA, Vick NA: Neuroradiological evaluation of lateral recess syndrome. Radiology 140: 97–107, 1981.

Olmarker K, Rydevik B: Pathophysiology of sciatica. Orthop Clin N Am 22: 223–234, 1991.

Pal GP, Routal RV: Mechanism of change in the orientation of the articular process of the zygapophyseal joint at the thoracolumbar junction. J Anat 195: 199–209, 1999.

Pal GP, Routal RV, Saggu SK: The orientation of the articular facets of the zygapophyseal joints at the cervical and upper thoracic region. J Anat 198: 431–441, 2001.

Tanaka N, Fujimoto Y, An HS, Ikuta Y, Yasuda M: The anatomic relation among the nerve roots, intervertebral foramina, and intervertebral discs of the cervical spine. Spine 25: 286–291, 2000.

Ward CV, Latimer B: Human evolution and the development of spondylolysis. Spine 30: 1808–1814, 2005.

SPINAL IMAGING

2

The basic aim of diagnostic imaging is to record a pattern of densities on a film, or illumination levels on a monitor, that corresponds to and conveys diagnostic information on the size, shape, pattern, and distribution of different tissues within a patient. Familiarity with both anatomy and radiologic anatomy of the spine is a prerequisite to understanding the various disorders and pathologies that affect the spine and its components. We dedicated the first chapter to describing anatomical details of the spine. This chapter is aimed toward introducing the main modalities currently in use for spinal imaging in medicine: X-rays, computed tomography (CT), and magnetic resonance imaging (MRI). We think it is useful to shed some light on the physics behind these modalities both so that the observer will better understand the image produced and to facilitate the choice of the optimal imaging necessary for the clinical problems encountered. Each of these modalities possesses advantages and disadvantages.

This chapter briefly describes the physics behind these modalities. A better understanding of the features in the image produced and their significance will help physicians evaluate the contribution of each of these modalities for detecting and diagnosing the broad spectrum of spinal disorders.

X-RAYS

As X-rays pass through the patient, they are attenuated; they are both absorbed and scattered within the patient. The amount of attenuation is dictated by the type of tissues present and by the X-ray beam energy. The X-rays that emerge from the patient arrive at the image receptor, where they are detected and recorded.

Image formation depends on a differential attenuation between tissues. The extent of this differential determines the amount of contrast between different tissues in the image formed. The amount of attenuation depends on the radiation energy and on three tissue characteristics: atomic number, density, and electrons per gram. Density

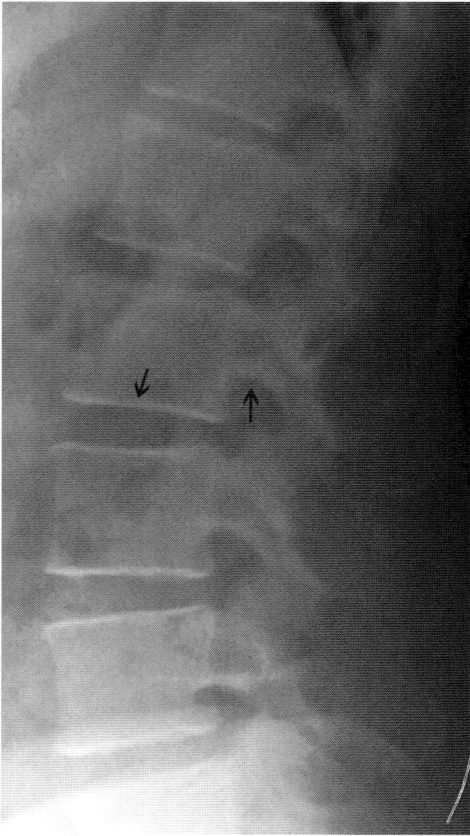

FIGURE 2-1
Plain X-ray showing the difference between the compact "white" cortical bone that surrounds the vertebral body as a thin pencil-like white line (downward arrow) and the trabecular spongy bone of lower density that appears grayish. The cortical bone that borders the pedicles (upward arrow) is usually thicker. Thin cortical bony borders envelop every element of the vertebra.

is one of the most important factors affecting attenuation, and radiographic image contrast is largely dependent on differences in tissue density. Bone (and metal) attenuates more X-rays than soft tissues and therefore will appear white on the film or screen. Different soft tissues will produce variable gray levels on the image, usually brighter than water, whereas air or gas, which are of low density, will appear black on the film or screen.

On an X-ray image the vertebrae appear as quadrangular structures with an outer layer of cortical bone that envelopes and surrounds the inner medullary portion composed of trabecular bone and bone marrow. Because the cortical bone is denser than the medullary, it appears as a white "pencil line" delineating the vertebral borders. The medullary component is more grayish, being a spongy structure of less density (Figure 2-1).

As was described in the previous chapter, each vertebra consists of multiple small elements. On a plain two-dimensional X-ray image all those small compartments or anatomical components are superimposed. Soft tissues of various densities that surround the spine are superimposed on the spine. Some of them, such as the airways in the cervical region and the lungs in the dorsal segments, contain gas that can superimpose over the cervical and dorsal spine and add to the confusion.

Air and gas in the lungs and the gastrointestinal track can produce difficulties for the observer trying to interpret plain films of the dorsal and lumbosacral spine (Figures 2-2A and 2-2B).

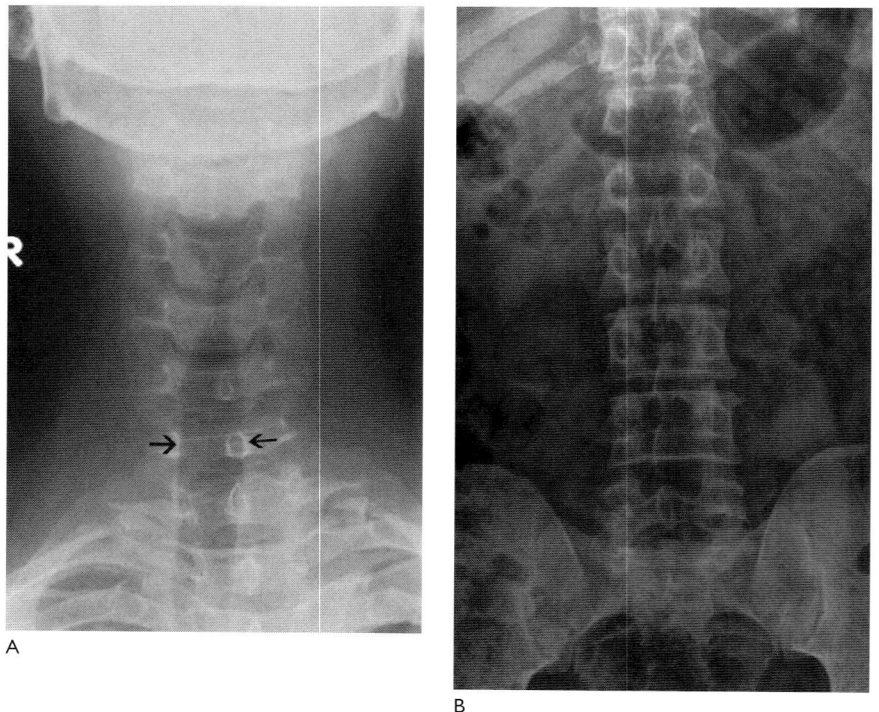

FIGURE 2-2
Plain X-rays of the cervical spine. (A) Air within the trachea appears as a dark structure (between the arrows) superimposed on the cervical spine in an AP projection. (B) Intestinal contents and air bubbles are superimposed on the lumbar spine in an AP view.

The cartilaginous intervertebral discs are not visible on a plain film, but their height can be estimated; they occupy the intervertebral spaces.

A plain film of the spinal column, taken in a lateral view, demonstrates the normal curvatures of the spine: the cervical and the lumbar lordosis and the thoracic kyphosis. A plain X-ray image of the normal spine taken in the anteroposterior (AP) direction delineates a straight column clearly showing the midline-positioned spinous processes (Figures 2-3A and 2-3B). Their alignment should be evaluated for rotational spinal injuries such as unilateral facet dislocation of the cervical spine.

A standard AP view is also the best view to study the cervical uncovertebral joints and their relationship to the neural foraminae (Figure 2-4). The AP view of the dorsal and lumbar spine shows the pedicles at each side of the vertebral bodies (Figures 2-5A and 2-5B). The pedicle size and shape as well as the interpedicular distance might point to a possibility of intraspinal space-occupying lesion (SOL). Their erosion might indicate a metastatic disease.

The lateral view demonstrates the different spinal curves: the cervical and lumbar lordosis and thoracic kyphosis. It better delineates

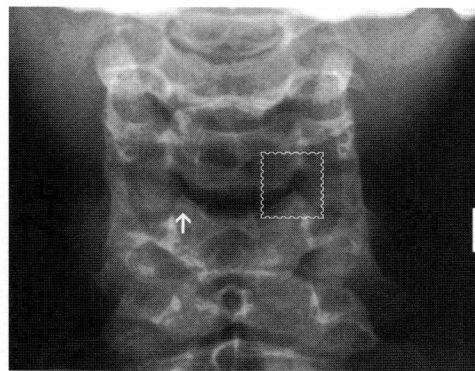

FIGURE 2-4
The uncovertebral joints of Luschka (rectangle) in the cervical spine as demonstrated on the AP projection on a plain film. The relation between the uncinate processes (arrow) and the neural foraminae can be evaluated at each level.

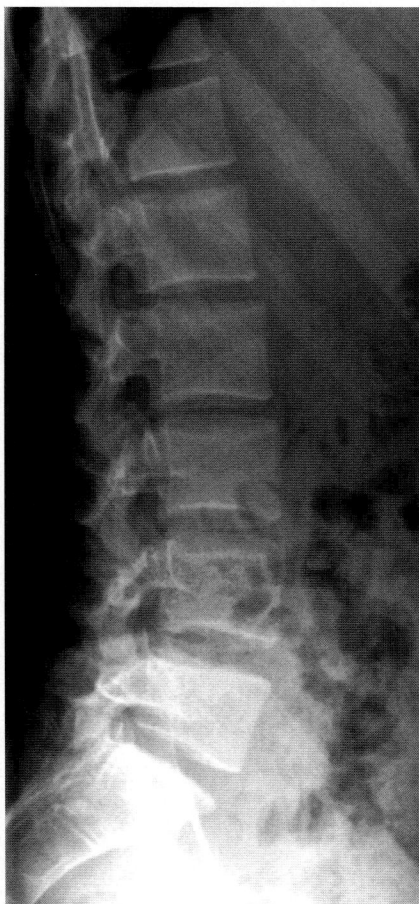
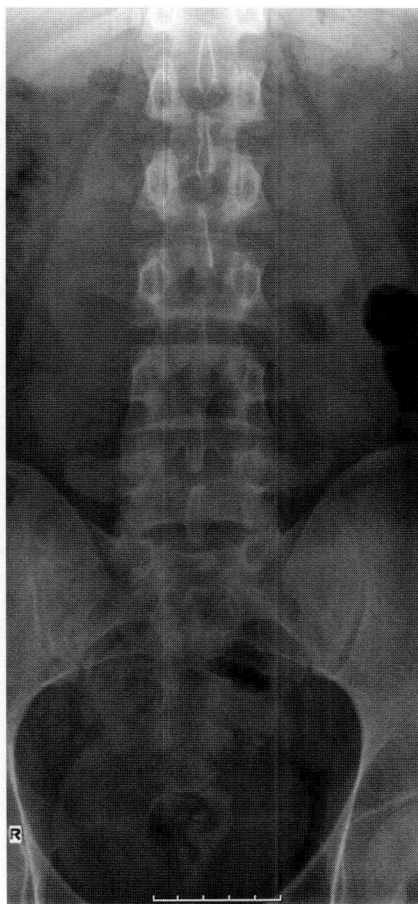

A   B

FIGURE 2-3
(A) Lateral view and (B) AP view of spinal plain films. Note that the normal spinal curvatures, the vertebral alignment, and the intervertebral spaces are better seen on the lateral view.

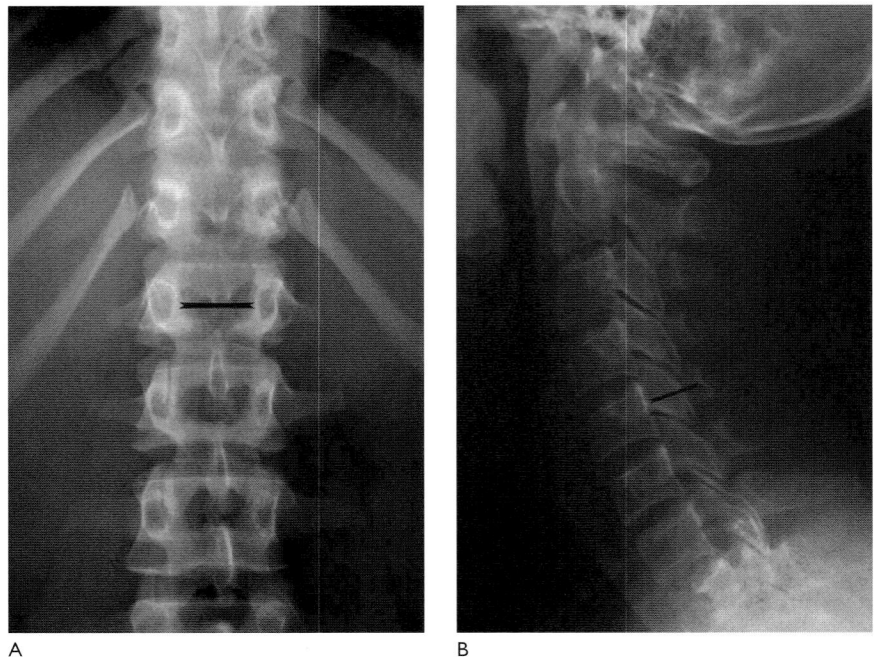

A   B

FIGURE 2-5
Spinal plain films. (A) The interpedicular distance (black line) measured on the thoraco-lumbar AP projection indicates the transverse width of the spinal canal. This distance increases gradually in the cranio-caudal direction. (B) The sagittal diameter of the spinal canal can be measured on the lateral projection by measuring the distance between the posterior aspects of the vertebral body and the spino-laminar line (black line).

the individual vertebral bodies and intervertebral spaces (compared with the AP view). It provides an excellent view of the odontoid process and its relationship to the anterior arch of the C1 vertebra (Figure 2-6A). The distance between the two should not exceed 3 mm in an adult and 5 mm in a child. On an AP view the odontoid process could be clearly seen only in an open mouth view (Figure 2-6B).

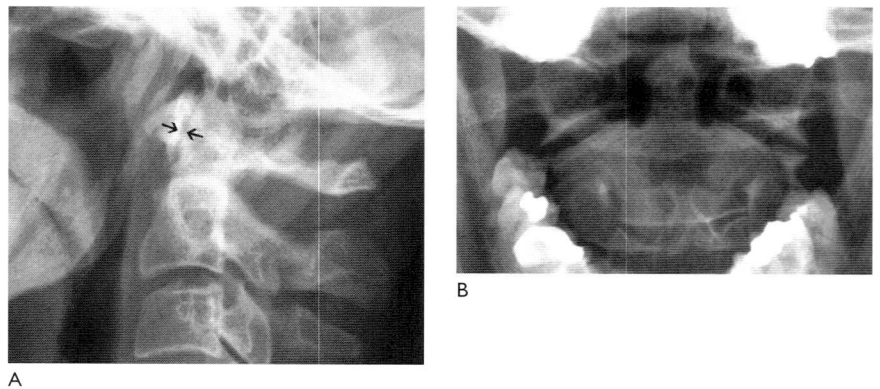

A

B

FIGURE 2-6
Plain films demonstrating the atlanto-axial complex. (A) Lateral projection allows measurements of the distance between the odontoid and the anterior arch of C1 (arrows). Note the large sagittal diameter of the spinal canal at this level. (B) Open mouth view demonstrating the relation between the odontoid and the lateral masses of the first cervical vertebra, the atlas.

The lateral view demonstrates the spinolaminar line as well as the posterior margins of the cervical facets (Figure 2-6B). A good view of the pre-vertebral soft tissue is provided.

The transverse width of the spinal canal can be roughly evaluated by the interpedicular distance on the anteroposterior view. Measuring, on a lateral view, the distance between the posterior surfaces of the vertebral bodies that represent the anterior border and the spinolaminar line, which represents the posterior border of the spinal canal, provides the sagittal diameter (Figure 2-5B). These measurements provide only a rough estimation, as there is a significant deviation between the object's actual size and its size on the film of about 20%.

The interspinous distance in the lateral view of the cervical spine is important in trauma patients.

Ossification of the posterior longitudinal ligament (OPLL) and diffuse idiopathic skeletal hyperostosis (DISH) can be easily recognized in the lateral view (see Chapter 4).

The lateral view of both thoracic and lumbar spine demonstrates the pedicles and the intervertebral foraminae, which are perpendicular to the long axis of the spinal column (Figures 2-7A and 2-7B). In the cervical spine the pedicles are obliquely oriented anteroposterior mediolaterally so that the intervertebral foraminae will be exposed

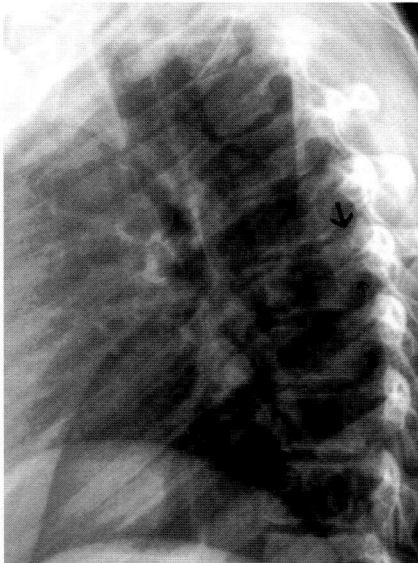

A

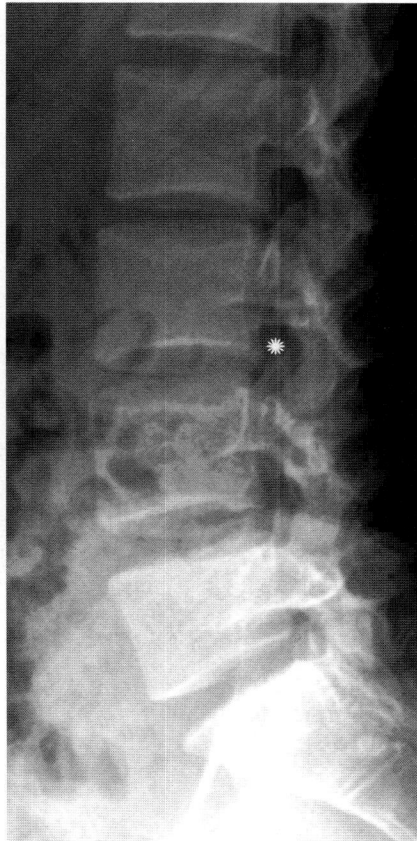

B

FIGURE 2-7
Plain films of the (A) thoracic and (B) lumbar spine. The pedicles (arrows) and the intervertebral foraminae between them (star) are demonstrated in the lateral projection.

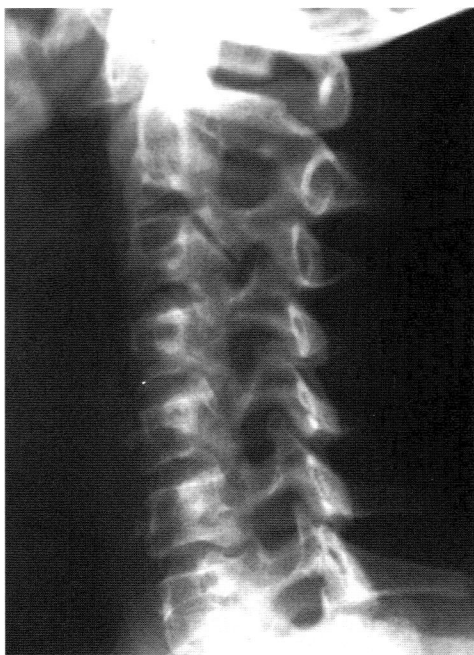

FIGURE 2-8
Plain x-rays of the cervical spine. An oblique view discloses the full extent of the pedicles and the round intervertebral foramina.

only in oblique projections. Oblique views of the cervical spine will therefore demonstrate both the pedicles, intervertebral foraminae, and the uncovertebral joints and facets (Figure 2-8).

Digital radiography should also be mentioned as it is now available and in use in modern imaging. It allows collection and storage of data on digital detectors and computers rather than on hardcopy films. It should be mentioned that digital images may be read on film, computer monitors, or video screens.

Advantages of Plain Radiographs

The advantages of plain X-rays are their high availability, quick turnaround time, and the ability to capture the spine in different positions such as flexion and extension views, thus having the possibility to evaluate the spine dynamically. Plain X-ray radiographs show the shape and the main anatomical components of the vertebrae as well as their alignment along the spinal column.

X-ray imaging is still an important tool in trauma assessment when fractures, dislocations, subluxations, and spondylolisthesis may be detected, although CT is now considered the modality of choice. Plain X-ray images are useful in the diagnosis of the following clinical problems:

- Cervical or lumbar instability (flexion or extension)
- Spondylolysis
- Rule out metal foreign bodies (prior to MRI)
- Cervical spine fracture
- Position of orthopedic devices

Plain films are also useful in studying the position of bone grafts, pedicle screws, plates, and cages. Trauma patients can be better assessed by a CT scan.

Disadvantages of Plain Radiographs

The disadvantages of plain radiographs are as follows:

- Low sensitivity for changes in the bony texture
- May not clearly show pathological changes, such as osteoporosis to a certain degree, intrinsic pathological foci, or defects within the medullary bone, unless they are prominent in size and extent
- Do not show the content of the spinal canal or detailed morphology of the tissues surrounding it.
- Lack of the possibility to expose the third dimension, which is easily demonstrated by CT or MRI.

MYELOGRAPHY

Myelography is an invasive procedure that has been largely abandoned for CT and MRI in most cases and is reserved at present for occasions when CT and MRI are unavailable. It is performed by injecting water-soluble contrast material containing iodine into the subarachnoid space by a spinal tap. The contrast enhances the cerebrospinal fluid (CSF) and delineates the dural sac and the nerve root sleeves emanating into the intervertebral foraminae (Figures 2-9A and 2-9B). Myelography, especially combined with CT in the so-called computerized assisted myelography (CAM), or myelo-CT, can be helpful for diagnosis of disc herniation, osteophytic impingement on cervical and lumbar roots, and cord compression. Some radiologists and surgeons insist on obtaining myelo-CT prior to surgery because it depicts finer details of the patho-anatomy. It is also helpful in detecting subarachnoid tumoral spread, drop metastasis, and arachnoiditis, as well as dilated vessels indicating vascular malformation when MRI is not available or is contraindicated (Figures 2-9C–F). Finally, CAM is sometime necessary to ascertain diagnoses such as prolapse or herniation of the spinal cord.

COMPUTED TOMOGRAPHY (CT)

Tomography was introduced to radiology during the 1930s. Whereas conventional radiological techniques produce summed images of an object, tomographic scanners rotate to divide the object and organize it into spatially consecutive, parallel image sections. The process, which was originally totally mechanical, has been improved upon by new technology. In computed tomography (CT), a computer stores a large amount of data—attenuation values—from a selected region of the body, making it possible to determine the spatial relationship of the radiation-absorbing structures within it. The computed tomogram consists of a matrix of attenuation values depicted in various shades of gray, thereby creating a spatial image of the scanned object. Attenuation is measured by detectors aligned behind the patient, opposite the X-ray source. The attenuation values measured by CT are reproducible. Important diagnostic information about tissues in the scanned regions of interest is obtained.

For technical realization of computed tomograms, the number and quality of data from individual picture elements, or the degree of spatial resolution, increases in proportion with the number of attenuation measurements taken from different angles.

There are basically four different types of CT scanning systems:

1. Single-detector rotate-translate systems (first generation). A fine X-ray beam scans the body through 180 steps of 1°. The intensity of the beam is measured by individual contralateral detector elements. After each angular increment, a (linear) translation is made as the beam traverses the body. A minimum of several minutes is required for scanning.

2. Multiple-detector rotate-translate systems (second generation). A detector array with 5 to 50 elements is located contralateral to the X-ray source. A pencil X-ray beam or a fan beam reduces the number of angular increments required

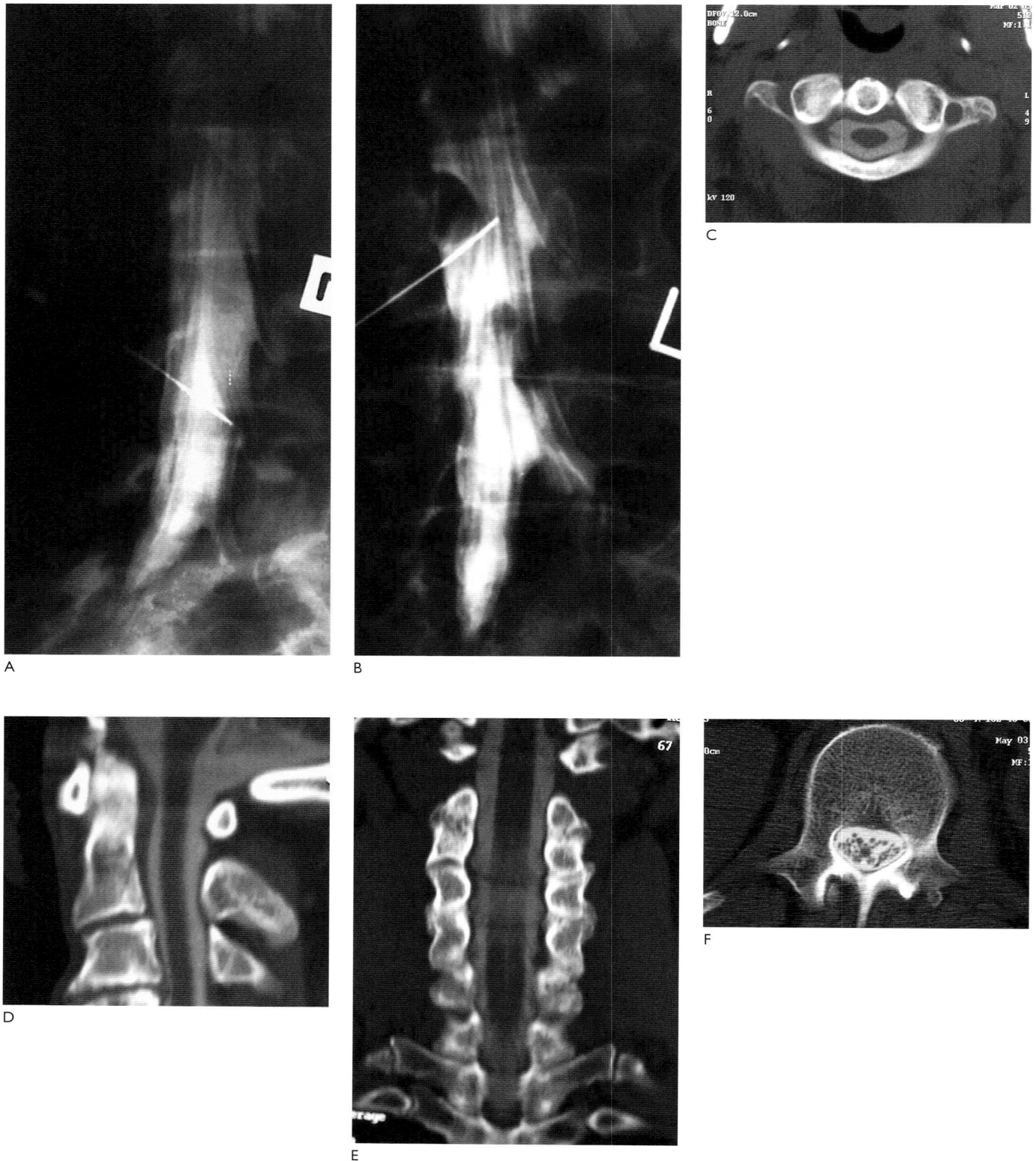

FIGURE 2-9

Lumbar myelography. (A) Oblique view of a normal myelogram. The cerebrospinal fluid (CSF) is enhanced following intrathecal injection of water-soluble, radio-opaque contrast material. The nerve roots are seen as elongated thread-like filling defects running through the enhanced CSF and emanating from the dural sac. Note the roots pushed away by the needle tip. (B) Drop metastasis are demonstrated as rounded filling defects of various sizes, scattered along the cauda equina in this pathological myelogram. (C) Myelo-CT at the atlanto-axial level showing the enhanced CSF in the subarachnoid space. Note the dark—non-enhanced—oval shape spinal cord in the center and bilateral horizontally oriented delicate roots. (D) Sagittal reconstruction of myelo-CT at the C1-C2 level. (E) Coronal reconstruction of myelo-CT through the whole cervical spine. (F) Axial cut through the tip of the conus medullaris at L1 level.

for scanning. Scans are made at steps of 10°, which corresponds to the angle of the fan beam. The minimum scan time ranges from 6 to 20 seconds.

3. Rotation scanner with movable detectors (third generation). A broad fan beam penetrates the test object and rotates around the body along with a detector array containing 200 to 1,000 detector units. The minimum scan time is 1 to 4 seconds.

4. Rotation scanner with stationary detectors (fourth generation). The angle of the fan X-ray beam covers the entire test object. The X-ray source rotates inside or outside a stationary ring detector array with 300 to 4,000 detectors in order to scan the test object. The scan time ranges from 3 to 8 seconds.

Short scanning times are desirable in spinal computed tomography, because motion artifacts can thereby be eliminated. Slow scanning systems with alternating, contrarotating movements are therefore being replaced by continuously rotating systems with faster scanning times. The attenuation values for each set of projections are registered in the computer, and the CT image is reconstructed by means of a complex computational process. The finite number of attenuation values corresponding to the scanned object is organized in matrix form. The translation of these numbers into various analogous gray levels creates a visual image of the scanned cross-sectional area. Due to their different absorptive capacities, different internal structures will be identifiable on the picture image. The size of the image matrix, more specifically the number of calculated picture elements, is dependent on the number of individual projections. Matrix size, therefore, also influences the quality of image resolution.

The smallest unit of a computed tomogram is the individual picture element, or pixel. A pixel represents a certain proportion of the total cross-sectional area or a tissue element the volume of which is determined by the slice thickness, matrix size, and diameter of the scanning field. Under these conditions, a picture element also represents a volume element, or *voxel*.

Each volume element is given a numerical value, an attenuation value, which corresponds with the average amount of radiation absorbed by the tissue in that picture element. CT density is directly linearly proportional to the attenuation coefficient, a tissue-dependent constant influenced by many factors. The attenuation coefficient quantifies the absorption of X-irradiation. In CT, attenuation values are measured in *Hounsfield units* (HU). The attenuation value of air and water (defined as −1,000 HU and 0 HU, respectively) represent fixed points on the CT density scale that remain unaffected by tube voltage. Depending on the effective radiation of the scanning device, the relationship of the attenuation of different tissue types to water attenuation will vary. Density values listed in the literature (Table 2-1) must therefore be considered as mere guidelines.

TABLE 2-1

CT Density of Spinal Structures on CT Measured in Hounsfield Units

Tissue Type	Hounsfield Units (HU)
Bone	1,000
Calcifications	100–200
Coagulated blood	50–75
Gray matter (CNS)	30–40
White matter	20–30
Cerebrospinal fluid	0
Fat	−30 to −100
Air	−1000

Each CT data value represents the arithmetic mean of all attenuation values measured in an individual volume element. The grayscale display of a scanned object alone provides some information on the relative density (radiodensity) of a structure on the image. Upon comparison with the surrounding tissue, the structure may be described as *isodense* (same density), *hypodense* (low density), or *hyperdense* (high density).

Image Variation

The attenuation values for image reconstruction, ranging from −1,000 HU to +1,000 HU, are conventionally depicted in numerous corresponding shades of gray. However, the human eye can distinguish only about 15 to 20 of these shades. If the entire density scale of 2,000 HU were to be displayed in a single image, the evaluator would be able to distinguish only a single shade of gray in the diagnostically important soft-tissue range. He or she could not visualize all densitometric nuances measurable by the computer, and important diagnostic information would be lost.

The *image window* was therefore developed as a means of producing vivid contrasts of even slight densitometric differences. The concept of the window makes it possible to expand the gray scale (*window width*) according to an arbitrarily set density range (25 to 1,000 HU). Attenuation values above the upper window limit appear white, and those below the lower limit are black on the image. The *window level* (center of the density scale) determines which attenuation values, and therefore which organ structures, are represented in the medium shades of gray.

The window adjustments must be set in accordance with the structures to be diagnosed. Narrow window widths provide high-contrast images; however, there is a danger that structures outside that window range may be inadequately demonstrated or overlooked. With broad window settings, minor density differences appear homogeneous and are thus masked. Resolution is thereby reduced.

Traditional CT Study of the Spine

Traditional CT study of the spine consists of multiple slices traversing the spinal elements in axial plains, perpendicular to the long axis of the spinal column, along its different curvatures—the cervical and lumbar lordosis and the dorsal and sacral kyphosis.

The slice thickness can be chosen to fit the desired resolution. It can go down to less than 1 mm in width, especially when multiplanar reconstructions (MPRs) are desired or needed. A smaller slice width will usually achieve better resolution, down to a certain limit. Each axial image through a vertebral body will demonstrate its shape, usually cylindrical. It contains cancellous medullary bone with trabeculae and marrow (Figure 2-10) covered by a thin layer of cortical bone delineating the vertebral body. Cortical bone delineating the posterior elements is

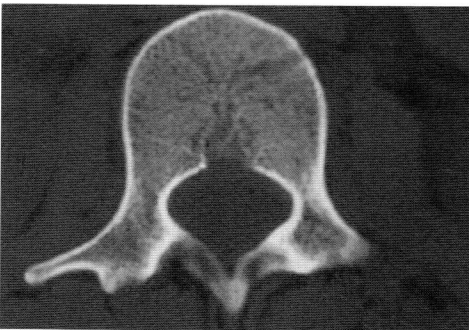

FIGURE 2-10
Axial CT cut through a lumbar vertebra showing the difference between dense compact cortical bone and the trabecular bone. Note the Y-shaped basivertebral venous plexus within the vertebral body.

thicker. At a disc level, the density of the cartilage and fibrous tissues will be lower than that of the bone yet higher—hyperdense—to that of the perivertebral muscles and of normal intraspinal components (Figure 2-11A). A normal lumbar intervertebral disc is slightly concave posteriorly in shape, except at L5-S1, where it appears rounded. The intraspinal normal epidural fat has a very low density on CT images as compared with all other spinal components. The epidural fat is more abundant at the lumbosacral level, where it is located mainly behind the dural sac, filling the triangular shape formed by the laminae, and in the lateral aspects of the spinal canal, medial to the intervertebral foramen (Figure 2-11B). The dural sac at the lumbosacral level is measured at about 0 HU and above in direct proportion to the relative amount of CSF. At the level of the dorsal spine the spinal cord appears as an oval-shaped structure of higher density surrounded by CSF. Remember that the cord tends to "take the side" of the concave aspect of the spine, or the "short way." So at the dorsal segment it will be anteriorly located and at the cervical segments it will be situated posterior within the spinal canal.

Modern CT systems can produce volumetric images so that reconstructions can be produced through the whole volume at any desirable plane with reasonable and good-contrast resolution. True sagittal and coronal images through the spine can be produced and enable evaluation of the alignment of the vertebrae and comparison of their shape and size, as well as evaluation of the width and shape of the spinal canal (Figures 2-12A and 2-12B).

The following are the major uses of CT in spinal imaging:

- Evaluation of acute spinal trauma
- Diagnosis of bony spinal stenosis
- Detection of degenerative spinal diseases
- Detection of calcification
- When MR is contraindicated or unavailable

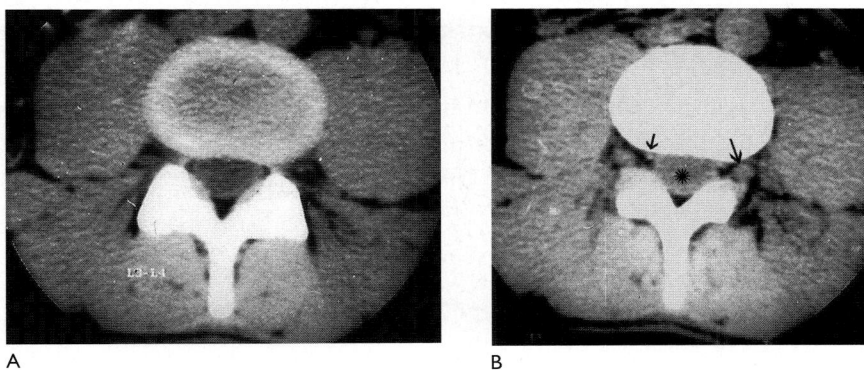

A

B

FIGURE 2-11
Axial CT slice through (A) the disc and (B) the vertebral body. The nerve roots on both sides are located within the intervertebral foramen (long arrow), the dural sac occupies most of the spinal canal (star), and epidural veins are visible (short arrow).

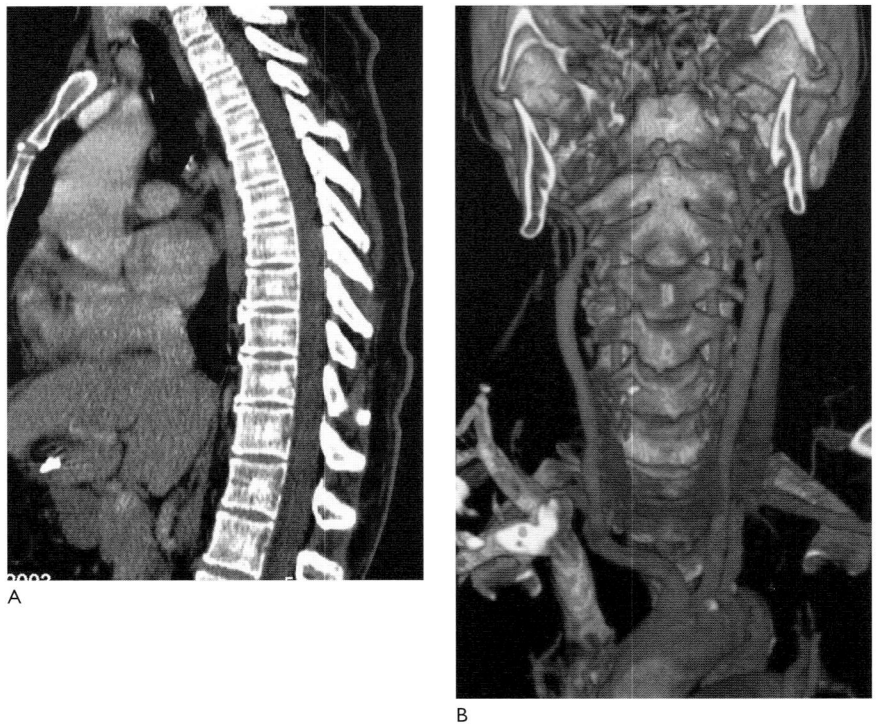

FIGURE 2-12
(A) Sagittal CT reconstruction of the dorsal spine. Sagittal diameter of the spinal canal and the discs' height can be more accurately measured and the endplates of the vertebral body are better assessed than on X-rays. (B) Three-dimensional reconstruction of the cervical spine including vertebrae, adjacent soft tissues, and the major blood vessels.

Contrast Agents in Spinal CT

Contrast agents can be used with CT studies in two fashions:

1. Intravenous injection of contrast material is indicated when pathologies such as primary or secondary tumors, or inflammatory processes are looked for, as they can enhance pathologic soft tissues within the bones or inside the spinal canal. The contrast agents used with CT contain Iodine. They harbor some contraindications as they can provoke hypersensitivity reactions and cause side effects.

2. Intra-thecal injection of contrast agents into the sub-arachnoid space is performed by a spinal tap to perform CT- Myelography or CAM (Figures 2-9C, 2-9D, 2-9E, and 2-9F).

MAGNETIC RESONANCE IMAGING (MRI)

MRI is an image modality based on an interaction between radiofrequency (RF) waves and hydrogen nuclei under the influence of a strong magnetic field. It is beyond the scope of this book to go into details of the physical principles of this imaging system. Several important facts, however, should be mentioned.

Magnets

Two main types of magnets are currently used in clinical imaging: superconductive magnets and permanent magnets. Their field strength is measured in Tesla, which is a unit of magnetic field strength that is equal to 10,000 gauss.

Superconductive magnets contain a spiral metal wire that carries electrical current and is wrapped around a cylindrical bore, thus creating a magnetic field oriented parallel to the axis of the supine patient body. These magnets require liquid helium and supercoolant liquid nitrogen, which keep the magnet cold enough to eliminate any resistance to the charge through the wire and maintain its superconductivity. The superconductive types are currently the most common in clinical and academic sites.

A *permanent magnet* is made of two bar magnets that generate a uniform magnetic field between them. This type of magnet does not require energy for maintaining its existence or strength. The patient lies supine between the two bars, and the magnetic field is oriented perpendicular to the axis of his body. These bars are composed of metallic alloys and contain iron; thus they are very heavy. For this reason these scanners are limited in field strength and reach a maximum of 0.5 Tesla or 5,000 gauss.

Coils

MRI systems contain gradient coils, which arrange the signals received from various locations within the body in the proper location in the image achieved. These coils are the main source of noise within the MRI system.

Radiofrequency receiver coils are used to receive magnetic signals from the region of interest within the body. Head and body coils both stimulate the imaged volume by transmitting radiofrequency waves and receive signals from it, while other coils are limited to receiving signals following stimulation by the body coil. These coils have limited coverage but a very high resolution and higher signal-to-noise ratio (SNR). In order to achieve high resolution without compromising the coverage, phased-array coils have been developed. One example is the modern spinal coil, which is composed of a linear array of coils electrically isolated from one another and each connected to a separate MR receiver, preamplifier, and digitizer. Each linear array covers a small segment of the spine but provides very high resolution. Signal is obtained simultaneously in order to cover as much of the spinal column as possible, and the created separate images are than combined to form one composed image of maximal coverage, SNR, and resolution.

Creating the MR Image

Under the influence of the strong magnetic field of the MR system, the hydrogen nucleus precesses at its own resonant frequency—the Larmor frequency, derived from its gyromagnetic ratio (a fundamental characteristic) and linearly related to the field strength.

Radiofrequency waves tuned to the Larmor frequency are transmitted repeatedly to the body being imaged for very short fractions of time measured in milliseconds. These bursts of energy are called *RF pulses*. Having the same frequency, the RF pulses can stimulate the hydrogen nuclei. Following the RF pulse the stimulated hydrogen nuclei tend to go back to the lower energy state and "relax" by two mechanisms. The first is termed T1 relaxation and the second T2 relaxation or T2 decay. An electrical signal is then received by an antenna—the receiving coil. All the signals derived from the volume imaged are then organized by the gradient coils to form an image.

Different tissues have different T1 and T2 relaxation times under the same magnetic field. The absolute T1 and T2 relaxation times change under the influence of different magnetic field strength but the relative differences remain (Table 2-2).

The differences in the relaxation times of different tissues are the key to the excellent contrast among them on the MR image created. To date MRI is the only imaging modality that has the ability to demonstrate and delineate clearly all spinal components and is therefore considered the best imaging modality of the spine.

Pulse Sequences

The radiofrequency waves are pulsed in a precise pattern to achieve the desired result:

Conventional spin-echo imaging. T1-weighted images (T1WI) are used for tissue discrimination. T2-weighted images (T2WI) are very sensitive to the presence of increased water and to differences in susceptibility between tissues. Usually both T1WI and T2WI are used in routine spinal imaging. The combination of signal intensities from the two sequences often allows some tissue specificity. Proton density–weighted images (PDWI) display contrast based on available mobile hydrogen proton concentration and are occasionally helpful for diagnostic specificity.

In order to emphasize T1 and T2 relaxation time effects, different pulse sequences have been developed. A spin echo pulse sequence consists of a 90-degree RF pulse that flips the longitudinal magnetiza-

TABLE 2-2

T1 and T2 Relaxation Times in Milliseconds (msec), for Different Tissues under the Influence of 0.5 and 1 Tesla Magnetic Field Strengths.

	0.5 T	0.5 T	1.0 T	1.0 T
Tissue	**T1 (msec)**	**T2 (msec)**	**T1 (msec)**	**T2 (msec)**
CSF	3000	2000	3000	2000
Gray matter	650	70	700	65
White matter	600	65	650	70
Fat	220	60	200	90
Muscle	540	50	600	40

tion of the tissue from the z-axis into the x-y plane. This is followed by a 180-degree pulse, which rephases the hydrogen protons that are dephased because of magnetic field distortions. By varying the time between the 90-degree pulses, termed repetition time (TR), and the echo time (TE), one can obtain T1WI and T2WI. Usually a short-TR and short-TE scan is T1-weighted, a long-TR long-TE scan is weighted toward T2 information, and a long-TR short-TE scan is weighted toward proton density (Table 2-3).

Another factor in scanning is the length of time before the 90-degree pulse that a 180-degree inversion pulse is placed—the inversion time (TI). This parameter can generate contrast and/or null the signal of a specific tissue in the spine, neck, or head when set to various values. Frequently used techniques in spinal imaging are fat suppression (STIR) and CSF suppression (FLAIR). The former technique is used in order to suppress the fat signal of the bone marrow, and the latter suppresses the high/bright signal deriving from the CSF, inverting it dark in T2-weighted sequences.

Fast spin echo (FSE). Fast spin echo (FSE) is used in order to achieve a more rapid T2WI. The FSE method can produce both proton density- and T2-like images in shorter scan time (up to 64 times or more) than the spin-echo images. The main difference between T2 FSE and T2 SE is the bright signal of fat tissue in the fast image, similar to that achieved with T1WI.

Gradient echo (GE). The magnetization vector of the proton is tipped off the z-axis toward the x-y plane in less than 90 degrees and a rephasing gradient pulse follows. Iron, hemosiderin, and other blood products, as well as calcium, are seen more readily in GE images. Therefore GE is valuable in post-trauma patients even months following the incidents.

Contrast Agents

The most common contrast agent used in MRI studies is gadolinium DTPA. Gadolinium is an earth element and a paramagnetic substance that causes shortening of T1 on the image. Its effect on T2 is negligible. It is injected intravenously in a peripheral vein, flows with the bloodstream, and accumulates in specific normal tissues of the spine such as the red bone marrow, dura, and blood vessels. It accumulates in pathological conditions such as lesions where the blood-brain barrier is absent or at a point of breakdown within the cord, in fibrous tissue within disc fissures, postsurgical scar tissue, and abnormal bone marrow infiltrated by primary or secondary tumors or affected by hematological disorders.

Because shortening of T1 brings about higher signal intensity on a T1WI, areas of gadolinium accumulation enhance; that is, they appear bright. To better depict these enhanced pathologies, a T1WI without contrast must precede that with contrast. The changes can then be assessed. Fat suppression can also help differentiate a bright enhancing lesion from normal bright fat. Similarly, the high intensity

TABLE 2-3

Typical Repetition Time (TR) and Echo Time (TE) for Pulse Sequences That Produce T1 Weighted Image (T1WI), T2 Weighted Image (T2WI), and Proton Density Weighted Image (PDWI).

Sequence	TR	TE
T1WI	<1,000 ms	<45 ms
T2WI	> 2,000 ms	> 60 ms
PDWI	> 2,000 ms	<45 ms

TABLE 2-4

Main Factors Influencing the Image Produced

Internal Factors	External Factors
T1	TR
T2	TE
PD	Flip angle
Flow	Contrast agents

of fatty tissue on T2 (FSE) might hide pathologies unless a fat suppression technique is applied.

MRI Features of the Spine

MRI is considered the best single imaging modality of the spine for its ability to demonstrate all of the spinal components—bone, discs, ligaments, fatty tissue, dura, CSF, neural tissue, and blood vessels—with superb contrast resolution.

Cortical bone and air both contain scarce water molecules and therefore scarce hydrogen protons. Hence they both present as a very low signal element on the MR image and therefore appear black in the image produced. The medullary bone has higher intensity in both T1- and T2-weighted images as compared with the cortical bone. The fibrous compact tissue of the outer annulus and the Sharpey's fibers have a low signal (dark) on both T1- and T2WI, whereas the nucleus pulposus, composed of fibrocartilaginous tissue with a mucoid matrix, has a high signal intensity on T2WI. In T1WI normal discs appear homogenous and the nucleus and annulus cannot be differentiated. (Figures 2-13A and 2-13B).

On axial sections, the roots of the filum terminale typically lie in a symmetric, crescent-shaped pattern with the lower sacral roots positioned dorsally and the lumbar roots positioned more anterolaterally. The most laterally positioned roots at each level are those about to

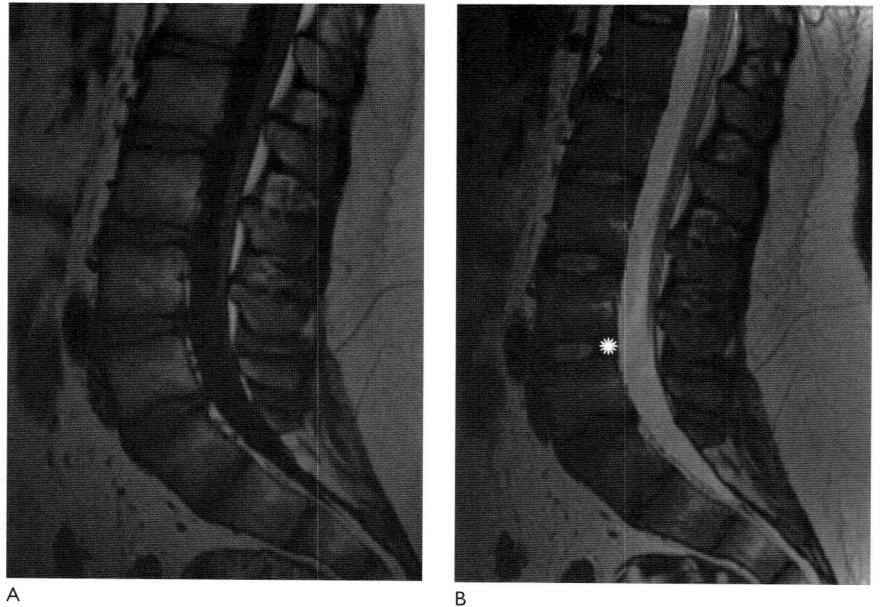

A   B

FIGURE 2-13
Sagittal T1 and T2 (FSE) MR images of the lumbar spine. (A) On T1WI the discs appear darker, of lower intensity than the vertebral bodies. Their texture appears homogenous on T1WI. (B) On fast T2WI the normal discs (nucleus pulposus) are of higher intensity than the vertebral bodies. The annulus fibrosus is darker (star) as shown at L4-L5 level and above. The disc at L5-S1 level is totally dark due to degenerative changes. Note the normal brightness (high intensity) of the CSF within the dural sac, similar to the fatty tissue in the epidural space.

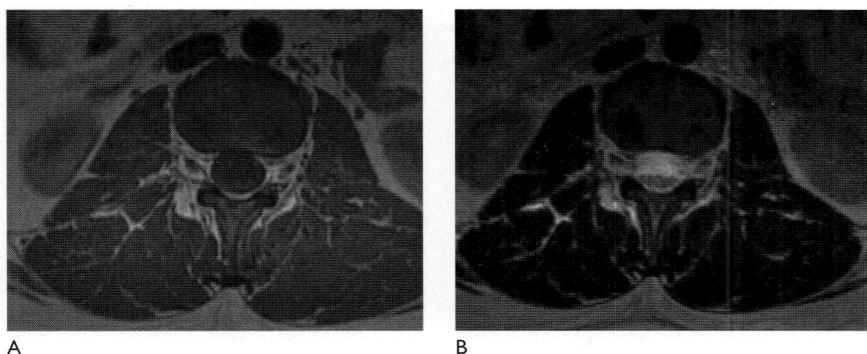

A   B

FIGURE 2-14

MR images of the lumbar spine, in axial views through the intervertebral foramimae at a level below the conus medullaris. The nerve roots (cauda equina) are located in the back of the dural sac. They appear (A) gray but brighter than CSF on T1-weighted images, and (B) dark in contrast to the high intensity of the CSF on T2WI.

exit the dural sac and pass through the intervertebral foramen. On T2-weighted images they look dark against the high-signal CSF, whereas on T1-weighted images they have moderate signal intensity and look gray as compared with the dark CSF (Figures 2-14A and 2-14B).

Using heavily T2-weighted spin-echo sequences results in MR "myelography effect" thus providing detailed definition of the thecal margins, nerve roots, and root sheaths that approaches conventional water-soluble lumbar myelograms and CT-myelography.

Sagittal T1- and T2-weighted images provide a good overview of the spinal structures. In T1-weighted images, however, the contrast between the discs, bone marrow, dural sac, CSF, and nerve roots is not as good as in T2-weighted images, in which the CSF is bright and thus provides a clearer background for the nerve roots and discs (Figures 2-15A and 2-15B). In T2-weighted images of normal discs the nucleus has a much brighter signal and can be easily differentiated from the darker annulus and the darker cortical bone. As the discs degenerate with age they lose height and desiccate. Thus they tend to lose the bright signal on T2-weighted images, resulting in a "black disc."

The spinal cord appears as a dark gray structure on T2 and is brighter than the CSF on T1-weighted images. Fatty tissue appears bright on both T1 and T2 (FSE) weighted images. The bone marrow signal depends on the patient's age. In younger individuals the red bone marrow appears darker on MRI whereas fatty (yellow) bone marrow, which is seen more frequently in older individuals, appears brighter. The basivertebral veins, the large, Y-shaped veins that provide venous drainage to the vertebral bodies, are commonly seen as bright lines entering the vertebral bodies on T2-weighted images. These veins drain into an extensive epidural venous system.

Disadvantages of MRI

MRI has certain disadvantages:

1. It has low sensitivity for calcium as compared to CT.
2. It has low sensitivity for subarachnoid hemorrhage.

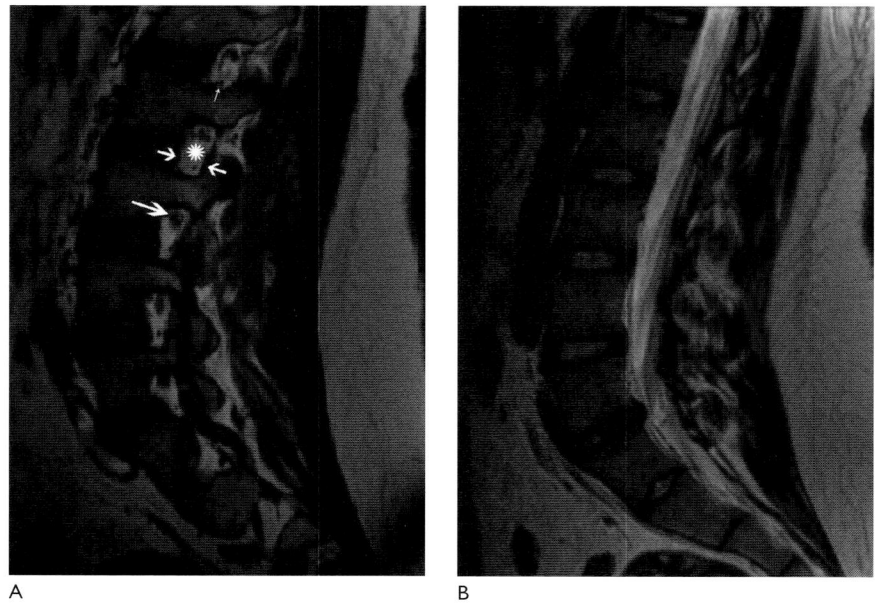

A   B

FIGURE 2-15

Sagittal MR images of the lumbar spine through the intervertebral foraminae (between short arrows). (A) The fat within the foramen (star) is of high intensity on the T1-weighted image. It provides a bright background to the low intensity of the exiting nerve root (long arrow). Note the radicular veins in the lower third of the foramen (vertical arrow). (B) On sagittal T2WI through the lateral recesses, the obliquely oriented nerve roots are demonstrated on their course toward the intervertebral foraminae.

3. Scan time is prolonged compared with CT.
4. Contraindications prevent certain patients from entering the MRI system.
5. Patients with claustrophobia cannot tolerate the study and need anesthesia.

Contraindications

Contraindications for MR imaging are dictated by the strong magnetic field in the system and by the electromagnetic radiation involved. They include both passive and active implants. The passive implants are usually made of metal, and the active include electromagnetic devices implanted in the body. At present absolute contraindications include cochlear implants, certain pacemakers, and electromagnetic devices such as neurostimulators and automatic cardioverters.

Most other implanted medical devices have become MRI-compatible during the past 20 years. Certain cardiac pacemakers have been recognized as safe under the MR system influence, and there is ongoing research to ascertain the compatibility of other active electromagnetic devices with MRI exposure. Nevertheless specific precautions are still needed prior to the patient's entrance into the MRI system. Exact details of any implants should be thoroughly checked.

Bibliography

Adams P, Eyre D, Rand Muir H: Biochemical aspects of development and aging of human lumbar intervertebral discs. Rheumatol Rehabil 16: 22–29, 1977.

Busong SC: Magnetic resonance imaging: Physical and biological principles. St. Louis, 1988, Mobsy year book.

Curry TS III, Dowdey JE, Christensen RC: Physics of diagnostic radiology, 4th edition. Murry William & Wilkins, 1990.

Grossman RI, Yousem DM: Neuroradiology the requisites, 2nd edition. Mosby, 2003.

Modic M, Massarik T, Ross J: Magnetic resonance imaging of the spine. Year book, 1989.

Newton TH, Potts DG: Computed tomography of the spine and spinal cord. Cladavel Press, 1983.

Osborne AG: Normal anatomy, chapter 19 in Diagnostic neuroradiology p 785–799. Mosby Year Book, 1994

Pech P, Haughton VM: Lumbar intervertebral disk: correlative MR and anatomic study. Radiology 156: 679–702, 1985.

Rothman SLG, Glenn WV: Multiplanar CT of the spine. Chapters 1–4, p. 1–112, chapters 16–17, p. 477–504. University Park Press, Baltimore. 1985.

St. Amour T., Hodges SC, Laakman RW, Tamas DE: MRI of the spine. Raven Press, 1993.

Stark DD, Bradley WG Jr.: Magnetic resonance imaging, 2nd edition. St Louis, 1992.

Van Den Hoof A: Histological age changes in the annulus fibrosus of the human intervertebral disk with a discussion of the problem of disk herniation. Gerontologia 9: 136–149, 1964.

Yamashita T, Minaki Y, Ozaktay AC, Cavanaugh JM, King AI: A morphological study of the human lumbar facet joint. Spine 21: 538–543, 1996.

DISC DISORDERS

3

DEGENERATIVE DISC DISEASE

Disc degeneration starts early in life and frequently progresses relentlessly. By the eighth decade the majority of individuals have diffuse disc degeneration throughout their spine. Although it is clear that disc degeneration is not synonymous with spine pain, it is well accepted that degenerative disc disease brings about a cascade of anatomic changes that play a major role in the pathophysiology of well-described clinical entities.

Pathogenesis

The pathogenesis of disc degeneration has not been completely elucidated. Multiple factors, working separately or in combination, contribute to disc degeneration. Being the largest avascular structures in the body, the discs depend on a tenuous nutritional supply that predisposes them to early degeneration. Heredity is another important factor that may contribute to disc degeneration under normal physiological conditions. Aging also plays a significant role in disc degeneration. Age-related vascular changes such as atherosclerosis and decreased vascular density, and vertebral endplate changes such as calcification, compromise discal nutrition and contribute to disc degeneration.

Mechanical factors such as repetitive trauma due to sports or occupation may also adversely affect the discs. Smoking has a negative impact on the metabolic processes within the discs, as nicotine-mediated vasoconstriction interferes with the discs' oxygen supply and nutrition.

During the degenerative process the disc undergoes both biochemical and biomechanical changes. Due to the compromised nutrition, increased lactic acid concentration, and low pH, the number of cells within the discs decreases and matrix synthesis diminishes. The proteoglycans and the water-retaining capacity of the disc decrease as well. Decreased discal height alters the load distribution in the motion segment and decreases the ability of the discs to withstand shear stress.

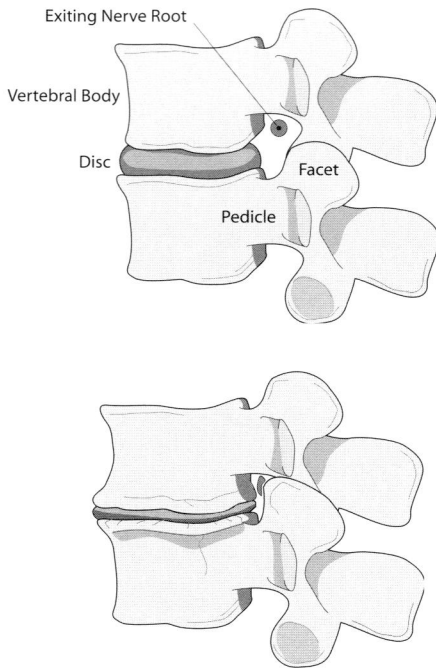

FIGURE 3-1
Schematic representation of normal lumbar spine (top) and the changes occurring secondary to degenerative disc disease. Note the severe neural foraminal narrowing due to disc thinning, disc bulging, or herniation and hypertrophy of the articular facets.

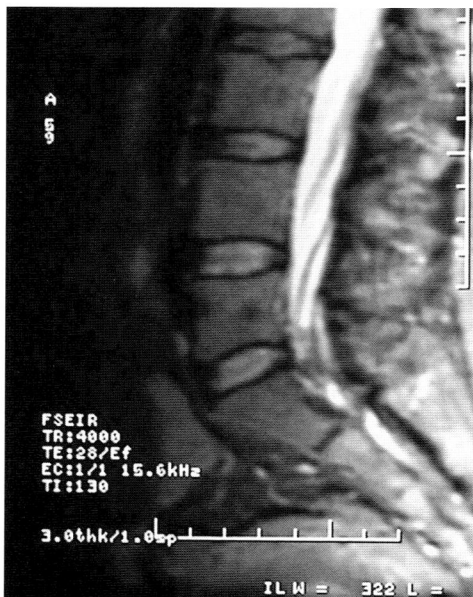

FIGURE 3-2
Sagittal MRI of the lumbar spine. Normal appearance of the intervertebral disc on T2-weighted image.

This may bring about anatomical changes in adjacent structures—vertebral bodies, facets (sclerosis), and ligaments—and result in segmental instability, spinal stenosis, and neural foraminal narrowing, which eventually lead to axial and radicular pain (Figure 3-1). At the same time, the integrity of the annulus fibrosus is compromised, and radial fissures appear that later develop into tears. Changes in the endplate region such as sclerosis and ossification may further compromise discal nutrition and oxygen supply, resulting in biochemical changes such as the release of inflammatory products into the disc, which can result in discogenic pain.

Clinical Presentation

The clinical significance of a "black disc" is still disputed in the literature. Severe multilevel degenerative changes are frequently observed in asymptomatic subjects. Often, however, patients present with axial pain without radicular symptoms, and with no instability, deformity, and tension signs such as straight leg raising and femoral stretch test. In these patients the degenerated disc is the likely cause of the symptoms. Imaging studies in these patients frequently demonstrate multilevel degenerative disc disease. The question then arises: which of the degenerative discs is responsible for the patient's symptoms? Discography can be obtained in order to determine which of the degenerated discs is symptomatic. This practice, however, has not been fully endorsed by all spine physicians and is still challenged as unreliable and, at times, potentially harmful.

When disc degeneration leads to spondylotic changes and/or instability, radicular symptoms frequently appear.

Imaging Studies

MRI: On T1-weighted images the signal of the nucleus and the annulus may look alike and also resemble the vertebral body signal. In healthy discs the nucleus pulposus and the annulus fibrosis can be easily differentiated using T2-weighted images: the nucleus pulposus appears brighter than the annulus fibrosus (Figure 3-2).

Fatty bone marrow infiltration occurs during the aging process, resulting in brighter vertebral signal whereas the disc signal becomes darker and more homogenous. The end result of this degenerative process is a "black disc," where the annulus and nucleus have the same dark signal (Figure 3-3). As the disc degenerates, nitrogen gas may accumulate within the disc and can be seen on X-rays, CT, and MRI (Figures 3-4A and 3-4B). The accumulation of gas within the substance of the disc is referred to as the "vacuum phenomenon" and is most prevalent in the lower lumbar discs (L4-L5-S1) and occasionally in the lumbar facet joints. The vacuum phenomenon is pathognomonic of the degenerative process. Occasionally gas may be seen within the spinal canal when gas-containing discal material herniates. On CT one can easily identify the gas within the canal, which attests to the presence of a disc fragment.

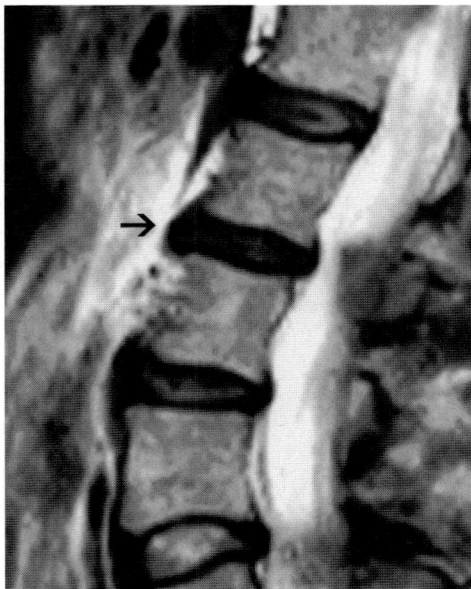

FIGURE 3-3

T2 sagittal MRI of the lumbar spine showing various stages of degenerative disc disease, as shown by the upper three black discs. The middle one is completely degenerated (arrow). The lowest disc retains a normal signal.

Over time, disc degeneration leads to abnormal loads that result in degenerative changes in the endplate region. Modic's classification of these changes has been well accepted and found to be reliable (Table 3-1, Figures 3-5A and 3-5B).

Management

Can anything be done to postpone or prevent disc degeneration or improve discs that have already degenerated? The answer to this is

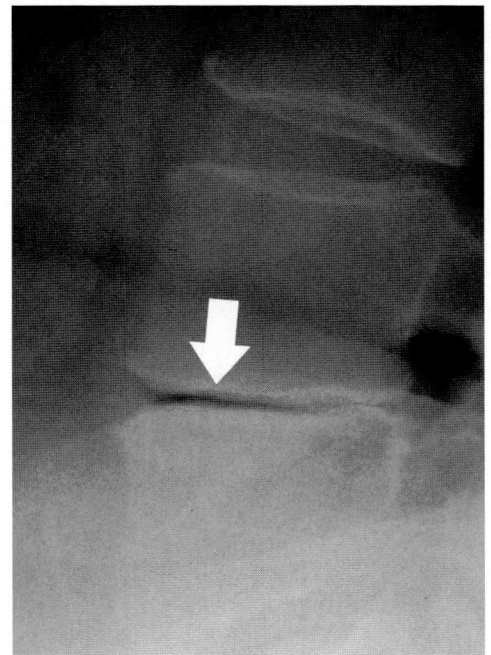

A

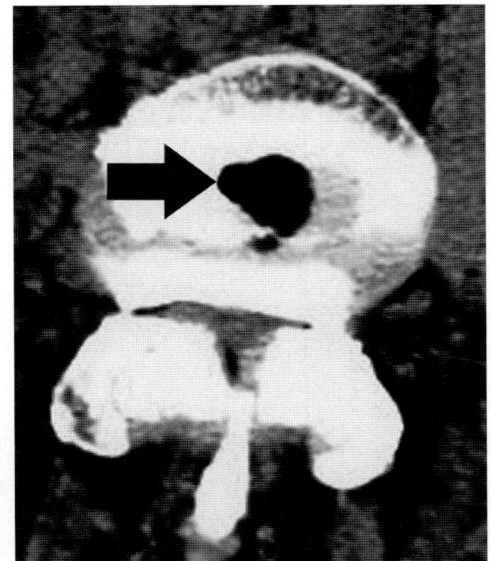

B

FIGURE 3-4

(A) Vacuum phenomenon in a degenerative lumbar disc, in a plain film. Note the traction spurs above and below the degenerated disc. (B) Vacuum phenomenon in a CT scan of a lumbar disc.

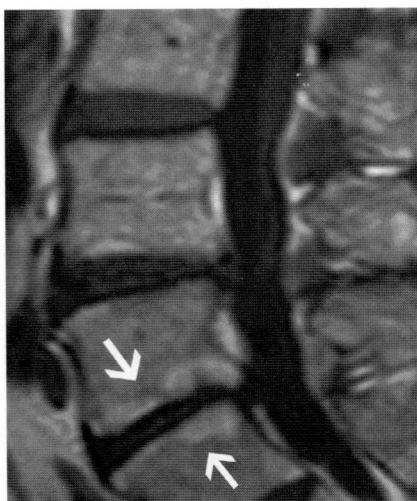

A

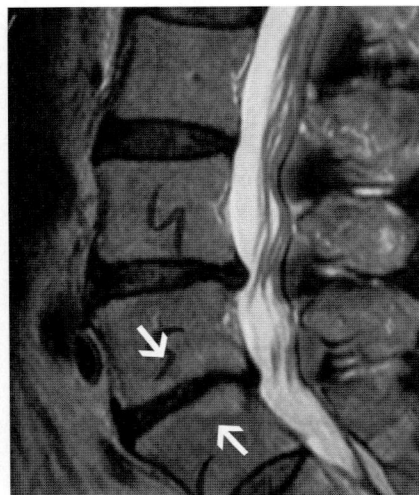

B

FIGURE 3-5

Modic type 2 changes. (A) Sagittal T1WI and (B) T2WI of the lumbar spine. In both images, the endplate region adjacent to the degenerated disc is hyperintense (arrows).

TABLE 3-1
Endplate MR Signal Changes as Described by Modic

	T1	**T2**	**Concomitant Histological Changes**
Modic type 1	Hypointense	Hyperintense	Granulation tissue within subchondral bone
Modic type 2	Hyperintense	Hyperintense or isointense	Fatty infiltration of adjacent bone marrow
Modic type 3	Hypointense	Hypointense	Endplate sclerosis

presently negative. It seems reasonable to recommend lifestyle changes such as smoking cessation, moderate levels of physical fitness, and avoidance of protracted unloading (immobilization, sedentary lifestyle) and static compressive loading. It is now apparent that the disc's metabolism is dependent on its mechanical environment; its nutrition benefits from intermittent loading, which results in fluid shifts in and out of the disc.

Intradiscal electrothermal treatment (IDET), consisting of a heat-emitting electrode that is introduced into the affected disc, may bring about pain relief in selected patients with discogenic pain. Patients who do not respond to conservative measures and have persistent severe pain frequently end up being treated with surgery. In many cases spine fusion is performed, with a reported success rate of 60–90%. This approach, however, predisposes the patient to adjacent level degeneration. Disc arthroplasty—disc replacement surgery—has been recently introduced. This approach may bring symptomatic relief while maintaining disc height and preserving spinal motion. More long-term studies are required, however, to better define the indications, long-term outcome, and complications of this type of approach.

Patients with radicular symptoms due to spondylotic changes may benefit from nonsteroidal anti-inflammatory drugs (NSAIDs), stabilization exercises, and selective nerve root blocks.

New experimental therapeutic approaches intended to reverse disc degeneration are being explored and developed. These include growth factors injections, gene therapy, and cell-based therapy. Exogenous growth factors have been shown to increase discal proteoglycan synthesis. Gene therapy, it is hoped, will target the cells within the discs and increase their metabolic activities so that they will be able to reverse degeneration. Cell-based therapy will transform marrow stromal cells into disc cells, which will then repair the damaged discs. These approaches seem promising but are still in the experimental stage.

HERNIATED DISCS

The "age of the disc" was heralded by Mixter and Barr in 1921 when, during surgery, they discovered what they initially thought to be a tumor and was found to be a herniated disc. Since that time the disc has taken a central role in spinal pathphysiology and symptomatology. The advent of CT and MRI, however, has clearly shown that quite frequently, even in the presence of a frank disc herniation, patients remain asymptomatic.

Pathophysiology

Currently most authors believe that annular tears, leading to disc herniation, occur secondary to repetitive stress, especially torsional stress, in a disc that has already undergone degenerative changes.

Annular tears initially appear in the outer layers of the annulus pulposus. Because these layers are innervated, it is reasonable to assume that these tears may elicit axial pain. The tears may progress to involve the whole annular width and subsequently may result in disc herniation. Nucleus pulposus herniation provokes a local inflammatory response, and when it is close to a nerve root, may involve and compress it and bring about radicular pain. Occasionally the herniated disc material loses its connection with the "mother" disc, resulting in a sequestrated disc. The separated piece may migrate in the canal cranially or caudally and at times may settle in the lateral recess or within the intervertebral foramen or, rarely, penetrate through the dura. There is ample documentation that extruded discs, even large ones, shrink in size over time and may, over two to three years, disappear altogether.

The direction of herniation, size of the herniated disc, and proximity to the neural elements will, to a large extent, determine the presence or absence of symptoms.

Posterolateral disc herniation will bring about radicular pain. The patient will complain of pain in the upper or lower extremity with or without axial (spine) pain.

Posteriorly directed herniations in the cervical or thoracic region may compromise the spinal cord and bring about progressive neurological deficits with bilateral long-tract signs. In the lower lumbar region posterior herniation of the same size may cause axial pain without any radicular symptoms. Large fragments, however, may compress the whole cauda equina and result in severe neurological compromise. "Pure" lateral herniations that end up in the intervertebral foramen frequently result in unremitting pain due to compression of the dorsal root ganglion (Figures 3-6A, 3-6B, and 3-6C).

Anteriorly directed herniations, however, are frequently seen on imaging studies without any clinical problems.

Clinical Presentation

In the cervical spine the C5-C6 disc is affected most often, followed closely by the C6-C7 disc. Patients affected at these levels frequently complain of numbness and pain in the lateral aspect of the forearm and hand. Herniated discs that compromise the C8 or T1 roots will lead to symptoms over the medial aspect of the arm, forearm, and hand. The pain may increase whenever the patient assumes the upright position or with head movements. Quite often, patients

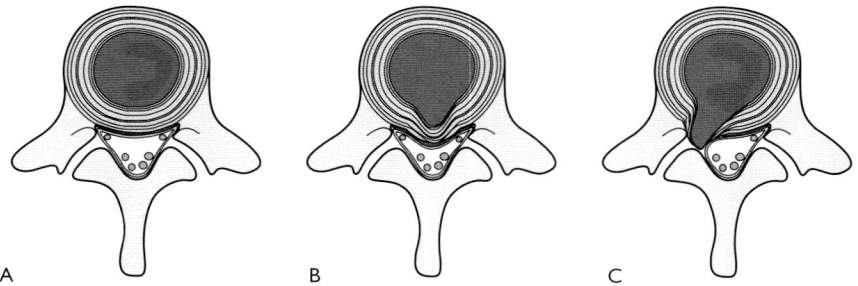

FIGURE 3-6
Schematic representation of (A) normal disc, (B) Central herniation, and (C) postero-lateral herniation into the lateral recess.

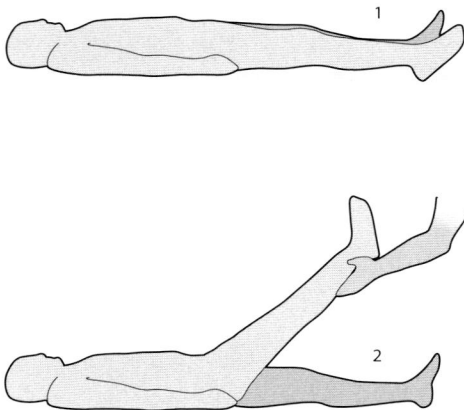

FIGURE 3-7
Straight leg raising test.

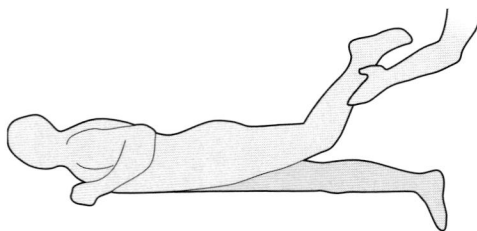

FIGURE 3-8
Femoral stretch test.

with cervical discs complain of pain in the interscapular region as well. Occasionally the pain may radiate into the chest—cervical angina. Weakness in myotomal distribution, numbness in dermatomal distribution, and reflex changes help localize the offending disc level. Posteriorly directed herniations, especially large ones, compress the spinal cord and lead to myelopathic symptoms: upper extremity weakness and atrophy and lower extremity spasticity.

In the lumbar region 90% of herniations occur at the L4-L5 and L5-S1 levels. These herniations bring about pain that is usually located below the knee region. The pain may be severe, burning, or throbbing. Typically it is worse sitting, somewhat better standing, and may be totally gone in the supine position. Some patients with severe pain prefer to remain standing during the interview process and refuse to sit down. The pain may or may not be accompanied by motor, sensory, and reflex changes. The straight leg raising test is positive in these patients. The well leg raising test, a test in which elevation of the nonpainful extremity elicits pain in the painful lower extremity, may be present as well (Figure 3-7).

Unlike patients with posterolateral herniation, who present with posture-dependent intermittent symptoms, patients with foraminal herniations frequently present with severe, constant pain that does not change even in the supine position. These patients frequently do not respond to conservative management and end up being treated with surgery. Posteriorly directed herniations frequently cause back pain without radicular symptoms and, as a result, may be more difficult to diagnose.

In the elderly population, as the lower lumbar discs have previously degenerated there is a tendency for higher lumbar disc (L1-L2, L2-L3, L3-L4) herniations. The clinical presentation in these patients is quite different than the one seen in lower lumbar herniations. The pain and sensory changes are located in the knee region, the anterior aspect of the thigh, or the hip and may simulate knee or hip pathology. Meticulous physical examination may help achieve the correct diagnosis. The Patrick test (passive flexion, abduction, external rotation of the hip) will be positive in hip arthritis eliciting groin pain whereas the femoral stretch test (reverse straight leg raising that is performed in the prone position with elevation of the lower extremity so that the hip goes into hyperextension while the knee is kept flexed) will elicit anterior thigh pain in patients with high lumbar herniations (Figure 3-8).

TABLE 3-2
Radicualr Changes in Upper Extremities

	Motor Changes	Sensory Changes	Reflex Changes
C5	Deltoid	Lateral aspect of arm	None
C6	Elbow flexors	Lateral aspect of forearm, thumb, index	Biceps jerk
C7	Elbow extensors	Middle finger	Triceps jerk

TABLE 3-3
Radicular Changes in Lower Extremities

	Motor Changes	Sensory Changes	Reflex Changes
L4	Quadriceps	Medial aspect of leg	Knee jerk
L5	Ankle dorsiflexors, hip abductors	Lateral aspect of leg, dorsum of foot	None
S1	Plantar flexors, hip extensors	Plantar aspect of foot	Ankle jerk

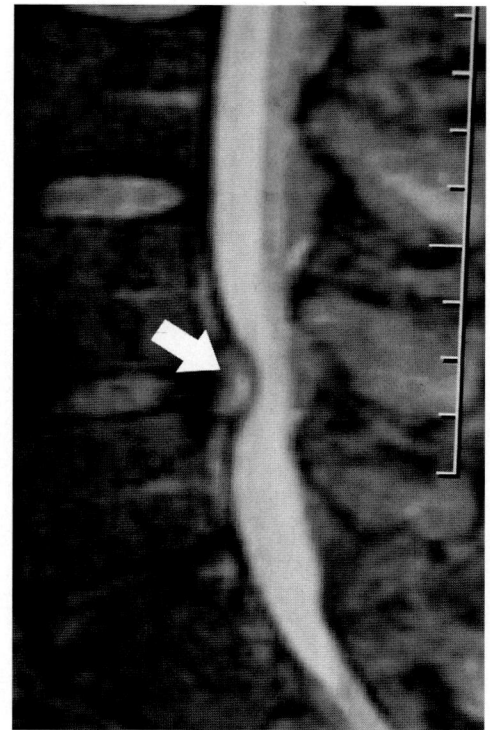

FIGURE 3-9
Sagittal T2-weighted MR image showing a high-intensity zone in a symptomatically herniated disc.

Thoracic disc herniations, although less common, are not rare and frequently involve the lower thoracic discs. They are frequently missed or diagnosed late because their pain referral pattern may confuse the inexperienced clinician. Patients usually present with axial and/or radicular pain that may be felt in the abdominal wall region or trunk, simulating intra-abdominal pathology. Not infrequently, small thoracic disc herniations are incidentally discovered on MRI films in the absence of any clinical symptoms.

Imaging Studies

Annular tears initially appear on MRI as high-intensity zones (HIZs) onT2-weighted images. These can be easily seen on sagittal and axial MRI cuts as small areas of increased signal and are usually found in the posterior or posterolateral aspects of the annulus (Figure 3-9). That region may enhance following contrast administration.

Herniated discs cannot be seen in plain films. When they herniate through the vertebral endplate, however, a situation that is frequently seen and believed to be secondary to endplate injury, they become visible. These herniations are called Schmorl's nodes. They are commonly seen in spinal X-rays as small circumscribed endplate defects that are continuous with the discs (Figure 3-10). Axial CT through such a node will show a soft tissue defect that is isodense and continuous with the disc and may be surrounded by sclerotic bony margins. MRI images will show basically the same picture. Bone marrow edema adjacent to a Schmorl's node will appear in the acute stage. It will appear hypointense on T1- and hyperintense on T2-weighted images (Figure 3-11).

Anterior herniations are commonly seen on imaging studies. They may lift the anterior longitudinal ligament and at times assume a rather larger size. On CT examination a soft tissue with density identical to that of the intervertebral disc will be seen extending anteriorly.

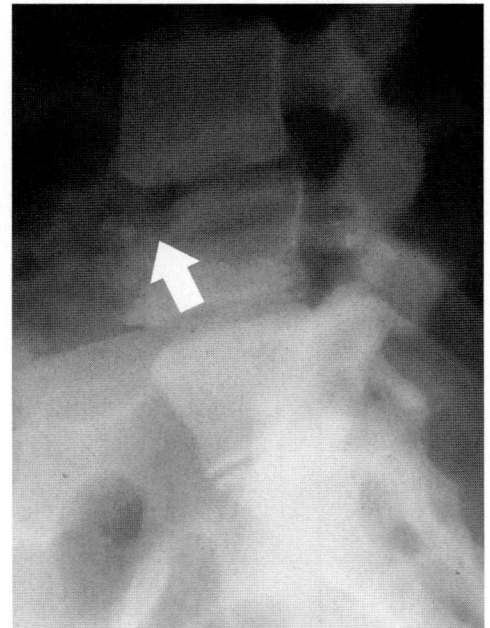

FIGURE 3-10
Anterior Schmorl's node on the upper endplate of L4 in a lateral plain film of the lumbar spine.

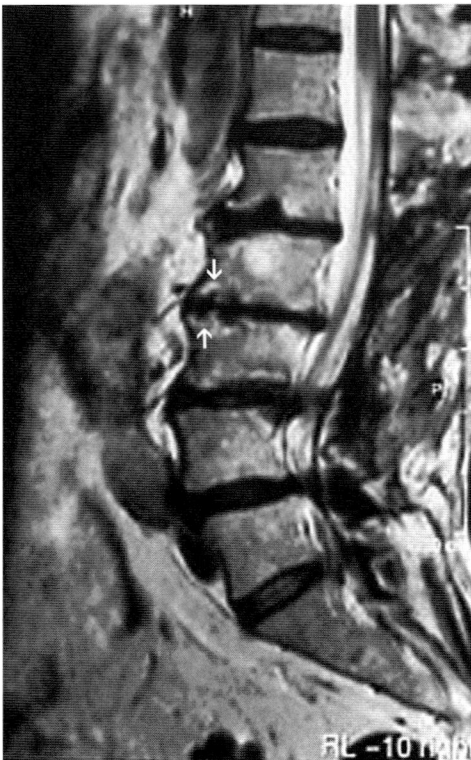

FIGURE 3-11
Sagittal T2WI showing Schmorl's nodes. Around some of them a small area of hyperintensity is seen (arrows).

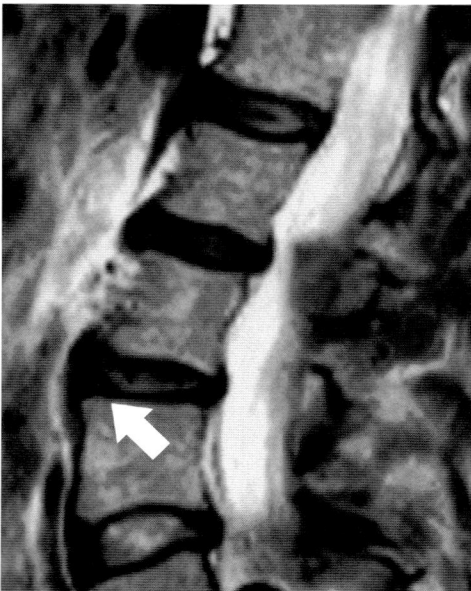

FIGURE 3-12
Sagittal T2WI of a degenerative spine. Note the anteriorly directed discal herniation (arrow).

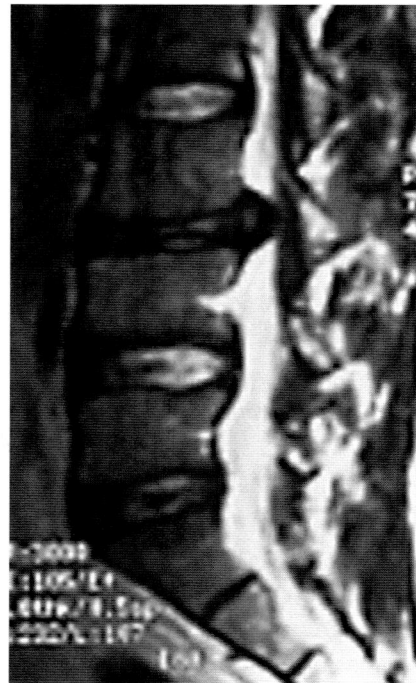

FIGURE 3-13
A large herniated disc at L3-L4 level obliterating the spinal canal.

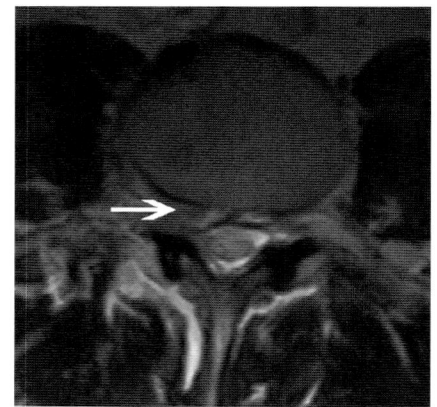

FIGURE 3-14
Right lateral disc herniation shown in post-contrast T1WI. Note the unenhanced disc fragment surrounded by a thin rim of enhanced fibrous tissue (arrow).

MRI examination will show the herniated disc to be isointense to the parent disc on T1-weighted images and isointense or hyperintense on T2-weighted films. On sagittal views the herniated disc may be seen lifting the anterior longitudinal ligament away from the anterior vertebral wall (Figure 3-12).

The direction of herniation can be easily determined on axial cuts. First one has to look for the facet joint in the particular axial image to ascertain that the cut is actually passing through the disc. The most common herniations, those that are directed posterolaterally, are fairly easily detected on CT and MRI studies. A herniated disc may be seen continuous with the "mother disc" or separated altogether from it (sequestered herniation) while retaining the same density and signal characteristic of the "mother disc" on CT and MRI studies (Figure 3-13). The herniated disc may deform the thecal sac, spinal cord, or roots. Following contrast administration the disc does not enhance.

Less frequently a "true" lateral disc herniation may occur. In a true lateral disc herniation, a piece of a disc herniates into the neural foramen, impinging on the exiting nerve root and compressing the dorsal root ganglion, which is located within the nerve root canal (Figure 3-14). This occurs more commonly at the L3-L4 level. Normally, the nerve roots are surrounded by fat within the neural foramen. This is clearly seen especially on MRI scans, in which the fat has a bright signal on T1-weighted images whereas the nerve root is darker (Figure

3-15). An extruded disc fragment within the foramen will appear dark as well and may be spotted as it eliminates part of the fatty tissue that normally surrounds the exiting nerve root.

At times the extruded piece may be small and difficult to spot. In such cases a thinly sliced CT scan (every 1–2 mm) and Myelo-CT of the suspected involved level may help in delineating the offending structure.

Postoperative patients who develop recurrent radiculopathy, at the same level as before surgery or at an adjacent level, will need an MRI examination with and without contrast. Contrast T1-weighted images are very helpful in differentiating radiculopathy due to postoperative scarring from radiculopathy due to residual or recurrent disc. Because the discs are avascular structures they do not enhance with contrast. The scar tissue, however, will enhance after contrast administration and will look brighter than the adjacent disc. The diagnostic yield can be further enhanced by obtaining contrast T1-weighted images with fat saturation. Fat suppression will allow the hyperintense scar tissue to stand out and become more visible.

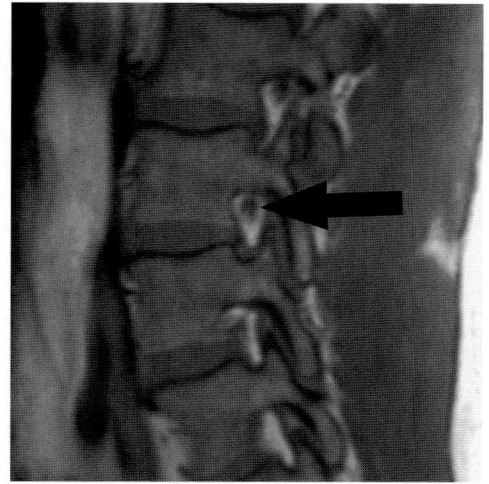

FIGURE 3-15
The dark nerve roots appear on a sagittal MR image (T1SE) surrounded by high-signal fatty tissue.

Management

Most patients with herniated discs respond to conservative care and have a positive outcome. It is expected that within three months more than 90% of herniated disc patients will feel significantly better. Anti-inflammatory drugs in combination with analgesic drugs help alleviate most of the symptoms. Cervical traction may prove beneficial in patients with C5-C6 and C6-C7 herniations. Cervical hyperextension and side bending should be avoided because these postures narrow the cervical foraminae and may bring about radicular pain. McKenzie exercises, which are specific sets of exercises that are administered by a trained physical therapist, are of paramount importance. They can lead to centralization of pain (from radicular to axial) and then can eliminate the pain altogether. Selected patients who do not respond to the above regime may benefit from a translaminar or transforaminal injection of steroids under CT guidance or fluoroscopy. Up to three injections may be administered over a period of several weeks. In addition, lifestyle modification is recommended: The patient is urged to stop smoking, refrain from long-distance driving, and incorporate physical therapy exercises into his or her daily routine.

Patients who do not respond to conservative care or who develop progressive neurological deficits should be referred for surgery.

CAUDA EQUINA SYNDROME

Cauda equina syndrome, a condition in which most or all of the lumbar nerve roots to both lower extremities are compressed by a very large disc herniation or any other large space-occupying lesion, is a medical emergency that should be promptly diagnosed and referred for surgical care without delay.

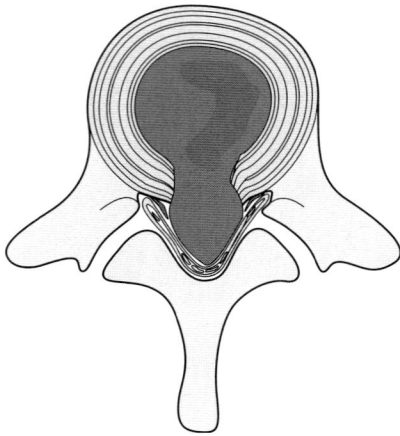

FIGURE 3-16
Schematic illustration of a huge central herniated disc filling the spinal canal and compromising the neural roots.

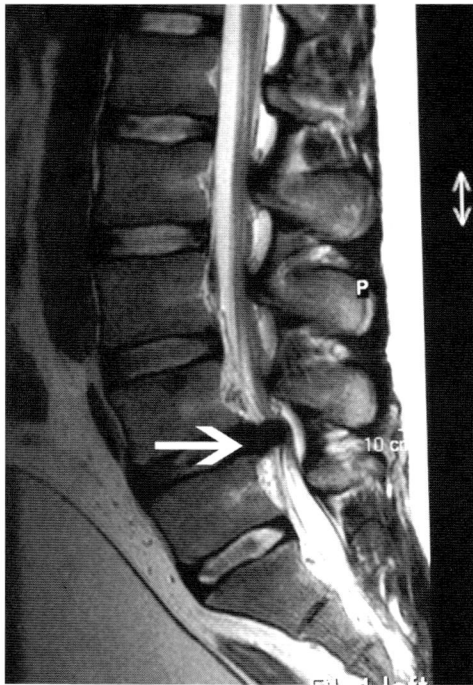

FIGURE 3-17
Sagittal T2WI showing a massive herniation at the L4-L5 level filling the spinal canal, compressing the dural sac, and abutting the posterior aspect of the spinal canal.

Clinical Presentation

Cauda equina patients usually present with backache accompanied by bilateral radicular symptoms. Severe pain may suddenly appear and radiate bilaterally to the buttocks, thighs, or legs. Perineal numbness may develop. The phrase *"Don't beat around the bush with numbness in the tush!"* is apt. The most common early urological manifestation of cauda equina syndrome is inability to empty the bladder rather than incontinence. Urinary retention is frequently overlooked, because the patient does not complain of it in the first few hours.

Whenever this diagnosis is entertained the patient should be referred for an immediate neuroradiological evaluation.

Imaging Studies

MRI, the procedure of choice, or CT myelography will reveal a very large disc herniation compressing or totally obliterating the thecal sac (Figures 3-16 and 3-17). At times, the herniated disc is very large, fills the whole spinal canal, and may, superficially, resemble the thecal sac on axial CT images. Unlike a normal thecal sac it does not contain any neural elements within it; it pushes the thecal sac posteriorly. This finding is referred to as *empty sac syndrome*.

Management

Prompt surgical decompression combined with removal of the herniated disc may preserve the cauda equina functions. Procrastination and delayed intervention may lead to permanent neurological deficits resulting in severe disability.

Bibliography

Ahn UM, Ahn NU, Buchowski JM, Garrett ES, Sieber AN, Kostuik JP: Cauda equina syndrome secondary to lumbar disc herniation: A meta-analysis of surgical outcomes. Spine 25: 1515–1522, 2000.

Anderson DG, Albert TJ, Fraser JK, Risbud M, Wuisman P, Meisel HJ, Tannoury C, Shapiro I, Vaccaro AR: Cellular therapy for disc degeneration. Spine 30 (17 Suppl): S14–S19, 2005.

Boden SD: The use of radiographic imaging studies in the evaluation of patients who have degenerative disorders of the lumbar spine. J Bone Joint Surg Am 78: 114–124, 1996.

Brain WR, Northfield D, Wilkinson M: The neurological manifestations of cervical spondylosis. Brain 75: 187–225, 1952.

Brodke DS, Ritter SM: Nonoperative management of low back pain and lumbar disc degeneration. J Bone Joint Surg Am 86: 1810–1818, 2004.

Buirski G, Silberstein M: The symptomatic lumbar disc in patients with low back pain: Magnetic resonance imaging appearances in both a symptomatic and control population. Spine 18: 1808–1811, 1993.

Buttermann GR: Treatment of lumbar disc herniation: Epidural steroid injection compared with discectomy. J Bone Joint Surg Am 86: 670–679, 2004.

Carragee EJ, Kim DH: A prospective analysis of magnetic resonance imaging findings in patients with sciatica and lumbar disc herniation. Correlation of outcomes with disc fragment and canal morphology. Spine 22: 1650–1660, 1997.

Carragee EJ, Paragioudakis SJ, Khurana S: 2000 Volvo award winner in clinical studies: Lumbar high-intensity zone and discography in subjects without low back problems. Spine 25: 2987–2992, 2000.

Cassinelli EH, Hall RA, Kang JD: Biochemistry of intervertebral disc degeneration and the potential for gene therapy applications. Spine J 1: 205–214, 2001.

Cooke PM, Lutz GE: Internal disc disruption and axial back pain in the athlete. Phys Med Rehabil Clin N Am 11: 837–865, 2000.

Debois V, Herz R, Berghmans D, Hermans B, Herregodts P: Soft cervical disc herniation. Influence of cervical spinal canal measurements on development of neurologic symptoms. Spine 24: 1996–2002, 1999.

Diaz JH: Permanent paraparesis and cauda equina syndrome after epidural blood patch for postural puncture headache. Anesthesiology 96: 1515–1517, 2002.

Ernst CW, Stadnik TW, Peeters CB, Osteaux MJC: Prevalence of annular tears and disc herniations on MR images of the cervical spine in symptom free volunteers. Eur J Radiol 55: 409–414, 2005.

Goupille P, Jayson MI, Valat JP, Freemont AJ: The role of inflammation in disk herniation-associated radiculopathy. Semin Arthritis Rheum 28: 60–71, 1998.

Hehng Y, Liew SM, Simmons ED: Value of magnetic resonance imaging and discography in determining the level of cervical discectomy and fusion. Spine 29: 2140–2145, 2004.

Inufusa A, An HS, Lim TH, Hasegawa T, Haughton VM, Nowicki BH: Anatomic changes of the spinal canal and intervertebral foramen associated with flexion-extension movement. Spine 21: 2412–2420, 1996.

Ito T, Takano Y, Nobuhiro Y: Types of lumbar herniated disc and clinical course. Spine 26: 648–651, 2001.

Jackson RP, Glah JJ: Foraminal and extraforaminal lumbar disc herniation: Diagnosis and treatment. Spine 12: 577–585, 1987.

Jones A, Clarke A, Freeman BJC, Lam KS, Grevitt MP: The Modic classification. Inter- and intraobserver error in clinical practice. Spine 30: 1867–1869, 2005.

Kankaanpaa M, Taimela S, Airaksinen O, Hanninen O: The efficacy of active rehabilitation in chronic low back pain. Effect of pain intensity, self-experienced disability, and lumbar fatigability. Spine 24: 1034–1042, 1999.

Lejeune JP, Hladky JP, Cotton A, Vinchon M, Christiaens JL: Foraminal lumbar disc herniation. Experience with 83 patients. Spine 19: 1905–1908, 1994.

Levicoff EA, Gilbertson LG, Kang JD: Gene therapy to prevent or treat disc degeneration: Is this the future? SpineLine March/April: 10–16, 2005.

Mehta TA, Sharp DJ: Acute cauda equina syndrome caused by a gas-containing prolapsed intervertebral disk. J Spinal Disord 13: 532–534, 2000.

Mitchell MJ, Sartoris DJ, Moody D, Resnick D: Cauda equina syndrome complicating ankylosing spondylitis. Radiology 175: 521–525, 1990.

Modic MT, Steinberg PM, Ross JS, Massaryk TJ, Carter JR: Degenerative disk disease: Assessment of changes in vertebral body marrow with MR imaging. Radiology 166: 193–199, 1988.

Ohmori K, Kanamori M, Kawaguchi Y, Ishihara H: Clinical features of extraforaminal lumbar disc herniation based on the radiographic location of the dorsal root ganglion. Spine 26: 662–666, 2001.

Olmarker K, Rydevik B: Pathophysiology of sciatica. Orthop Clin N Am 22: 223–234, 1991.

O'Neill C, Alamin T, Weinstein SM: The utility of provocation discography in the evaluation and treatment of chronic low back pain: A state of the art debate. SpineLine March/April: 17–25, 2005.

Peng B, Wu W, Hou S, Li P, Zhang C, Yang Y: The pathogenesis of discogenic low back pain. J Bone Joint Surg Br 87: 62–67, 2005.

Prasad SS, O'Malley M, Caplan M, Shackleford IM, Pydisetty RK: MRI measurements of the cervical spine and their correlation to Pavlov's ratio. Spine 28: 1263–1268, 2003.

Rao R: Neck pain, cervical radiculopathy, and cervical myelopathy. Pathophysiology, natural history and clinical evaluation. J Bone Joint Surg Am 84: 1872–1881, 2002.

Rhode RS, Kang JD: Thoracic disc herniation presenting with chronic nausea and abdominal pain. A case report. J Bone Joint Surg Am 86: 379–381, 2004.

Rydevik B, Brown MD, Lundborg G: Pathoanatomy and pathophysiology of nerve root compression. Spine 9: 7–15, 1984.

Shapiro S: Medical realities of cauda equina syndrome secondary to lumbar disc herniation. Spine 25: 348–351, 2000.

Slipman CW, Lipetz JS, Jackson HB, Rogers DP, Vresilovic EJ: Therapeutic selective nerve root block in the nonsurgical treatment of atraumatic cervical spondylotic radicular pain: A retrospective analysis with independent clinical review. Arch Phys Med Rehabil 81: 741–746, 2000.

Tsitouridis I, Sayegh FE, Papapostolou P, Chondroamtidou S, Goustsaridou F, Emmanouilidou M, Sidiropoulou MS, Kapetanos GA: Disc-like herniation in association with gas collection in the spinal canal: CT evaluation. Eur J Radiol 56: 1–4, 2005.

Uhlenbrock D, Henkes H, Weber W, Felber S, Kuehne D: Degenerative disorders of the spine, pp. 159–268 in Uhlenbrock D: MR imaging of the spine and spinal cord. Georg Thieme Verlag, 2004.

Wood KB, Blair JM, Aepple DM, Schendel MJ, Garvey TA, Gundry CR, Heitoff KB: The natural history of asymptomatic thoracic disc herniations. Spine 22: 525–530, 1997.

Wong AK, Leong CP, Chen CM: The traction angle and cervical intervertebral separation. Spine 17: 136–138, 1992.

ACQUIRED SPINAL STENOSIS

4

Acquired spinal stenosis is very common in the elderly. It usually affects two spinal regions: the cervical and the lumbar. The basic underlying pathophysiological mechanisms leading to canal narrowing in the cervical and lumbar regions are the same. The resulting clinical manifestations, however, are quite different. The clinical symptoms depend on the degree of stenosis (how much space is left for the neural elements), the location of stenosis (central versus lateral stenosis), and the number of levels that are involved. Not uncommonly patients develop stenosis at both the cervical and the lumbar regions simultaneously.

CERVICAL SPONDYLOTIC MYELOPATHY

The major clinical/pathological complication of cervical spondylosis is cervical spondylotic myelopathy (CSM).

Pathophysiology

Degenerative changes in the vertebral bodies, discs, and ligaments lead to hypertrophy, calcification, and ossification, resulting in encroachment on the space that separates these structures from the cord (Figures 4-1A and 4-1B). As the space left for the spinal cord is

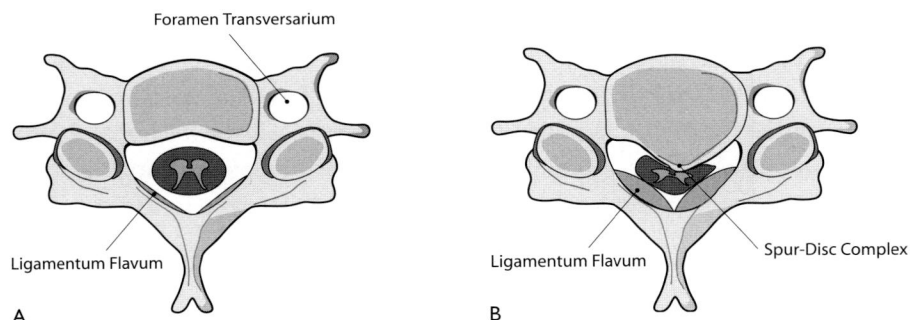

FIGURE 4-1
Schematic illustration of (A) a normal cervical spine and (B) a degenerated cervical spine in which the cord is compressed by a posteriorly directed disc herniation and anteriorly bulging of hypertrophied ligamenta flava.

encroached upon, several mechanisms can lead to cord pathology and dysfunction. The spinal cord can be damaged due to compression as well as ischemia. The latter can develop due to anterior spinal artery compression, which may lead to ischemic changes at several adjoining levels. Over an extended period of time the cord undergoes pathological changes (demyelination, meylomalacia, atrophy) that may eventually become irreversible.

Clinical Presentation

CSM evolves slowly. The predominant symptoms occur due to lower motor neuron symptoms in the upper extremities, and upper motor neuron symptoms in the lower extremities. Weakness and atrophy of the small muscles of the hands result in fine motor coordination deficits: handling keys, manipulating buttons, and writing become awkward and clumsy. This may be accompanied by numbness in both hands. Upper motor neuron symptoms such as spasticity and increased reflexes develop in the lower extremities. The toes may become upgoing. Clinically this translates to gait dysfunction. The patient may stumble and fall. Quite often it is a close family member that identifies early on the changes in the patient's gait. Most patients retain control of their sphincters for a long time. Pain does not play a major role in the clinical picture of CSM. Most patients may have had neck pain in the past but at the time of diagnosis pain is not a major complaint. The clinical picture just described is very similar to that seen in the early stages of amyotrophic lateral sclerosis (ALS). Because the latter condition is universally fatal, every patient suspected of ALS should be referred for a CT or an MRI examination of the cervical spine to rule out cervical myelopathy.

LUMBAR SPINAL STENOSIS

Lumbar spinal stenosis, the most common spinal disorder in the elderly, consists of clinical signs and symptoms, which result from narrowing of the spinal canal.

Pathophysiology

Lumbar spinal canal narrowing results from degenerative thickened facets, hypertrophy of the ligamentum flavum, bulging discs, or degenerative spondylolisthesis (Figure 4-2). It has been shown that the hypertrophied ligamentum flavum loses its elastic fibers and may become calcified or, at times, ossified. Reduced elasticity may lead to bulging of the ligamenta flava into the spinal canal even in the standing position.

Clinical Presentation

Lumbar spinal stenosis often presents with low back and bilateral lower extremity pain. Walking brings about pain in the buttocks, thighs, or legs—neurogenic claudication. The pain may become severe

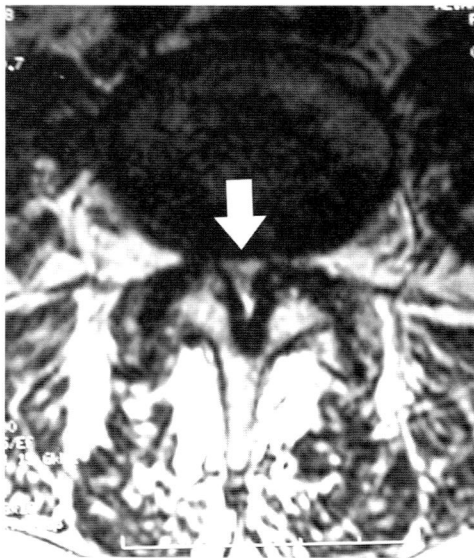

FIGURE 4-2
Severe lumbar spinal canal stenosis (arrow). Hypertrophied facets combined with degenerative spondylolisthesis (note the anterior positioning of the inferior articular facets) lead to decreased transverse canal diameter and severely narrowed lateral recesses.

TABLE 4-1

Neurogenic versus Vascular Claudication

	Neurogenic Claudication	**Vascular Claudication**
Age	Elderly	Elderly
Distance traveled before symptoms	Variable	Fixed
Peripheral pulses	Present	Absent
Symptom relief obtained with	Sitting	Standing

TABLE 4-2

Clinical Differences between Spinal Stenosis and Herniated Disc

	Spinal Stenosis	**Herniated Disc**
Age	Elderly	Young
Laterality of symptoms	Bilateral	Unilateral
Straight leg raising	Negative	Positive
Sensory changes	Fleeting, changing	Fixed
Motor changes	Absent to fleeting	Fixed
Reflex change	Changing	Fixed

and forces the patient to stop ambulating. Following a short period of rest, especially if the patient sits down or stoops forward, walking can be resumed. Some patients notice that they can ambulate farther when they walk uphill whereas downhill walking precipitates symptoms rather early. The pain may be sharp or may feel as if vices or bands have been applied to the legs. Frequently, the pain is concentrated around the calves. This may be accompanied by fleeting numbness and paraesthesia. These symptoms may appear unilaterally or bilaterally and are not stable in nature. The patient remains totally asymptomatic while sitting or lying down. Quite frequently the physical examination remains entirely normal. Not infrequently decreased reflexes or areflexia may be found, a common finding also in healthy elderly subjects. The straight leg raising test remains negative. Infrequently motor weakness may be found.

Neurogenic claudication and vascular claudication may be difficult to differentiate. At times, both conditions may occur simultaneously. Table 4-1 summarizes the similarities and differences between the two conditions. Differentiation between spinal stenosis and herniated disk is presented in Table 4-2.

Imaging Studies

In cervical and lumbar stenosis the X-rays may show multilevel disc degeneration accompanied by anterior and posterior osteophytes,

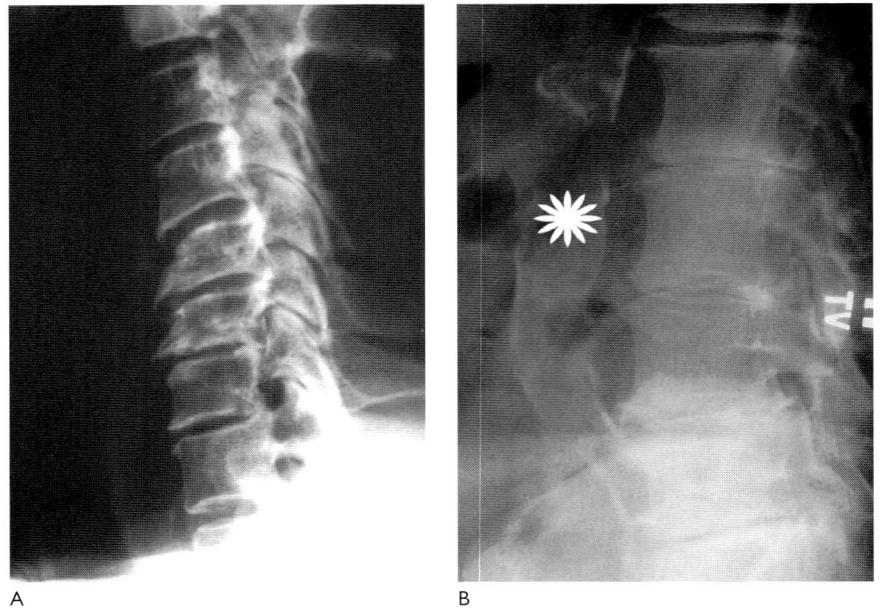

A   B

FIGURE 4-3

Lateral plain films demonstrating anterior and posterior osteophytes. (A) At C4 through C6 the intervertebral spaces are decreased with reversal of the cervical lordosis. (B) In lateral plain films of the lumbar spine narrowed intervertebral spaces are noted with small anterior and posterior osteophytes. Note the extensively calcified abdominal aorta (star).

facet hypertrophy, and segmental instability (Figures 4-3A and 4-3B). Degenerative instability may seem absent or mild on static plain films. Flexion and extension films, however, may reveal the degree of instability and provide an explanation for the clinical symptoms (Figures 4-4A and 4-4B). In the cervical region there may be straightening of the

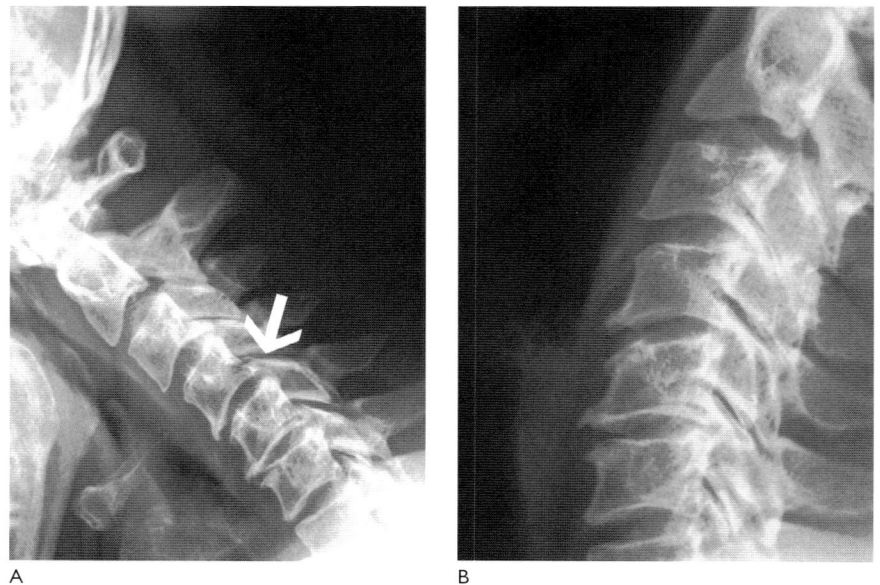

A   B

FIGURE 4-4

Flexion and extension lateral plain films of the cervical spine demonstrating instability due to degenerative disc disease. A subluxation is noted at C4-C5 in (A) flexion view (arrow) with full correction on extension (B).

cervical lordosis or, quite commonly, reversal of the cervical lordosis —cervical kyphosis. A congenitally narrow cervical canal is a significant risk factor for the development of myelopathy once degenerative changes occur. The Torg-Pavlov ratio can be obtained by dividing the sagittal diameter of the cervical spinal canal by that of the vertebral body as obtained in lateral spine films. In normal individuals the ratio is one. A ratio of 0.8 or less helps identify patients with a high risk of developing this disease (Figure 4-5). In the lumbar region degenerative scoliosis is quite commonly seen. Oblique films of the cervical spine and lateral films of the lumbar spine frequently show single or multi-level neural foraminal narrowing. A posterior disc height of less than 4 mm or foraminal height of less than 15 mm is an indicator of potential foraminal stenosis.

Spinal MRI is most useful in delineating the location and extent of stenosis. Both modalities will clearly show the severity of the disease and delineate the anterior and posterior structures that are the cause of the stenosis. In the cervical region the canal is frequently encroached upon by posteriorly directed ridges, calcified herniated discs, and hypertrophic and, at times, ossified posterior longitudinal ligament. From the back the canal may be encroached upon by hypertrophic facets and thickened ligamenta flava (Figures 4-6A and 4-6B). In the lumbar spine hypertrophic facets and thickened ligamenta flava are the most common offending structures. Not infrequently facet cysts play a role in symptom production (Figures 4-7A and 4-7B). The spinal canal may be further compromised by degenerative unstable segments.

In the cervical region, facet hypertrophy in combination with uncovertebral joint hypertrophy compromise the neural foraminae and lead to nerve root dysfunction. MRI of the cervical spine, in sagittal and axial cuts, will provide invaluable information about the spinal cord. Quite frequently an increased cord signal is seen on T2-weighted images of the compressed segments. The increased signal represents

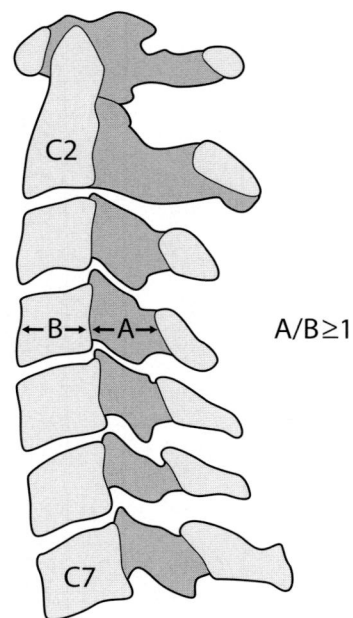

FIGURE 4-5
Schematic lateral view of the cervical spine. The canal diameter (A) is compared to the vertebral diameter (B).

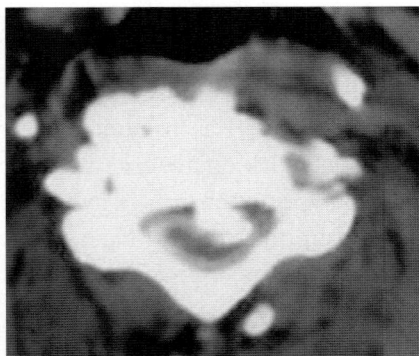

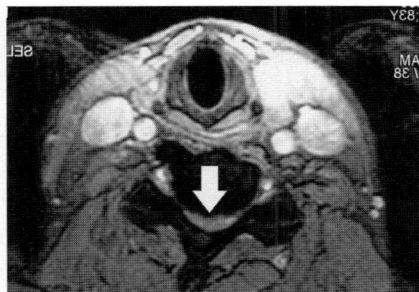

FIGURE 4-6
(A) CT myelography showing central-left ossified posterior longitudinal ligament (OPLL) impinging on the dural sac and the cord. (B) Axial T2WI MR image in another patient demonstrating posteriorly directed "hard disc" (arrow) compromising the neural canal.

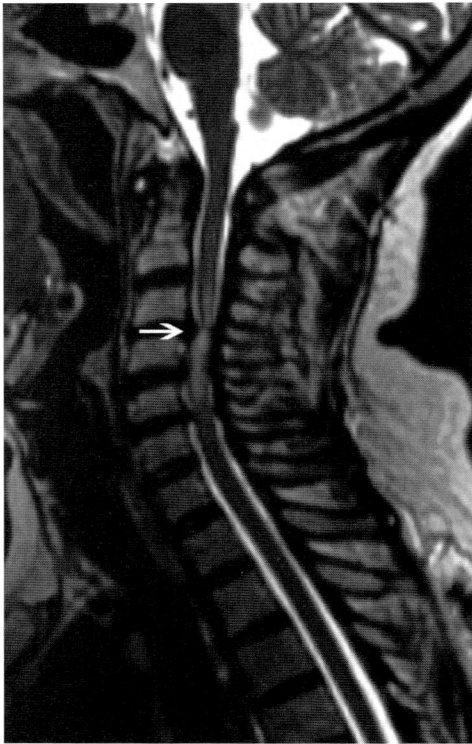

FIGURE 4-8
Sagittal T2-weighted MRI depicting disc herniations at C3-C4 and C4-C5 intervertebral spaces compressing the cord posteriorly toward the hypertrophied ligamenta flava. There is severe cord compression at C3-C4 (arrow). The cord signal is increased due to meylomalacia or gliosis.

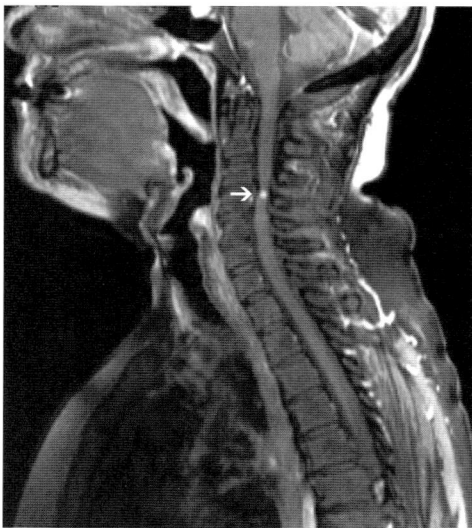

FIGURE 4-9
T1-weighted sagittal MR image post–gadolinium administration showing enhancement at the C3-C4 level within the compressed cord.

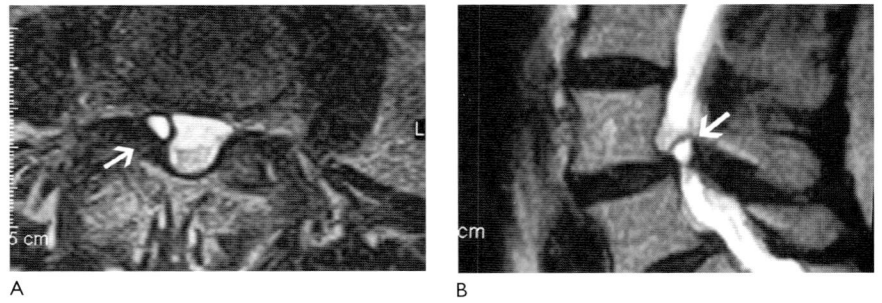

A   B

FIGURE 4-7
Axial (A) and sagittal (B) T2-weighted MRI of the lumbar spine showing a facet joint synovial cyst (arrow) bulging into the spinal canal. Note that the facet signal is similar to that of the CSF and it does not enhance with gadolinium.

cord edema, demyelination, or gliosis (Figure 4-8). In the acute and subacute phases enhancement may appear following contrast administration (Figure 4-9). On T2 axial cuts the increased signal may be diffuse and difficult to discern without the respective sagittal images. At times, the increased signal appears in two symmetrical discrete spots akin to "cobra eyes" (Figures 4-10A and 4-10B). Longstanding compression can result in severe cord atrophy, which may be a bad prognostic sign. In late stages the atrophic cord appears homogenous with no difference between white and gray matter.

Progressive degenerative changes in the lumbar region result in canal shape change. Normally, the lumbar canal is oval in shape. Degenerative changes lead to narrowing of the canal in the sagittal diameter, coronal diameter, or both. Eventually it may become trefoil-shaped with apparent, severe thecal sac compression (Figures 4-11 and 4-12). Some patients develop severe stenosis at one level, usually at the L4-L5 level, and some at multiple levels.

Management

The management of spinal stenosis includes conservative and surgical measures. Patients with mild to moderate cervical stenosis are instructed to avoid cervical hyperextension as it decreases the anteroposterior diameter of the canal. Rather than drinking directly from a bottle, the patient is urged to drink with a straw. The patient is told to avoid overhead activities and to adjust his work environment (such as seat height or monitor height) so that hyperextension is avoided. Chin-tuck and isometric neck exercises are emphasized. Analgesic and anti-inflammatory medications may provide some relief. Protracted use of cervical collars is not recommended.

Lumbar stenosis patients are taught to perform pelvic tilt, William flexion, and lumbar stabilization exercises. They are instructed to avoid hyperextension (arching) of the back and to incorporate flattening of the lumbar lordosis by pelvic tilt exercises in their daily routine. Analgesic and anti-inflammatory medications are prescribed. These may provide temporary relief. Epidural steroid injections usually provide only part-time relief but should be tried prior to surgery.

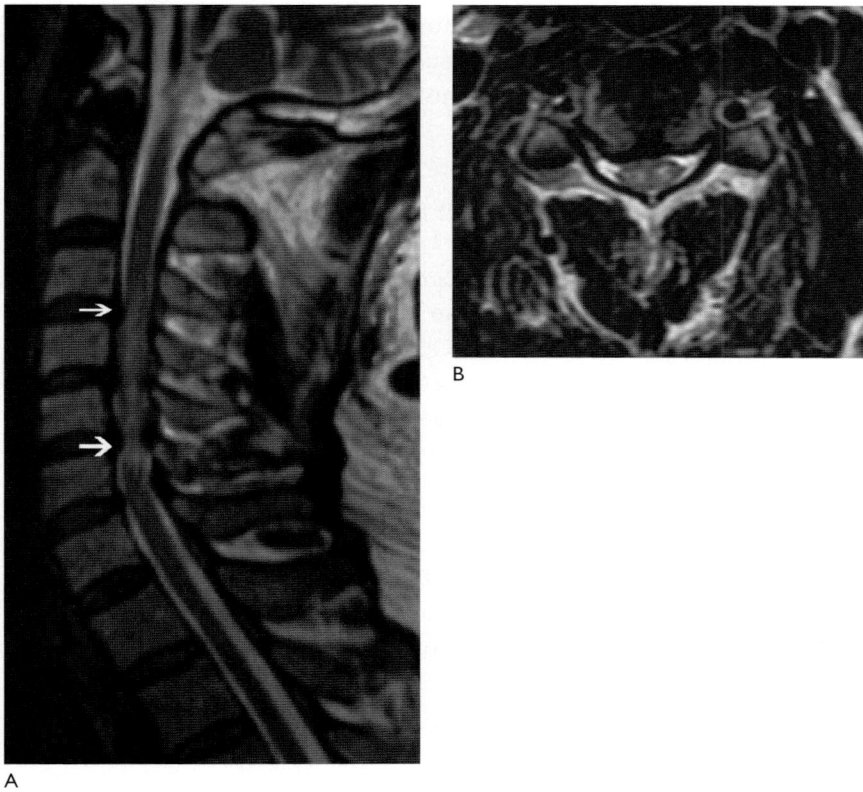

A

B

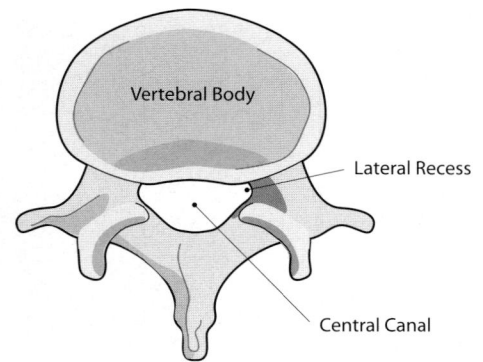

FIGURE 4-11
Schematic drawing of normal lumbar spinal canal shape.

FIGURE 4-10
(A) Cord edema/myelomalacia at C3 through C6 levels is easy to depict in the sagittal T2-weighted images. (B) Axial T2-weighted image showing the "cobra eyes" sign.

Decompressive surgery is recommended in patients with progressive neurological loss or patients whose quality of life is affected to a great extent. The timing of surgery in patients with cervical myelopathy is of paramount importance and quite challenging. Procrastination in the face of clear neurological deterioration may result in permanent disability. When evidence for cord compression, cord signal changes, or cord atrophy is present the patient may not regain lost function even after adequate decompression. Patients with up to three myelopathic levels can be safely operated on in an anterior approach. Patients with more extensive disease involving four or five levels may fare better with the posterior approach as the rate of complications of the anterior approach rises in such extensive disease. Cervical laminoplasty may be the procedure of choice for patients with extensive multilevel disease who are operated on in the posterior approach.

Lumbar stenosis patients whose symptoms interfere with their quality of life should be referred for decompression. Wide laminectomies and facetectomies may provide permanent relief. Stabilization with pedicle screws bilateral lateral fusion allows early mobilization.

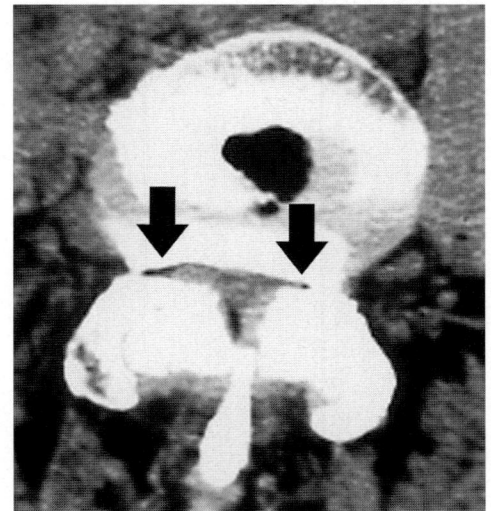

FIGURE 4-12
Axial CT slice demonstrating severe narrowing of the spinal canal in both the sagittal and coronal diameters. Note the severe tre-foil shaped stenosis of both lateral recesses (arrows).

DEGENERATIVE ADULT SCOLIOSIS

Not infrequently, mostly in elderly females in the sixth or seventh decades, multilevel degenerative lumbar scoliosis and stenosis is

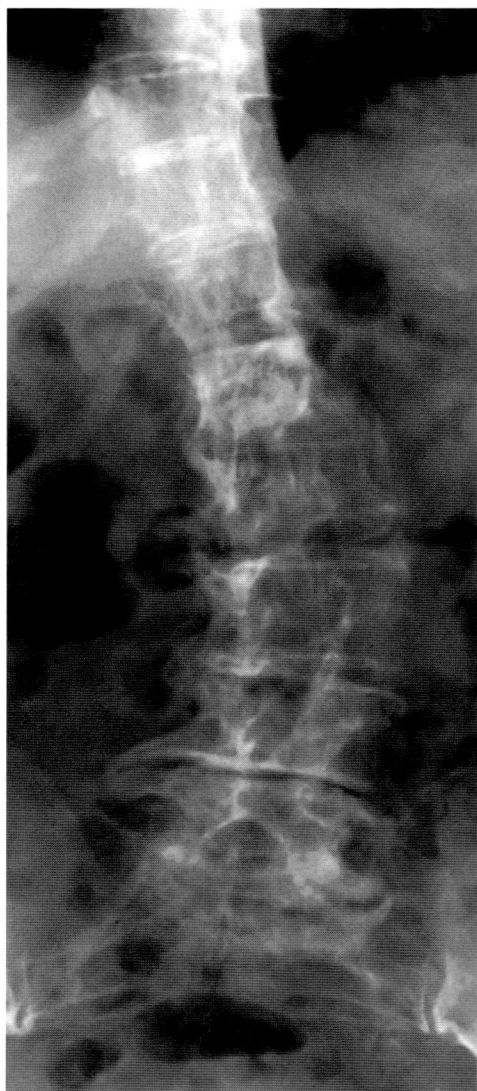

found (Figure 4-13). This is a de novo scoliosis, as it did not exist earlier. Degenerative adult scoliosis usually consists of a short curve, often spanning from L1 to L4 or L5. The curve may be severe, up to 70–80 degrees.

The scoliotic vertebrae rotate, forming what is termed *corkscrew deformity*. The vertebral bodies may develop antero and lateral listhesis at several levels as well (Figure 4-14). Presently it is not known why certain patients with multilevel degenerative disc disease develop scoliosis whereas others with the same level of disc degeneration do not.

CT images clearly show the extent of central, lateral recess and foraminal stenosis in these patients (Figure 4-15). MRI will document the scoliosis and accompanying spinal stenosis. Disc herniations, at higher lumbar levels, may be spotted as well.

Management

Managing patients with degenerative adult scoliosis is quite a challenge. It is frequently difficult to identify the pain generator in patients with multilevel disease. Furthermore, because of advanced age, the presence of comorbidities, and consumption of multiple medications, management decisions have to be carefully made. Quite often surgery is not an option. Conservative care is not simple. As many medications cannot be administered at the usual dosage because of reduced kidney function and consumption of multiple other medications, special attention should be given to the choice of drug and dosage selection. Judicious use of analgesic, anti-inflammatory, and narcotic drugs is called for. When necessary, facet blocks and epidural steroid injections can provide short-term relief. Radiofrequency ablation of the nerves to the facets may provide long-term relief in some patients.

FIGURE 4-13
Degenerative dorso-lumbar scoliosis on plain film (AP view). Note the rotatory component, severe multilevel disc degeneration, and osteophytes.

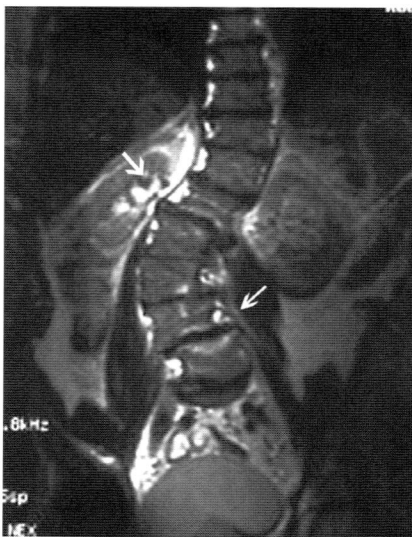

FIGURE 4-14
Degenerative lumbar scoliosis in an 82-year-old man with severe axial pain. Note the lateral listhesis (arrows) at several levels on this coronal T1-weighted image.

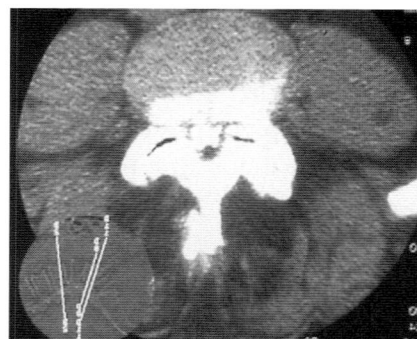

FIGURE 4-15
Axial CT slice of a lumbar vertebra. Note the obliterated lateral recess due to the severe stenosis. Facet arthropathy with vacuum phenomenon in both facet joints is noted.

OSSIFICATION OF THE POSTERIOR LONGITUDINAL LIGAMENT

Ossification of the posterior longitudinal ligament (OPLL) is a progressive disorder most commonly observed in the cervical region. The ossified ligament may lead to cervical stenosis, cord compression, and myelopathy. OPLL was originally described in Japanese people but later was found to occur in Caucasians as well. It is more common in males and usually presents in the fifth decade.

This idiopathic condition affects primarily the cervical region but may involve the thoracic region as well. The posterior longitudinal ligament gradually ossifies and thickens. It grows posteriorly into the spinal canal, gradually taking more space and eventually leading to spinal cord compression. Most patients remain asymptomatic for quite some time. When the ossified ligament occupies 60% or more of the anteroposterior diameter of the spinal canal myelopathic symptoms appear. Occasionally the condition is discovered incidentally on X-rays, CT, or MRI.

Imaging Studies

Lateral cervical spine films may show sclerosed and thickened bone mass posterior to the vertebral bodies. Frequently no mass is detected posterior to the discal space. The ossified ligament can be easily missed unless the ossification is extensive. In the latter case a flowing ossified posterior longitudinal ligament is seen. Of note, the facet joints are not fused (Figure 4-16).

The condition can be easily spotted and its severity assessed on axial CT that can be aided by sagittal reformation (Figure 4-17). The MRI scan will show a hypointense ossified ligament on T1- and T2-weighted images (Figure 4-18). It is possible to evaluate the cord condition only on MRI scans.

Management

When OPLL is discovered in an asymptomatic patient whose physical examination is normal, the patient should be monitored and followed periodically. Patients with myelopathic symptoms should be referred for surgical decompression and stabilization. Surgical intervention should not be delayed; symptom duration of over one year or sphincter involvement are indicators of poor prognosis.

DIFFUSE IDIOPATHIC SKELETAL HYPEROSTOSIS

Diffuse idiopathic skeletal hyperostosis (DISH), also known as ankylosing hyperostosis or Forestier disease, is a common degenerative condition that affects the elderly. It may be more common in diabetics and affects males more frequently. It is seen mostly in people of Caucasian origin. In many instances it is found as an incidental discovery. At times, however, it may cause symptoms. DISH most commonly affects the thoracic spine, but in many patients the cervical and lumbar regions may be affected as well.

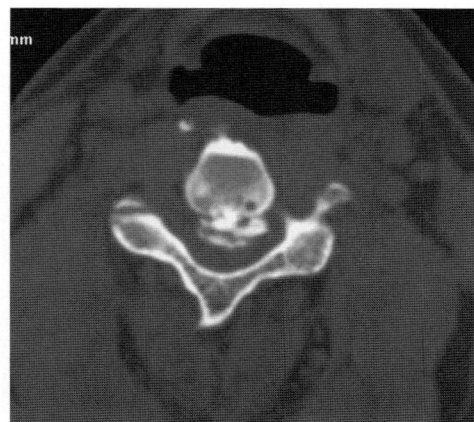

FIGURE 4-16
An ossified posterior longitudinal ligament encroaching on the spinal canal on an axial CT scan of a cervical vertebra.

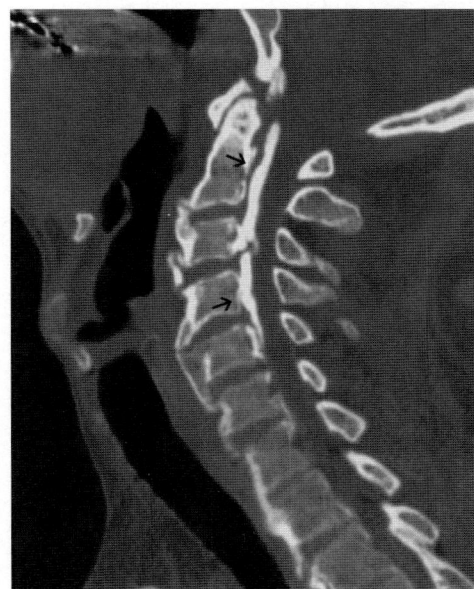

FIGURE 4-17
Sagittal CT reconstruction of the cervical spine demonstrating ossification of the posterior longitudinal ligament extending throughout the cervical spine (arrows). The ossification reaches up to the clivus level.

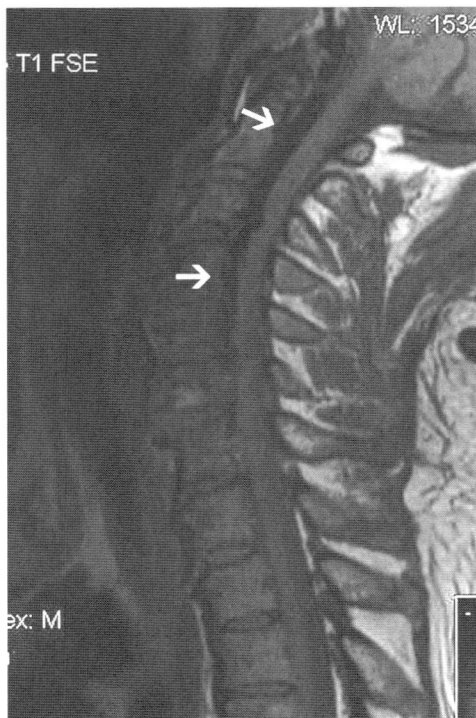

FIGURE 4-18
Sagittal T1-weighted MR image of the cervical spine. The ossified ligament appears as a thick low-signal structure (dark) behind the vertebral bodies (arrows). The ligament protrudes into the spinal canal, causing cord compression.

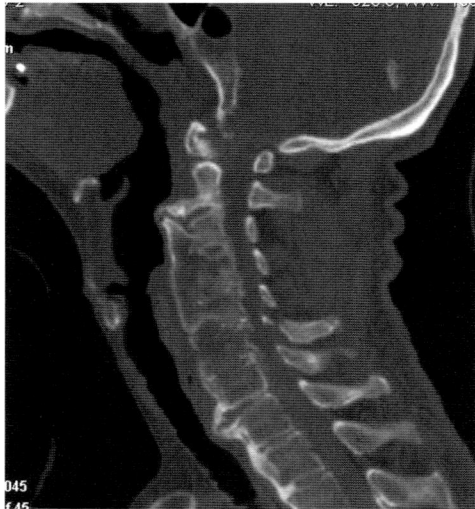

FIGURE 4-19
(A) Cervical plain film lateral view showing the anterior hyperostosis/flowing osteophytes spanning from C3-C4 to C6-C7. Note spared intervertebral spaces. (B) AP view of the dorsal spine. Note flowing osteophytes on the right side (arrow) while the left side is spared.

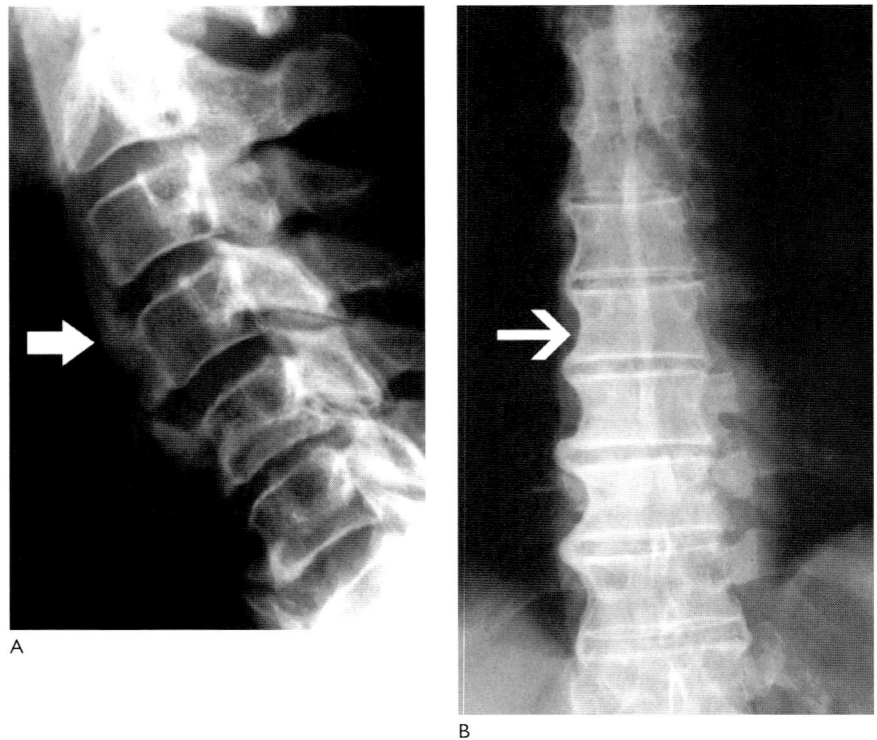

FIGURE 4-20
Sagittal reconstruction of cervical CT, showing marked anterior hyperostosis extending throughout the cervical spine. Note the low density of the hyperostotic elements from C2 to C6 due to fatty bone marrow. The osteophytes at C7 to T2 are hyperdense.

Imaging Studies

X-rays reveal flowing osteophytes formed in the anterior and lateral aspects of the vertebral bodies. These are sometimes large and extensive especially in the cervical region. The osteophytes usually involve more than four spinal levels. In the thoracic region the osteophytes are more prominent on the right side. It is believed that the pulsating aorta prevents extensive ossification on the left side. Unlike ankylosing spondylitis, the facets and the sacroiliac joints are not involved in DISH. The disc spaces are usually normal as well (Figures 4-19A and 4-19B).

The CT examination will easily detect the ossification of the anterior longitudinal ligament (Figure 4-20). The ossified area will appear on MRI as hypointense on T1- and T2-weighted images. When bone marrow develops within the ossified ligament the signal may be hyperintense on T2-weighted images (Figures 4-21A and 4-21B). Fused segments tend to show less spondylotic changes than nonfused segments.

Management

There is no specific treatment for this condition. The patient should be reassured of its benign character and provided with analgesic medication when necessary. Patients with severe dysphagia may require excision of the osteophytes.

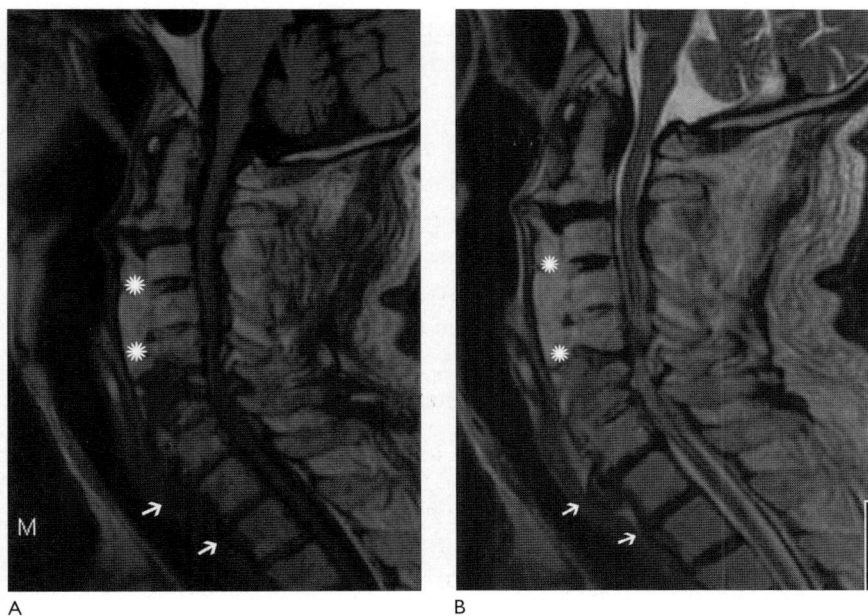

FIGURE 4-21
MRI of the cervical spine of the same patient as in Figure 4-20. Note the severe stenosis. Marked high intensity of the fatty bone marrow within the hyperostotic osteophytes (stars) is seen in both T1WI (A) and T2WI (FSE) (B) images. At the lower spinal segments (arrows) the osteophytes appear dark because they are devoid of fatty tissue.

EPIDURAL LIPOMATOSIS

Epidural lipomatosis (EL) is an uncommon but not a rare condition that frequently leads to spinal stenosis.

Pathophysiology

EL occurs due to excessive epidural accumulation of fatty tissue. It is most frequently encountered in the thoracic region, especially in the mid-thoracic section. Less commonly it is seen in the lower lumbar and sacral regions. In the thoracic region the fat usually accumulates posteriorly to the cord, whereas in the lumbar region it may be circumferential, surrounding the thecal sac.

The condition occurs in both genders, usually in the fourth or fifth decades. Most commonly it is found in patients on chronic exogenous steroid treatment, following epidural steroid injections, in patients with endocrine disorders that result in endogenous increased steroid production (Cushing's disease, hypothyroidism), in extremely obese individuals, and in HIV patients on protease inhibitors (which may cause lipodystrophy with central accumulation of fatty tissue). Not infrequently, idiopathic cases in healthy non-obese individuals are encountered.

Clinical Presentation

The most common symptoms include backache and, less frequently, radicular pain. Some patients present with intermittent claudication or unilateral radiculopathy simulating spinal stenosis or herniated disc, respectively. In patients with significant cord or thecal sac compression bilateral lower extremity weakness, reflex changes, sensory changes, and even urinary dysfunction may occur.

Imaging Studies

X-rays are usually negative. Osteoporosis and compression fractures may be seen in patients on long-term steroids. The CT scan will demonstrate low attenuation mass typical for the excessive, epidurally deposited, fatty tissue. In cases with severe thecal sac compression axial cuts will show a dural sac deformation in stellar, trifid, or Y shapes. This has been coined the Y sign and can also be seen on axial cuts in MRI examination. It has been proposed that the Y shape found in severe cases of epidural lipomatosis is brought about by the presence of meningovertebral ligaments that anchor the outer surface of the dura mater to the osteofibrous walls of the lumbar spinal canal.

MRI, the study of choice in these patients, will show a hyperintense soft tissue compressing the thecal sac on T1-weighted images. The cauda equina will clearly appear as dark crowded strands on the background of the hyperintense fatty tissue (Figures 4-22A and 4-22B). Fat suppression will change the signal to hypointense. On T2-weighted images the fat will appear with intermediate signal intensity.

The fatty tissue will not enhance after contrast administration. This helps in the differentiation of EL from tumors such as lymphoma.

Management

The management of patients with EL is determined by the etiology, the presenting symptoms, and the findings on clinical examina-

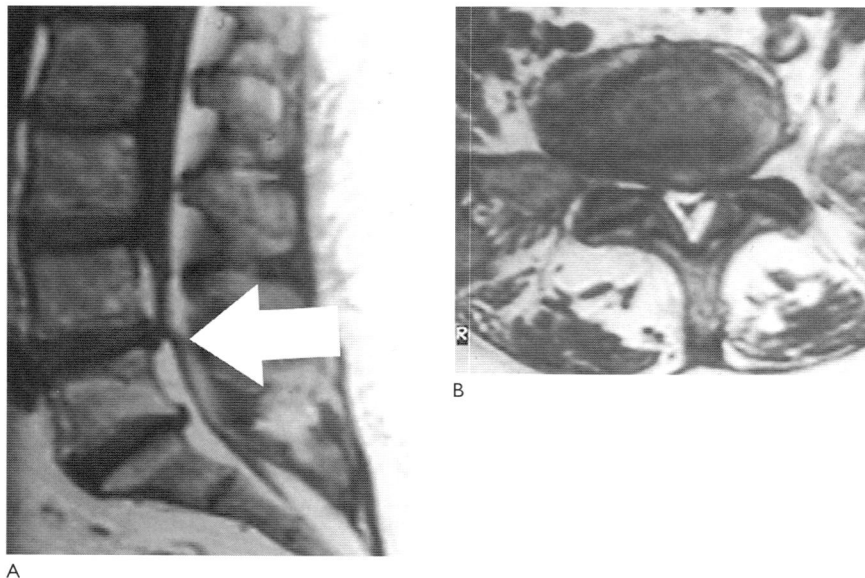

A

B

FIGURE 4-22

MRI of the lumbosacral spine. (A) Sagittal T1WI showing the dural sac severely compressed and narrowed from L4 downward. Note that it is pushed away from the spinolaminar line and the vertebral bodies by an abundant high-intensity fatty tissue. (B) On the axial cut the compressed dural sac (low-intensity signal) is of Y-shaped form.

tion. Not infrequently epidural lipomatosis is discovered as an incidental finding on imaging studies and does not merit special attention. In symptomatic patients elimination of risk factors such as exogenous steroids may bring some relief. Weight loss may lead to epidural fat reduction and clinical improvement in obese patients. When progressive neurological deficits are encountered or in patients with cauda equina syndrome surgical intervention is required. Laminectomy combined with fat debulking may bring about pain relief.

Bibliography

Arnoldi C, Brodsky A, Cauchoix H, Crock HV, Dommisse GF, Edgar MA, Gargano FP, Jacobson RE, Kirkaldy-Willis WH, Kurihara A, Langenskiold WH, Macnab I, McIvor GW, Newman PH, Paine KW, Russin LA, Sheldon J, Tile M, Urist MR, Wilson WE, Wiltse LL: Lumbar spinal stenosis and nerve root entrapment syndromes: Definition and classification. Clin Orthop 115: 4–5, 1976.

Atlas SJ, Keller RB, Robson D, Deyo RA, Singer DE: Surgical and nonsurgical management of lumbar spinal stenosis. Spine 25: 556–562, 2000.

Bernhardt M, Hynes RA, Blume HW, White III AA: Current concepts review: Cervical spondylotic myelopathy. J Bone Joint Surg Am 75: 119–128, 1993.

Brain WR, Northfield D, Wilkinson M: The neurological manifestations of cervical spondylosis. Brain 75: 187–225, 1952.

Cersosimo MG, Lasala B, Folgar S, Micheli F: Epidural lipomatosis secondary to indinavir in an HIV-positive patient. Clin Neuropharmacol 25: 51–54, 2002.

Chen CJ, Lyu RK, Lee ST, Wong YC, Wang JJ: Intramedullary high signal intensity on T2-weighted MR images in cervical spondylotic myelopathy: Prediction of prognosis with type of intensity. Radiology 221: 789–794, 2001.

Ehara S, Shimamura T, Nakamura R, Yamazaki K: Paravertebral ligamentous ossification: DISH, OPLL, OLF. Eur J Radiol 27: 196–205, 1998.

Epstein NE: Ossification of the cervical posterior longitudinal ligament: A review. Neurosurg Focus 5: 540–545, 1998.

Epstein NE: Ossification of the yellow ligament and spondylosis and/or ossification of the posterior longitudinal ligament of the thoracic and lumbar spine. J Spinal Disord 12: 250–256, 1999.

Epstein NE: Laminectomy for cervical myelopathy. Spinal Cord 41: 317–327, 2003.

Fast A: Low back disorders: Conservative management. Arch Phys Med Rehabil 69: 880–891, 1988.

Fast A, Robin GC, Floman Y: Surgical treatment of lumbar spinal stenosis in the elderly. Arch Phys Med Rehabil 66: 149–151, 1985.

Fritz JM, Delitto A, Welch WC, Erhard RE: Lumbar spinal stenosis: A review of current concepts in evaluation, management, and outcome measurements. Arch Phys Med Rehabil 79: 700–708, 1998.

Fujimura Y, Yukimi N, Nakamura M, Toyama Y, Suzuki N: Long term follow-up study of anterior decompression and fusion for thoracic myelopathy resulting from ossification of the posterior longitudinal ligament. Spine 22: 305–311, 1997.

Herkowitz HN, Sidbu KS: Lumbar spine fusion in the treatment of degenerative conditions: Current indications and recommendations. J Am Acad Orthop Surg 3: 123–135, 1995.

Jenis LG, An HS: Lumbar foraminal stenosis. Spine 25: 389–394, 2000.

Kerr R: Diffuse idiopathic skeletal hyperostosis (DISH). Orthopedics 8: 1428–1434, 1985.

Kuhn MJ, Youssef HT, Swan TL, Swenson LC: Lumbar epidural lipomatosis: The Y sign of thecal sac compression. Comput Med Imaging Graph 18: 367–372, 1994.

Law MD, Bernhardt M, White III AA: Evaluation and management of cervical spondylotic myelopathy. Instr Course Lect 44: 99–110, 1995.

Leroux JL, Legeron P, Moulinier L, Laroche M, Mazieres B, Blotman F, Arlet J: Stenosis of the lumbar spinal canal in vertebral ankylosing hyperostosis. Spine 17: 1213–1218, 1992.

Lisai P, Doria C, Crissantu L, Meloni GB, Conti MA, Achene A: Cauda equina syndrome secondary to idiopathic spinal epidural lipomatosis. Spine 26: 307–309, 2001.

Liu H, Ishihara H, Kanamori M, Kawaguchi Y, Ohmori K, Kimura T: Characteristics of nerve root compression caused by degenerative lumbar spinal stenosis with scoliosis. Spine J 3: 524–529, 2003.

Matsumoto M, Toyama Y, Ishikawa M, Chiba K, Suzuki N, Fujimura Y: Increased signal intensity of the spinal cord on magnetic resonance images in cervical compressive myelopathy. Spine 25: 677–682, 2000.

Morio Y, Teshima R, Nagashima H, Nawata K, Yamasaki D: Correlation between operative outcomes of cervical compression myelopathy and MRI of the spinal cord. Spine 26: 1238–1245, 2001.

Olivieri I, Fiandra E, Muscat C, Barozzi L, Tomassini C, Gerli R: Cervical myelopathy caused by ossification of the posterior longitudinal ligament in ankylosing spondylitis. Arthritis Rheum 39: 2074–2077, 1996.

Ono K, Yonenobu K, Miyamoto S, Okada K: Pathology of ossification of the posterior longitudinal ligament and ligamentum flavum. Clin Orthop 359: 18–26, 1999.

Parke WW: The significance of venous return impairment in ischemic radiculopathy and myelopathy. Orthop Clin N Am 22: 213–221, 1991.

Postacchini F, Gumina S, Cinotti G, Perugia D, DeMartino C: Ligamenta flava in lumbar disc herniation and spinal stenosis. Light and electron microscopic morphology. Spine 19: 917–922, 1994.

Prassad SS, O'Malley M, Caplan M, Shackleford IM, Pydisetty RK: MRI measurements of the cervical spine and their correlation to Pavlov's ratio. Spine 28: 1263–1268, 2003.

Resnick D, Niwayama G: Radiographic and pathologic features of spinal involvement in diffuse idiopathic skeletal hyperostosis (DISH). Radiology 119: 559–568, 1976.

Resnick D, Shaul SR, Robins JM: Diffuse idiopathic skeletal hyperostosis (DISH): Forestier's disease with extraspinal manifestation. Radiology 115: 513–524, 1975.

Saifuddin A: The imaging of lumbar spinal stenosis. Clin Radiol 55: 581–594, 2000.

Sairyo K, Biyani A, Goel V, Leaman D, Booth R, Thomas J, Gehling D, Vishnubhotla SL, Long R, Ebraheim N: Pathomechanism of ligamentum flavum hypertrophy: A multidisciplinary investigation based on clinical, biomechanical, histologic, and biologic assessments. Spine 30: 2649–2656, 2005.

Sampath P, Bendebba M, Davis JD, Ducker TB: Outcome of patients treated for cervical myelopathy. A prospective, multicenter study with independent clinical review. Spine 25: 670–676, 2000.

Suen AW, Suen PW, Mroz TE, Wang JC: Update on the management of ossification of the posterior longitudinal ligament. Contemp Spine Surg 4: 73–80, 2003.

Suri A, Chabbra RP, Mehta VS, Gaikwad S, Pandey RM: Effect of intramedullary signal changes on the surgical outcome of patients with cervical spondylotic myelopathy. Spine J 3: 33–45, 2003.

Uhlenbrock D, Henkes H, Weber W, Felber S, Kuehne D: Degenerative disorders of the spine, pp. 159–268 in Uhlenbroch D: MR imaging of the spine and spinal cord. Georg Thieme Verlag, 2004.

Vince G, Brucker C, Langmann P, Herbold C, Solymosi L, Roosen K: Epidural spinal lipomatosis with acute onset of paraplegia in an HIV-positive patient treated with corticosteroids and protease inhibitor: Case report. Spine 30: E524–E527, 2005.

Wada E, Yonenobu K, Suzuki S, Kanazawa A, Ochi T: Can intramedullary signal change on magnetic resonance imaging predict surgical outcome in cervical spondylotic myelopathy? Spine 24: 455–461, 1999.

Yonenobu K: Cervical radiculopathy and myelopathy: When and what can surgery contribute to treatment? Eur Spine J 9: 1–7, 2000.

Yuan PS, Albert TJ: Nonsurgical and surgical management of lumbar spinal stenosis. J Bone Joint Surg Am 86: 2320–2330, 2004.

Yue WM, Tan SB, Tan MH, Koh DCS, Tan CT: The Torg-Pavlov ratio in cervical spondylotic myelopathy. A comparative study between patients with cervical spondylotic myelopathy and a nonspondylotic, nonmeylopathic population. Spine 26: 1760–764, 2001.

SPONDYLOLYSIS AND SPONDYLOLISTHESIS

5

The term *spondylolysis* means breakage within the vertebrae. Spondylolysis refers to a unilateral or bilateral fatigue fracture that occurs in the pars interarticularis (the osseous bridge between the superior and inferior articular facets). About 6% of adults age 18 and older may have bilateral spondylolysis. The condition occurs most frequently at L5, with decreased incidence in L4 and even lower incidence at other sites. It is more common in males and appears in the first or second decades of life, mostly during adolescence. Spondylolysis is thought to occur due to repeated stress that leads to a "fatigue fracture" of the pars interarticularis. This region corresponds with the neck of the "Scottie dog" on oblique films of the lumbar spine (Figure 5-1).

Spondylolysis usually develops in an adolescent engaged in sport activities that involve repetitive lumbar flexion and extension, such as

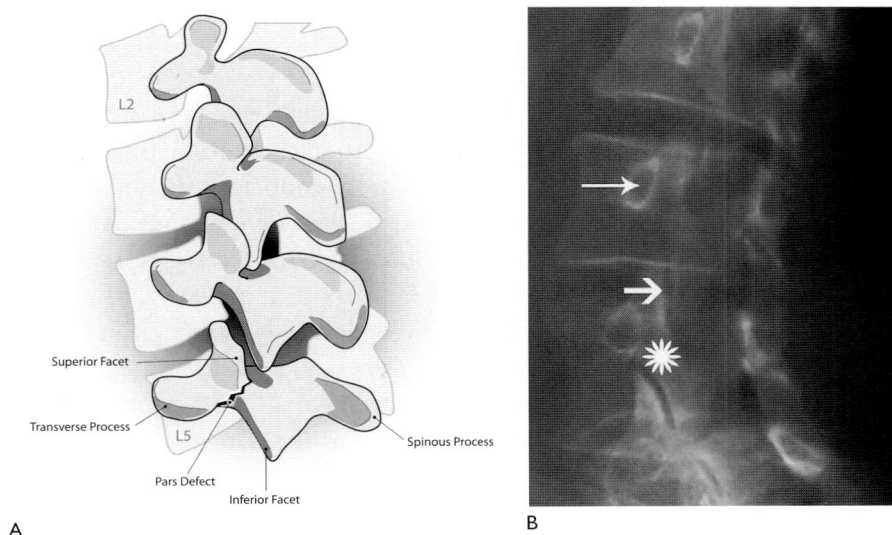

A   B

FIGURE 5-1
(A) Schematic drawing of an oblique view of the lumbar spine. (B) Plain film of the same region. The Scottie dogs are apparent in the oblique view. The pedicle (long arrow), the facet (short arrow), and the pars interarticularis (star) are well visualized.

dancing, martial arts, or weight lifting. Genetics also play a role in this condition. It is infrequently seen in people of African descent whereas in northern Inuit people spondylolysis occurs in about 50% of individuals. Spondylolytic spondylolisthesis (vertebral slip) usually occurs at the L5-S1 region and much less frequently at L4-L5. Not all the factors leading to the development of a slip in young adults with bilateral pars defects have been fully elucidated. Forward slippage tends to occur more frequently in young females with a trapezoid-shaped L5 vertebral body and dome-shaped sacrum, and in patients with vertebral slip angle of greater than 50%. The pars defects decrease the ability of the motion segment to withstand anteriorly directed shear forces and thus lead to an increased mechanical stress at the vertebral growth plate. Hence, most of the slip progression occurs while the spine is immature and still growing and not after the spine has matured.

CLINICAL PRESENTATION

Spondylolysis patients usually present with activity-related axial pain. The pain is of gradual onset rather than sudden. While the neurological examination remains normal, many patients have tenderness over the spine and very tight hamstrings.

Patients with spondylolytic spondylolisthesis may complain of back pain and radicular pain, especially when there is a high degree of slippage. The radicular pain may be caused by nerve root stretching or nerve root compression secondary to reduction of foraminal height or horizontal deformation of the neural foramen or due to exuberant bony callus that forms around the isthmic defect. Physical examination may detect shortened hamstrings, increased lumbar lordosis, and radicular findings when a nerve root is compromised.

IMAGING STUDIES

In the initial stages, when the fracture is forming, the plain films may be negative. Bone scan, however, which can detect areas of bone turnover (i.e., bone deposition even before the actual fracture has developed), may be positive and thus is an important diagnostic tool at the early stages of the condition. Single photon emission computed tomography (SPECT) may be the most sensitive test for detecting impending pars defects, as bone under stress with increased osteoblastic activity due to remodeling will have increased activity and appear hot. Later on, when the defect is established and is large enough, it can be spotted on various projections on plain films (Figure 5-2).

CT scan is the most sensitive method for detection of spondylolysis, whether it is unilateral or bilateral. The defects can be easily spotted in an axial cut (Figure 5-3). Sagittal reformats demonstrate the defect clearly. The key to identification of the defect is that it is separate from the facet joints. In the acute stage MRI may show, especially on T2-weighted images, increased signal around the pars defect due to bone marrow edema. Subsequently, focally decreased signal may be

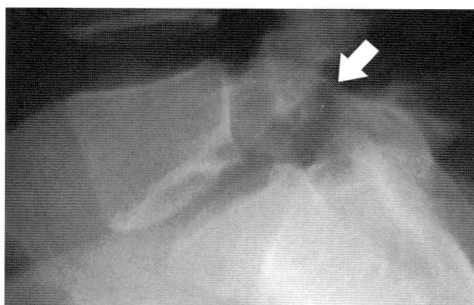

FIGURE 5-2
Lateral plain film of the L5-S1 region. The bony defect in the pars interarticularis is large enough to be detected (arrow). Note a stage one slip-spondylolisthesis of L5 over S1.

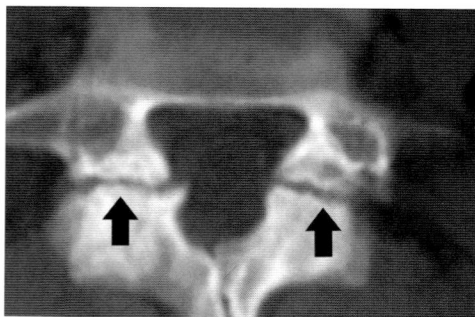

FIGURE 5-3
Axial CT image showing bilateral bony defects (arrows). Note that the sagittal canal diameter is elongated.

seen on sagittal and axial images. T1-weighted images with fat suppression may demonstrate the bony cleft (Figure 5-4). MR is an insensitive technique for pars interarticularis defects and spondylolysis detection. The reasons are basically that the slice thicknesses of the MR sagittal sequences are relatively thick, and the fracture does not have great contrast. Frequently the cuts are not centered on the fracture and it can thus be easily missed. In routine studies the axial images are often performed with the intention of visualizing disc and spinal canal anatomy rather than pars defects.

A simple and well accepted grading system for spondylolisthesis has been devised by Myerding and is named after him. The upper endplate of the vertebra below the slipping vertebra is divided into quarters. Grade 1 slip is when the vertebra above slips forward up to 25% of the diameter of the endplate below. Grade 2 is slippage of between 25% and 50%, grade 3 between 50% and 75%, and grade 4 over 75% (Figure 5-5). At times, L5 slips forward all the way and "falls" in front of S1. This condition is termed spondyloptosis.

Lateral X-rays clearly demonstrate the degree of slippage. In longstanding cases, bone remodeling and sclerosis may be seen, especially at the sacral dome (Figures 5-6A and 5-6B). In advanced L5-S1 spondylolisthesis AP views may disclose an inverted "Napoleon's hat." The hat's brim is made of the transverse processes of the L5 vertebra (Figure 5-7).

CT studies, especially on sagittal reformation, and sagittal MRI views can easily determine the degree of slippage. It should be noted that the forward slippage that occurs in the spinous processes secondary to the vertebral slip is found one level above the spondylolytic vertebra. Because the spinous process of the spondylolytic vertebra is not carried forward with the slipping vertebral body as it is separated from it by the pars defects, the "gap" in the posterior elements occurs one

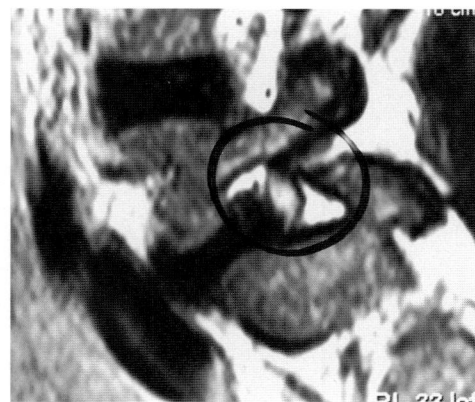

FIGURE 5-4
A close-up MR image through a spondylolytic defect.

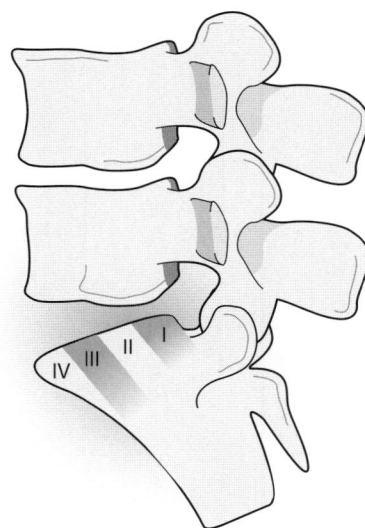

FIGURE 5-5
Schematic demonstration of Meyerding's classification of spondylolisthesis.

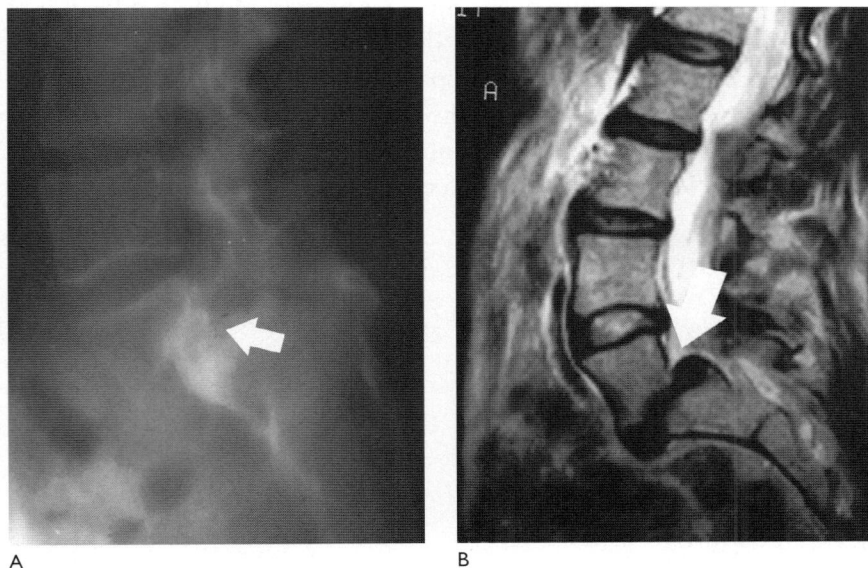

FIGURE 5-6
(A) Plain lateral film showing grade two-to-three slip. Note sclerotic endplates of the involved vertebrae. (B) Sagittal T2WI MRI showing grade two slip (arrow).

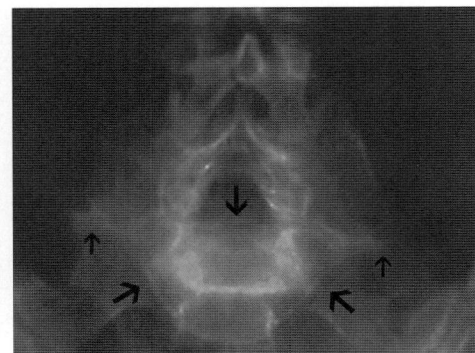

FIGURE 5-7
Plain film AP view showing an inverted "Napoleon hat."

level higher. In axial CT and MRI, especially on T2-weighted images, the spinal canal seems to be elongated in the AP diameter (Figures 5-8A and 5-8B). The neural foramen may have an altered shape, and the perineural fat may be reduced or missing altogether. Direct impingement of the nerve root may be seen.

MANAGEMENT

When a youngster is diagnosed while the pars is in the process of breaking—negative X-rays, positive bone scan—an attempt to heal the fracture may be made by stopping symptom-provoking activities (sports activities) and prescribing a brace for a period of up to 6 months.

Grade 1 and 2 slips can be managed conservatively. The patients are instructed to avoid activities involving hyperextension (lifting, dancing, martial arts) and are instructed to perform William's flexion exercises. Analgesic and anti-inflammatory medications may be prescribed. Patients with high-degree slippage (grade 3 and up), especially when accompanied by neurological symptoms, could be referred for surgery. Decompression and stabilization may offer permanent symptom relief.

ADULT SPONDYLOLYSIS

The pathogenesis of low back pain in an adult with bilateral spondylolysis, who was asymptomatic before, is intriguing. Finding pars defects in adults with low back pain may not have clinical relevance. It can be safely assumed that these defects have been there all along and something else, rather than the spondylolysis itself, may be the source of the new symptoms. The same applies to low grade isthmic slips.

In recent years it has been appreciated that middle-aged patients with bilateral longstanding pars defects or minimal slippage may develop progressive vertebral slippage, spondylolisthesis, which can get worse over the years. The pathophysiology of spondylolisthesis in an adult with a mature spine is complex. It is believed that disc degeneration at the level of the pars defects compromises the ability of the

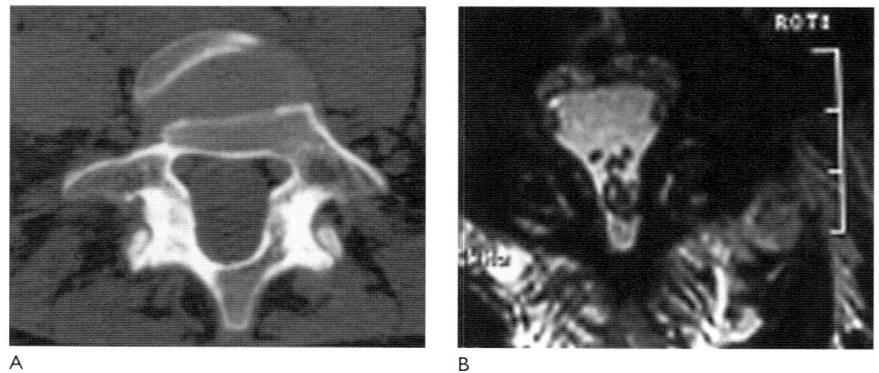

FIGURE 5-8
Axial CT (A) and T2WI MR (B) showing an elongated spinal canal and dural sac in the sagittal diameter.

spine to withstand anterior shear stress and contributes to the vertebral slippage. It seems that the integrity of the disc at the spondylolysis level plays a key role in the stability of that segment. Although conservative care can offer temporary relief to these patients, most respond well to surgical care.

DEGENERATIVE SPONDYLOLISTHESIS

Degenerative spondylolisthesis is a common condition. It occurs in the fifth or sixth decades, mostly in women. It almost always occurs at the L4-L5 level but occasionally is seen higher up in the lumbar spine. Degenerative spondylolisthesis rarely progresses beyond stage one.

The etiology of degenerative spondylolisthesis is multifactorial. Predisposing factors include generalized joint laxity, pregnancy, sagittal facet orientation at L4-L5, and sacralization of the fifth lumbar vertebra. Disc degeneration leads to altered load distribution in the motion segment. These biomechanical changes combined with slackening of the stabilizing ligaments (due to the decreased discal height) and changes in the facet joints lead to the development of segmental instability and degenerative slip.

Clinical Presentation

Initially patients present with mechanical low back pain predominantly during standing and walking. As the degenerative processes progress, radicular symptoms may develop. With time, neurogenic claudication becomes debilitating. Patients are prevented from functional walking due to severe discomfort and pain in both lower extremities. The latter condition appears to be due to lumbar stenosis that is formed when degenerative changes involving the facets, vertebral body, and ligaments occur and is aggravated by the vertebral slip (Figure 5-9).

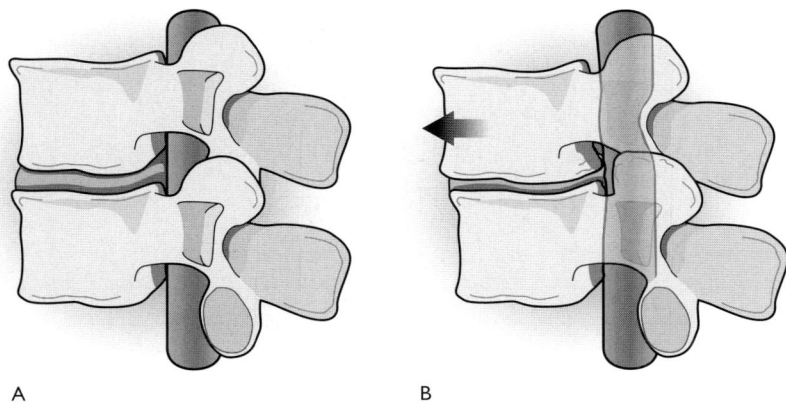

A   B

FIGURE 5-9
Schematic drawing of a degenerative spondylolisthesis with deformation and stenosis of the spinal canal and the intervertebral foramen (B) as compared to the normal alignment and normal disc hight (A). There is discal height loss and diffuse bulge in the degenerated spine, leading to thecal sac compression.

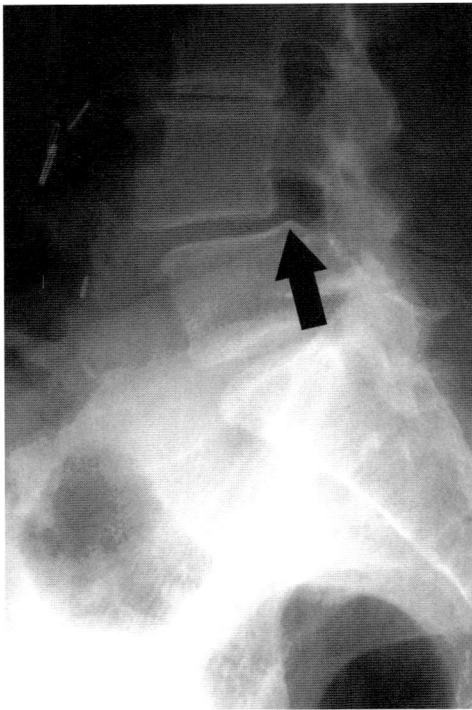

FIGURE 5-10
Lateral plain film showing degenerative spondylolisthesis at L4-L5.

TABLE 5-1
Comparison between Spondylolytic and Degenerative Slip

	Spondylolytic Spondylolisthesis	Degenerative Spondylolisthesis
Age	Young	Middle aged
Level	Predominantly at L5-S1	Common at L4-L5
Gender	More common in males	More common in females
Slip progression	Common	Limited, up to 30%

Imaging Studies

Plain lateral films usually show degenerative disc disease and vertebral slip at L4-L5. It is not uncommon to find anterior or posterior slippage in vertebrae above L4. No pars defects are seen (Figure 5-10). Facet arthropathy and vacuum phenomenon are frequently found. Traction spurs are present at the L4 or L5 vertebral bodies. Unlike osteoarthritic spurs, which emanate from the vertebral body corner, traction spurs originate 1–2 mm away from the vertebral corner, at the attachment point of the anterior longitudinal ligament. Traction spurs are usually parallel to the vertebral endplate (Figures 5-11A and 5-11B).

Lateral flexion and extension views help determine the degree of instability. Frequently, they show increased forward slippage and vertebral body tilt during flexion. Both, the slip and vertebral tilt are frequently reduced during extension (Figures 5-12A and 5-12B).

CT and MR images will clearly demonstrate the degenerative changes, the vertebral slip, and the intact pars (Figure 5-13).

Management

No specific treatment is presently available for degenerative disc disease. Analgesic medications and anti-inflammatory drugs usually

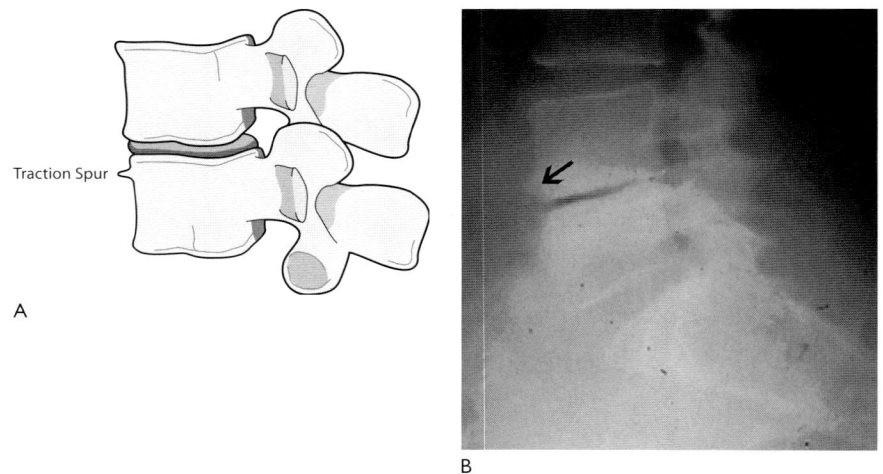

FIGURE 5-11
(A) Schematic drawing of a traction spur typically located 1–2 mm away from the vertebral corner. (B) Lateral plain film of the lumbar spine showing a traction spur in the L4 vertebra. Note vacuum phenomenon within the disc between L4 and L5.

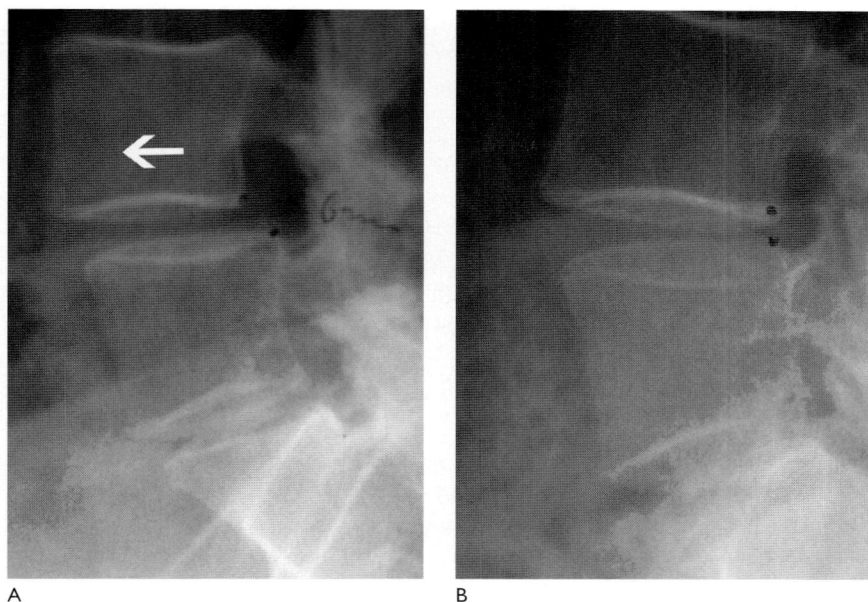

FIGURE 5-12
Lateral plain films of the lumbosacral spine in (A) flexion and (B) extension. Note degenerative slip at L4-L5 during flexion (A), which is reduced in extension (B).

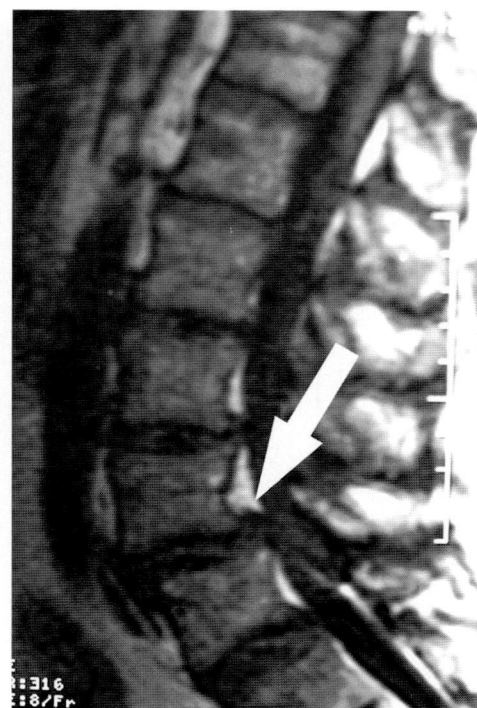

FIGURE 5-13
Sagittal T1WI MRI demonstrating L4-L5 degenerative spondylolisthesis secondary to disc degeneration. Note that the disc seems to bulge posteriorly into the spinal canal, called pseudobulge, as it remains attached to the higher endplate of the lower vertebra (arrow).

provide symptomatic relief. Activity modification—minimizing time spent in painful postures—can be helpful as well.

Stabilization exercises combined with pelvic tilt exercises may prove helpful for those patients willing to spend the time to master these exercises and incorporate them in their daily routine. Fitness exercises, especially those performed in the pool (balneotherapy), may also offer temporary symptomatic relief. Radiofrequency neurotomy of arthritic, painful facets can bring significant long-term relief in selected patients. Patients with severe unremitting pain and neurogenic claudication could be referred for surgery. Decompression with stabilization and fusion should be considered in these patients. The future role of disc arthroplasty in this condition is still to be determined.

Bibliography

Bell DF, Ehrlich MG, Zaleske DJ: Brace treatment for symptomatic spondylolisthesis. Clin Orthop 236: 192–198, 1988.

Boden SD, Riew KD, Yamaguchi K, Branch TP, Schellinger D, Wiesel SW: Orientation of the lumbar facet joints: Association with degenerative disc disease. J Bone Joint Surg Am 78: 403–411, 1996.

Bono CM: Low-back pain in athletes. J Bone Joint Surg Am 86: 382–395, 2004.

Buetler WJ, Fredrickson BE, Murtland A, Sweeney CA, Grant WD, Baker D: The natural history of spondylolysis and spondylolisthesis: 45-year follow-up evaluation. Spine 28: 1027–1035, 2003.

Collier BD, Johnson RP, Carrera GF, Meyer GA, Schwab JP, Flatley TJ, Isitman AT, Hellman RS, Zielonka JS, Knobel J: Painful spondylolysis or spondylolisthesis studied by radiography and single-photon emission computed tomography. Radiology 154: 207–211, 1985.

Deutman R, Diercks RL, de Jong TE, van Woerden HH: Isthmic lumbar spondylolisthesis with sciatica: The role of the disc. Eur Spine J 4: 136–138, 1995.

Ebraheim NA, Xu R, Darwich M, Yeasting RA: Anatomic relations between the lumbar pedicle and the adjacent neural structures. Spine 22: 2338–2341, 1997.

Edelson JG, Nathan H: Nerve root compression in spondylolysis and spondylolisthesis. J Bone Joint Surg Br 68: 596–599, 1986.

Floman Y: Progression of lumbosacral isthmic spondylolisthesis in adults. Spine 25: 342–347, 2000.

Fredrickson BE, Baker D, McHolick WJ, Yuan HA, Lubicky JP: The natural history of spondylolysis and spondylolisthesis. J Bone Joint Surg Am 66: 699–707, 1984.

Gregory PL, Batt ME, Kerslake RW, Scammell BE, Webb JF: The value of combining single photon emission computerized tomography and computerized tomography in the investigation of spondylolysis. Eur Spine J 13: 503–509, 2004.

Hammerberg KW: New concepts on the pathogenesis and classification of spondylolisthesis. Spine 30: S4–S11, 2005.

Jinkins JR, Rauch A: Magnetic resonance imaging of entrapment of lumbar nerve roots in spondylolytic spondylolisthesis. J Bone Joint Surg Am 76: 1643–1648, 1994.

Kim KW, Chung JW, Park JB, Song SW, Ha KY, An HS: The course of the nerve root in the neural foramen and its relationship with foraminal entrapment or impingement in adult patients with lumbar isthmic spondylolisthesis and radicular pain. J Spinal Disord Tech 17: 220–225, 2004.

Lundin DA, Wiseman DB, Shaffrey CI: Spondylolysis and spondylolisthesis in the athlete. Clin Neurosurg 49: 528–547, 2002.

Mardjetko SM, Connolly PJ, Shott S: Degenerative lumbar spondylolisthesis: A meta-analysis of literature 1970–1993. Spine 19(suppl): 2256–2265, 1994.

Matsunaga S, Sakou T, Morizono Y, Masuda A, Demitras AM: Natural history of degenerative spondylolisthesis: Pathogenesis and natural course of the slippage. Spine 15: 1204–1210, 1990.

Pneumaticos SG, Esses SI: Scoliosis associated with lumbar spondylolisthesis: A case presentation and review of the literature. Spine 3: 321–324, 2003.

Pucher A, Jankowski R, Nowak S: Surgical treatment of degenerative lumbar spondylolisthesis. Neurol Neurochir Pol 39: 114–119, 2005.

Sairyo K, Katoh S, Ikata T, Fujii K, Kajiura K, Goel VK: Development of spodylolytic olisthesis in adolescents. Spine J 1: 171–175, 2001.

Sengupta DK, Herkowitz HN: Degenerative spondylolisthesis: Review of current trends and controversies. Spine 15: 30(suppl): S71–S81, 2005.

Standaert CJ, Herring SA: Spondylolysis: A critical review. Br J Sports Med 34: 415–422, 2000.

Ward CV, Latimer B: Human evolution and the development of spondylolysis. Spine 30: 1808–1814, 2005.

Wiltse LL, Newman PH, Macnab I: Classification of spondylolysis and spondylolisthesis. Clin Orthop 117: 23–29, 1976.

Wiltse LL, Widell EH Jr., Jackson DW: Fatigue fracture: The basic lesion in spondylolisthesis. J Bone Joint Surg Am 57: 17–22, 1975.

Wiltse LL, Winter RB: Terminology and measurement of spondylolisthesis. J Bone Joint Surg Am 65: 768–772, 1983.

SPINAL INFECTIONS

6

PYOGENIC VERTEBRAL OSTEOMYELITIS AND DISCITIS

Spinal infections are not commonly seen in general practices. Unfortunately, however, they are not rare and quite often are diagnosed late. Predisposing factors include diabetes, intravenous drug abuse, septicemia, and compromised immunity as seen in HIV, malignancies, chronic steroid consumption, and malnutrition. Delayed diagnosis has detrimental effects as the infection tends to spread and results in irreversible damage to the vertebral bodies, discs, and ligaments. This frequently results in significant morbidity and, at times, mortality.

Pyogenic infections usually occur in patients over 50 years old. Many patients do not appear systemically ill in the initial stages of the disease and remain afebrile with a normal white blood cell count for quite some time. More than 50% of infections involve the lumbar spine, and the causative agent will turn out to be staphylococcus aureus. Immunocompromised patients, however, will often have gram-negative infections such as pseudomonas or klebsiella. In most patients following interventional procedures or surgery, the bacteria reach the vertebral bodies via the arterial system or through venous dissemination. A common source of infection in elderly males is the lower urinary tract.

Clinical Presentation

Patients usually present with severe, longstanding axial pain that does not go away with rest. Local tenderness, muscle spasm, and limited spinal range of motion are frequently observed. Only a small percentage of patients develop motor or sensory deficits. Thus, every patient with persistent, unremitting pain should undergo a work-up that includes complete blood count with differential, C-reactive protein or sedimentation rate, bone markers, and serum and urine protein electrophoresis. Initially, plain X-rays and bone scan should be obtained. When infection is suspected repeated blood cultures and

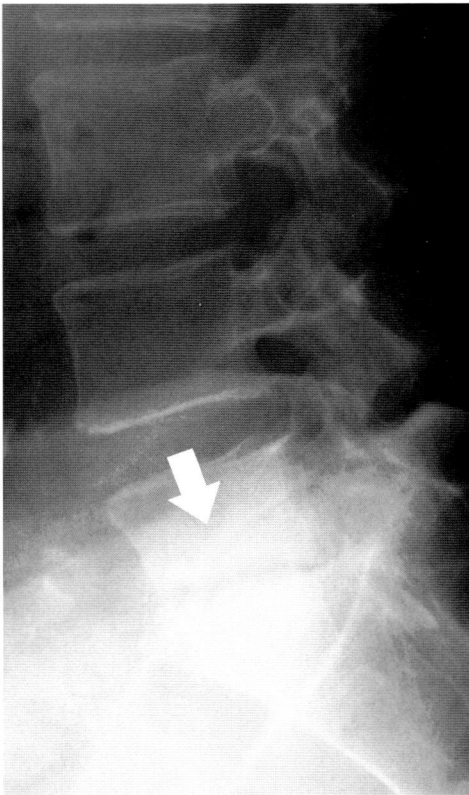

FIGURE 6-1
Lateral plain film of the lumbar spine of a 65-year-old man with severe low back pain of three months duration. Note blurring and irregularity of the sclerotic endplates and severe disc space narrowing . Patient responded to antibiotic treatment.

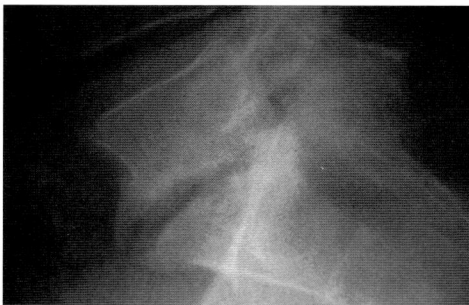

FIGURE 6-2
Same patient as in Figure 6-1 two years later. Lateral plain films show bony sclerosis at the endplates that appear now with sharper delineation and bridging osteophytes adding stability to the affected region.

CT or MRI studies may help establish the correct diagnosis. Negative blood cultures in the presence of imaging abnormalities suspicious of infection will necessitate closed biopsy for organism identification and broad-spectrum antibiotics.

Imaging Studies

Plain radiographs have a very low sensitivity and specificity in the initial stages of infection and thus are unreliable and do not exclude spinal infection when they are found to be normal. Early findings on plain films include blurring of the vertebral endplate region, followed within a short period of time by disc space narrowing (Figure 6-1). Bone scan at this stage will show increased uptake at the affected region. As the infection progresses, the disc space may be completely lost and bony erosions will appear in the adjacent vertebral bodies. The vertebral bodies may look moth-eaten and eventually may collapse. Sclerotic new bone formation may appear at a later stage (Figure 6-2).

CT scan is more sensitive than plain radiographs but is not specific enough and thus is not as helpful as MRI. It will show disruptions in the vertebral cortex and erosions in the vertebral bodies. The erosions will be irregular and darker (hypodense) than healthy bone. Infected discs may appear hypodense as well. Soft tissue images may help detect swelling and pus collection in the surrounding soft tissues (i.e., muscles). This will appear as a hypodense area within the muscle substance with clear demarcation lines. Rarely, gas may be seen in the infected areas. Epidural abscess may be detected on postcontrast CT scans as an enhancing epidural mass compressing the thecal sac.

MRI, the diagnostic modality of choice, is highly sensitive and specific and may confirm the presence of infection at an early stage of the disease. T1-weighted images will show decreased signal in the involved vertebral bodies, especially at the endplate region. As a result, the disc and the bone signal may appear similar in intensity. The endplate margins may look fuzzy, and interruption of cortical continuity may be seen. T2-weighted images will show increased signal of both the disc and the affected vertebral body (Figures 6-3A and 6-3B). In late stages of osteomyelitis, when bone sclerosis occurs, T2-weighted images will show decreased signal due to the obliteration of the bone marrow and increased production of bone. The presence of gas within the vertebral body will result in decreased signal on T1- as well as T2-weighted images. Following contrast administration, the affected discs and bones will show clear enhancement even at the early stages of the disease (Figure 6-4).

TABLE 6-1
Characteristic MRI Signal Changes in the Presence of Infection

T1	T2	Postcontrast T1
Decreased vertebral body signal	Increased discal and vertebral body signal	Enhancement of affected disc and bone

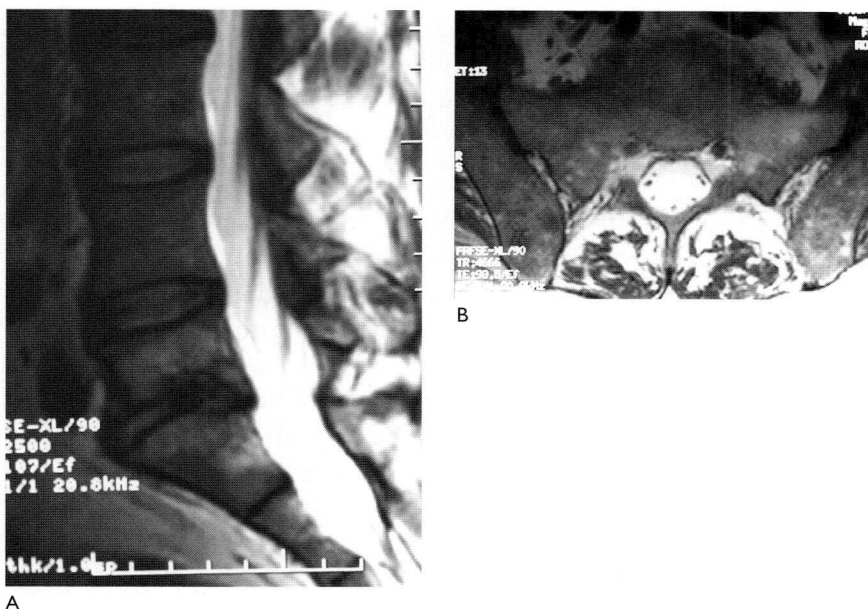

A

B

FIGURE 6-3
(A) Sagittal and (B) axial T2WI MR images of the same patient in the initial stages of infection. Inhomogeneous increased signal is seen with the L5 and S1 vertebrae. The posterior halves of the endplates are ill-defined or obscure.

The paraspinal structures should be carefully reviewed as abscesses can form within the soft tissues. These may be isointense to muscle on T1-weighted images and hyperintense on T2-weighted images. Paraspinal abscesses may be best visualized in postcontrast T1-weighted images with fat suppression. Soft tissue abscesses will enhance mostly peripherally as the necrotic core remains hypointense (Figures 6-5 and 6-6).

Management

In order to obtain a successful outcome early identification of the offending agent should be obtained. Early intravenous administration of antibiotics will lessen the incidence of epidural abscess formation, instability, and neurological deficits. Nutritional supplementation is of high importance as spinal infections frequently occur in patients with premorbid nutritional deficits, and the infection itself is a highly catabolic condition. The intravenous drugs should be administered for a period of at least 4–6 weeks and followed by orally administered antibiotics. C-reactive protein is more sensitive than sedimentation rate and should be frequently obtained to monitor response to treatment.

Epidural Abscess Formation

When the infective process is allowed to continue it may spread posteriorly into the spinal canal and compress the dural sac and/or the neural elements. Epidural collection of pus may quickly organize as an abscess within the spinal canal and lead to severe neurological deficits in about 30% of patients.

Epidural abscess (EA) is more common in the sixth and seventh decades, especially in immunocompromised, diabetic, and septicemic

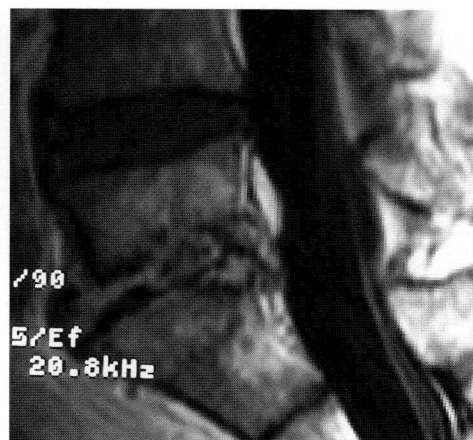

FIGURE 6-4
Sagittal T1WI with contrast shows enhancement in the vertebral bodies and the intervening disc. Most of the disc has been destroyed.

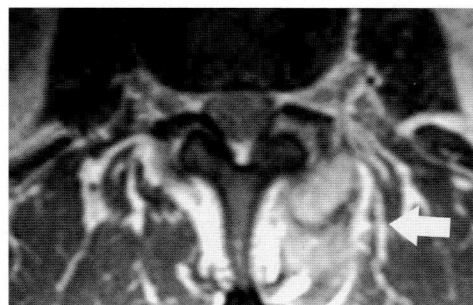

FIGURE 6-5
Axial T1WI showing facet infection on the left side. The infection has spread to the soft tissue and has formed an abscess within the paraspinal muscles (arrow). Courtesy Dr. N. Haramati.

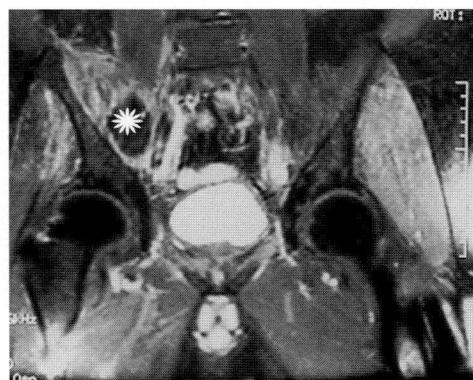

FIGURE 6-6
Coronal T2-weighted MRI with fat suppression showing a soft tissue abscess within the right ilio-psoas muscle (star). Note that the abscess is hypointense and is surrounded by a white rim. The patient had local pain, held the hip joint in flexion, and did not allow hyperextension of that joint.

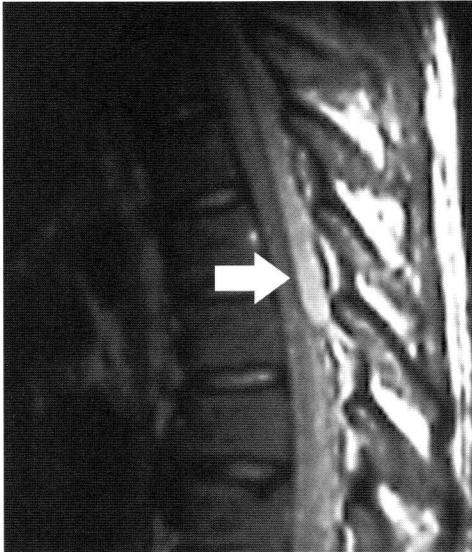

FIGURE 6-7
Sagittal T2WI MRI showing an elongated mass dorsal to the spinal cord. The mass is hyperintense to the cord and represents epiduritis / an epidural abscess.

patients, and following spinal procedures and surgery. Most epidural abscesses occur in the low thoracic or lumbar regions. Cervical abscesses are less common but have a poorer outcome.

Clinical Presentation

Patients present with subacute to acute axial pain. At times, the complaints may be similar to those seen in patients with herniated discs. The patients may be febrile and have a high sedimentation rate and leukocytosis. In some patients radicular symptoms or sudden, progressive neurological deterioration may be the first clue to the presence of an epidural abscess. Within a short period of time the patient develops paralysis with loss of bladder and bowel control. In these cases an emergency MRI with contrast should be obtained.

Imaging Studies

The MRI will show a collection of substance that is hypointense to the spinal cord on T1-weighted images and hyperintense to the cord on T2-weighted images.

Following contrast administration the periphery of the collection will enhance, whereas the core of the abscess will not enhance (Figure 6-7). Frequently, the neural elements also enhance following contrast administration.

Management

The abscess should be surgically drained under coverage of broad-spectrum antibiotics. Once the offending agent has been identified, a more specific antibiotic can be administered for at least eight more weeks. Consultation with infectious diseases specialists is of paramount importance in order to achieve a positive outcome.

TUBERCULOUS OSTEOMYELITIS (POTT'S DISEASE)

The incidence of tuberculous spondylodiscitis (TBS) has increased in the last few decades. Tuberculosis is more commonly found in poor people, people living in overcrowded environments such as prisons, and in patients with AIDS, especially those with a CD4 T-cell count between 50 and 200 cells. Drug-resistant tuberculosis is a major therapeutic challenge that, unfortunately, is frequently seen in major hospitals throughout the world.

In a significant number of TBS patients the source of the infection is not evident but is assumed to originate from a small locus of infection within the lungs. Usually the infection reaches the spine via the arterial system and settles in the anterior portion of the vertebral bodies in the subchondral region. The disease appears mostly in the thoracic spine and less frequently in the thoraco-lumbar junction. In the majority of patients several contiguous levels may be involved. Occasionally the affected levels are not contiguous and, at times, one-level disease may be observed.

Clinical Presentation

The onset of symptoms is rather insidious. Pain may appear in the thoracic region in a girdle-like distribution and may be accompanied by local tenderness. The pain persists and the patient may become febrile. This may be accompanied by night sweats, especially when concomitant pulmonary tuberculosis is present. Weight loss may be documented. Most patients are diagnosed late. The evolution of symptoms is slower in TBS than in pyogenic osteomyelitis, and the reported pain may be milder for quite some time. Weeks to months may pass before the diagnosis is established. Diagnosis delay may result in disease progression leading to vertebral body collapse, kyphotic deformity (gibbus), abscess formation, spinal instability, and neurological deficits due to spinal cord compression.

Imaging Studies

X-rays may remain negative for weeks and thus are not helpful in the early stage of the disease. Later on the vertebral body may show osteopenia, osteolysis, and sclerosis. The endplate may be eroded and the disc space reduced. These radiological changes do not differentiate TB spondylitis from other infections. In later stages of the disease there may be total vertebral body collapse with fusion across the disc space due to reactive new bone formation. A kyphotic deformity—gibbus—may be formed. When two adjacent vertebral bodies are affected, the intervertebral disc may be deprived of its nutrition and tend to lose its height (Figures 6-8 and 6-9). Calcifications in the paravertebral soft tissues are typical of this disease.

CT examination will clearly show vertebral body erosions, destruction, and sequestration (depending on infection duration). Bone fragments may appear within the spinal canal or in the soft tissues (Figures 6-10A and 6-10B). CT with contrast may help delineate

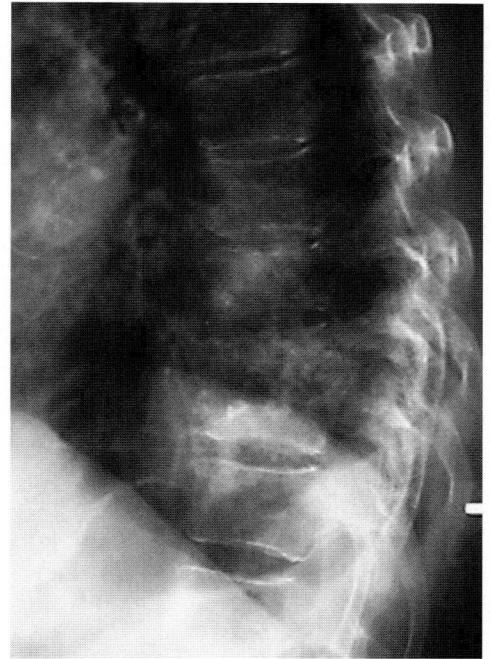

FIGURE 6-8
Lateral plain spine film showing osteopenia, osteolysis with relative preservation of the intervertebral disc in the early stages of TB infection of the spine.

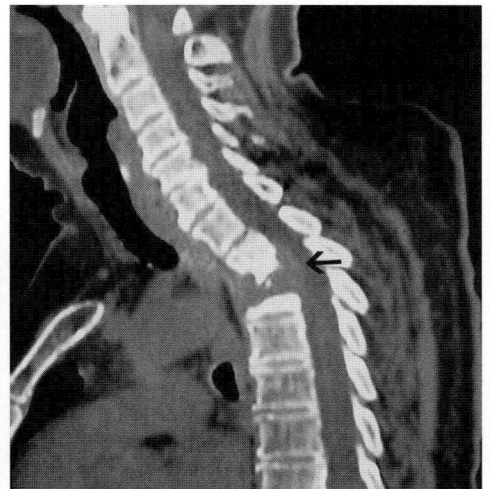

FIGURE 6-9
Reformatted sagittal CT image of the spine showing destruction of T2 vertebral body with gibbus formation and soft tissue density protruding into the canal (arrow). Courtesy Dr. J. Houten.

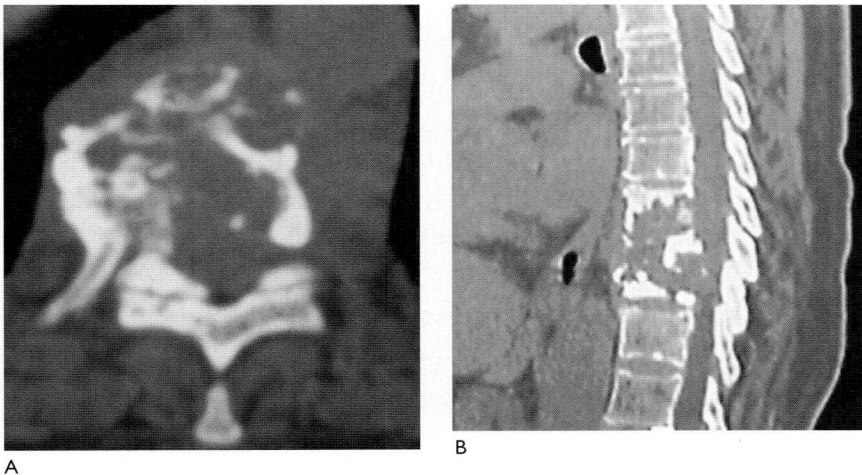

A

B

FIGURE 6-10
(A) Axial and (B) sagittal reformatted CT cut through the thoracic spine shows extensive destruction of 3 consecutive vertebral bodies affected by TB. Note the penetration of the causative material through the anterior cortex into the retroperitoneal soft tissues and the posterior cortex into the vertebral canal. Courtesy Dr. J. Houten.

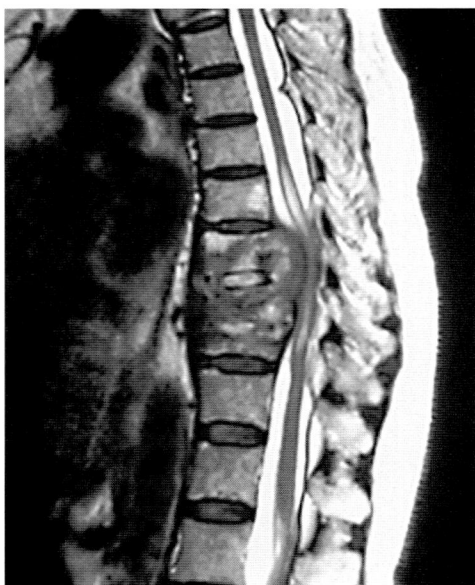

FIGURE 6-11
Sagittal T2-weighted MR image showing destruction of three thoracic vertebrae with abscess formation and spinal cord compression. Note the
increased signal within the vertebral body above
the abscess. Courtesy Dr. J. Houten.

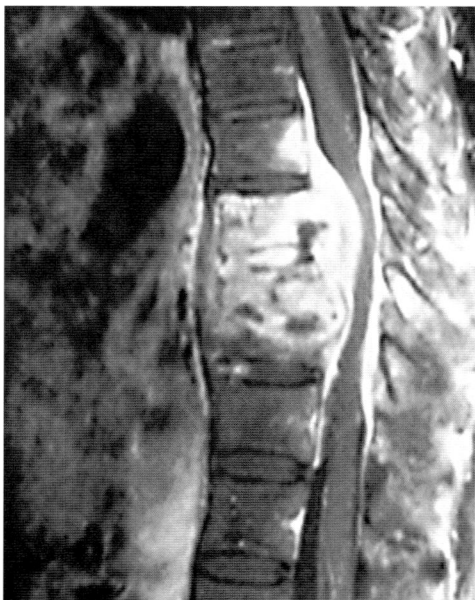

FIGURE 6-12
Sagittal T1WI with contrast discloses the
full extent of the infectious process: There is
marked enhancement of the infiltrated, thick
epidural fat anterior and posterior to the dural
sac along 6 segments—at, above and below
the infectious core. Encasement of the dural
sac and the cord by the enhancing infiltration
is demonstrated. Note the involvement of a
fourth vertebra located above, with sparing of
the disc between them.

TABLE 6-2
Differences between Pyogenic and Tuberculous Osteomyelitis

Pyogenic Osteomyelitis	Tuberculous Osteomyelitis
More common in lumbar spine	More common in thoracic spine
Early involvement of Intervertebral discs	Sparing or late involvement of discs
Spinal deformity less common	Spinal deformity (gibbus) common
Small paraspinal abscesses, less common	Large paraspinal abscesses, common
Rapid progression, often severe pain	Slow progression, mild pain
High ESR	ESR may remain normal
Subligamentous spread uncommon	Subligamentous spread more common

the soft tissue abscesses. The abscesses may be prevertebral, paravertebral, or epidural.

On MRI the affected vertebral bodies will appear hypointense
on T1-weighted images and hyperintense on T2-weighted images,
especially in the subchondral region. No enhancement of the discs
is seen in the early stages of the disease. This helps differentiate TB
spondylitis from pyogenic spondylitis. Paraspinal abscesses appear
hypointense on T1WI and hyperintense on T2WI. Diffuse enhancement may appear on T1WI following contrast administration. Axial
cuts are very important in assessing spinal cord integrity (Figures 6-11,
6-12, and 6-13).

The prognosis of TBS is related to the time of diagnosis. Early
diagnosis and treatment result in preservation of spinal alignment and
prevention of neurological complications. Late identification of the
disease may result in instability, gibbus formation, and abscesses with
potentially severe neurological deficits.

Management

Anti-tuberculous medications should be administered for at
least one year. Initially four drugs are administered: isoniazid, rifam-
picin, ethambutol, and pyrazinamide. Close monitoring with repeated
neurological examinations, imaging, and laboratory tests is performed.
Drug-resistant patients would benefit from second-line drugs.

ACUTE TRANSVERSE MYELITIS

Acute transverse myelitis (ATM) is a clinical syndrome in which
damage to the cord is thought to occur via an immune mediated process without any evidence of cord compression. It can occur at any age
and affects both genders to the same extent.

ATM may occur only once or may appear in a relapsing, recurrent
form. When it occurs as an isolated event without an apparent reason
it is called idiopathic ATM. It may, however, occur within the con-
text of a systemic disease (lupus, Sjogren's syndrome, antiphospholipid
syndrome) in which multiple body systems are affected, following an

infection (parainfectious myelopathy), neoplastic disease, vaccination, radiation therapy (delayed transverse myelitis), or as part of a multifocal neurological disorder (multiple sclerosis, neuromyelitis optica). Regardless of its cause, ATM results in weakness or paralysis, sensory deficits, sphincter control problems, and autonomic dysfunction. The clinical outcome varies, depending on the etiology of ATM.

This chapter will deal with the idiopathic form of ATM only.

Clinical Presentation

Initially patients present with acute neck or back pain, which is followed within hours or days by progressive neurological deficits. Within a period of up to three weeks, and usually over several days only, the patients develop the full-blown picture: sensory changes including sensory level or paraesthesia and muscle paralysis or weakness. These can quickly evolve to complete paraplegia or quadriplegia, depending on the cord region that is affected. The sphincters are commonly involved as well. The signs and symptoms are bilateral but are not necessarily symmetrical. The thoracic cord is the area most frequently affected. In the initial stages the physical examination will detect lower motor neuron findings, such as areflexia and hypotonia. Severe atrophy of the involved muscles develops within days. The diagnosis is established by excluding other known causes of myelopathy such as multiple sclerosis, anterior spinal artery infarction, infectious myelitis, cord tumors, and vascular malformations. Cerebrospinal fluid examination will detect pleocytosis. No oligoclonal bands are documented in the spinal fluid.

Imaging Studies

Plain films are not helpful in this condition. Brain imaging remains normal throughout the disease. CT examination may disclose cord swelling. There may be focal or diffuse enhancement following contrast administration. The examination of choice is MRI. T1-weighted images may detect hypointense cord enlargement. The hypointensity usually involves more than two vertebral levels. The spinal cord will be hyperintense on T2-weighted images. The hyperintensity tends to occupy over two-thirds of the cross-sectional area of the cord and is frequently centrally located. Following contrast administration there is clear contrast enhancement in both axial and sagittal T1-weighted images. The enhancement may be moderate, nodular, or diffuse, and tends to involve an area smaller then the hyperintense area as seen on T2-weighted images (Figures 6-14A and 6-14B). Contrast enhancement is more frequently found in the subacute stage. Because multiple sclerosis is frequently considered in these patients, an MRI of the brain should be obtained as well.

Management

During the acute stage, most patients are managed with systemic steroids with variable responses. There is no conclusive evidence in

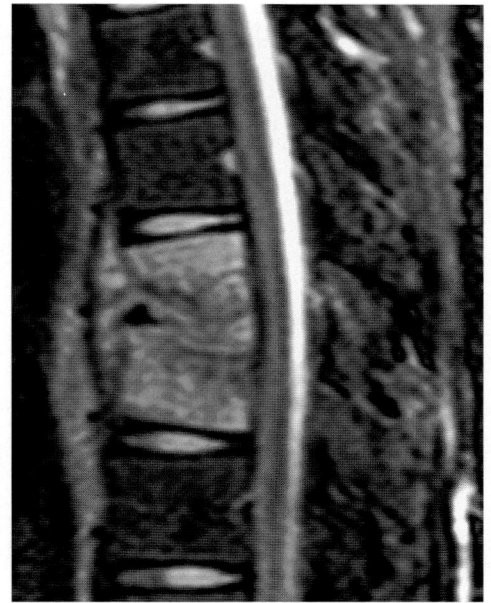

FIGURE 6-13
Sagittal T2WI with fat suppression clearly showing involvement of two adjacent vertebral bodies in another patient. Courtesy Dr. J. Houten.

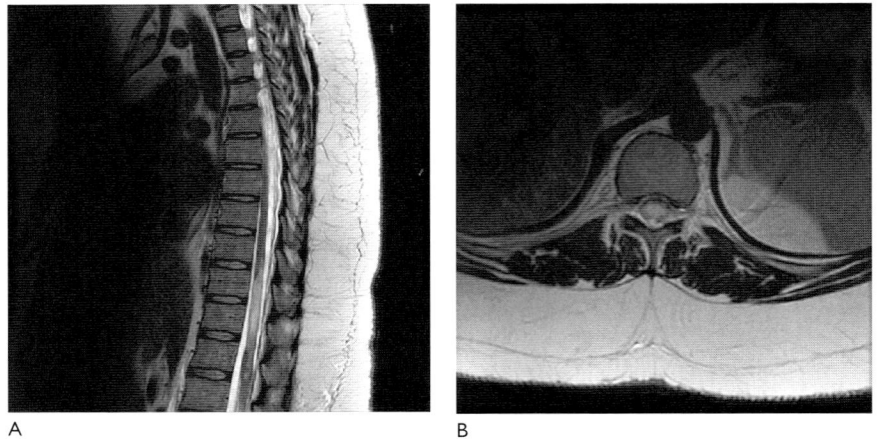

A   B

FIGURE 6-14
(A) Sagittal and (B) axial T2WI of the thoracic spine showing multisegmentary epiduritis behind the spinal cord with Note the increased cord signal indicating edema
and myelopathy.

the literature, however, that steroids have a positive influence on the
outcome. In most patients the outcome remains unpredictable. Some
patients improve, whereas others, especially those with early, severe
involvement, remain permanently disabled.

Bibliography

Almeida A: Tuberculosis of the spine and spinal cord. Eur J Radiol 55: 193–201, 2005.

Bezer M, Kucukdurmaz F, Aydin N, Kocaoglu B, Guven O: Tuberculous spondylitis of the lumbosacral region. Long term follow-up of patients treated by chemotherapy, transpedicular drainage,
posterior instrumentation, and fusion. J Spinal Disord Tech 18: 425–429, 2005.

Campi A, Filippi M, Comi G, Martinelli V, Baratti C, Rovaris M, Scotti G: Acute transverse
myelopathy: Spinal and cranial MR study with clinical follow-up. Am J Neuroradiol 16: 115–123,
1995.

Carragee EJ: Pyogenic vertebral osteomyelitis. J Bone Joint Surg Am 79: 874–880, 1997.

Choi KH, Lee KS, Chung SO, Park JM, Kim YJ, Kim HS, Shinn KS: Idiopathic transverse myelitis: MR characteristics. Am J Neuroradiol 17: 1151–1160, 1996.

Cree BAC, Wingerchuk DM: Acute transverse myelitis: Is the "idiopathic" form vanishing? Neurology 65: 1857–1858, 2005.

Dagirmanjian A, Schils J, McHenry M, Modic MT: MR imaging of vertebral osteomyelitis revisited. Am J Radiol 167: 1539–1543, 1996.

Desai SS: Early diagnosis of spinal tuberculosis by MRI. J Bone Joint Surg Br 76: 863–869,
1994.

De Seze J, Lanctin C, Lebrun C, Malikova I, Papeix C, Wiertlewski S, Pelletier J, Gout O, Clerc
C, Moreau C, Defer G, Edan G, Dubas F, Vermersch P: Idiopathic acute transverse myelitis:
Application of the recent diagnostic criteria. Neurology 65: 1950–1953, 2005.

De Seze J, Stojkovic T, Breteau G, Lucas C, Michon-Pasturel U, Gauvrit JE, Hachulla E, Mounier-
Vehier F, Pruvo JP, Leys D, Destee A, Hatron PY, Vermersch P: Acute myelopathies: Clinical,
laboratory and outcome profile in 79 cases. Brain 124: 1509–1521, 2001.

Govender S: Review article: Spinal infections. J Bone Joint Surg Br 87: 1454–1458, 2005.

Hadjipavlou AG, Mader JT, Necessary JT, Muffoletto AJ: Hematogenous pyogenic spinal infections and their surgical management. Spine 25: 1668–1679, 2000.

Jain R, Sawhney S, Berry M: Computed tomography of vertebral tuberculosis: Patterns of bone
destruction. Clin Radiol 47: 196–199, 1993.

Jeffrey DR, Mandler RN, Davis LE: Transverse myelitis: Retrospective analysis of 33 cases, with differentiation of cases associated with multiple sclerosis and parainfectious events. Arch Neurol 50: 532–535, 1993.

Kerr DA, Aeytey H: Immunopathogenesis of acute transverse myelitis. Curr Opin Neurol 15: 339–347, 2002.

Kim KK: Idiopathic recurrent transverse myelitis. Arch Neurol 60: 1290–1294, 2003.

Kim NH, Lee HM, Suh JS: Magnetic resonance imaging for the diagnosis of tuberculous spondylitis. Spine 19: 2451–2455, 1994.

Maiuri F, Iaconetta G, Gallicchio B, Mano A, Briganti F: Spondylodiscitis: Clinical and magnetic resonance diagnosis. Spine 22: 1741–1746, 1997.

Nene A, Bhorjraj S: Results of nonsurgical treatment of thoracic spinal tuberculosis in adults. Spine J 5: 79–84, 2005.

Oostveen JCM, Van de Laar MAFJ: Magnetic resonance imaging in rheumatic disorders of the spine and sacroiliac joints. Semin Arthritis Rheum 30: 52–69, 2000.

Patzakis MJ, Rao S, Wilkins J, Moore TM, Harvey PJ: Analysis of 61 cases of vertebral osteomyelitis. Clin Orthop 264: 178–183, 1991.

Rath SA, Neff U, Schneider O, Richter HP: Neurosurgical management of thoracic and lumbar vertebral osteomyelitis and discitis in adults: A review of 43 consecutive surgically treated patients. Neurosurg 38: 926–933, 1996.

Reihsaus E, Waldbaur H, Seeling W: Spinal epidural abscess: A meta-analysis of 915 patients. Neurosurg Rev 23: 175–204, 2000.

Ross JS, Brant-Zawadzki M, Moore KR, Crim J, Chen MZ, Katman GL: Infections, pp. 1–61 in Ross JS, Brandt-Zawadzki M, Moore KR, Crim J, Chen MZ, Katman GL: Diagnostic imaging, vol. III: Spine. Amirsys, 2004.

Schwartz ST, Spiegel M, Ho Jr. G: Bacterial vertebral osteomyelitis and epidural abscess. Semin Spine Surg 2: 95–105, 1990.

Sharif H: MR in managing spine infections. Am J Radiol 158: 133–145, 1992.

Tang HJ, Lin JH, Lui YC, Li CM: Spinal epidural abscess: Experience with 46 patients and evaluation of prognostic factors. J Infect 45: 76–81, 2002.

Transverse myelitis consortium working group: Proposed diagnostic criteria and nosology of acute transverse myelitis. Neurology 59: 499–505, 2002.

Turgut Tali E: Spinal infections. Eur J Radiol 50: 120–133, 2004.

Weinstein MA, Eismont FJ: Infections of the spine in patients with human immunodeficiency virus. J Bone Joint Surg Am 87: 604–609, 2005.

Wisnesky RJ: Infectious disease of the spine: Diagnostic and treatment considerations. Orthop Clin N Am 22: 491–501, 1991.

SPINAL CYSTS

7

Spinal cysts are not uncommon. They are frequently seen as an incidental finding on imaging studies obtained for other reasons and have no clinical significance. At times, however, they may cause axial and/or radicular pain and bring about significant morbidity.

SYNOVIAL CYSTS

Synovial cysts are most commonly found in the lumbar spine, mostly at the L4-L5 level. They usually develop in patients with degenerative disc disease, facet arthropathy, and degenerative spinal stenosis. Quite frequently degenerative spondylolisthesis or facet joint instability is also found at the level of cyst formation. The latter findings, it is thought, support the notion that increased segmental motion plays a role in the pathogenesis of these cysts.

Typically the cysts occupy the posterolateral aspect of the spinal canal, are adjacent to the facet joints, and are attached to the facet joint capsule. They contain serous or gelatinous fluid and measure up to two centimeters in diameter.

Clinical Presentation

The patients, usually females in the sixth decade, present with back pain and radicular pain. The pain is frequently intermittent and is often mechanical in nature. It may be worse standing but may persist in other postures as well. The pain does not respond to conservative management and usually persists. On rare occasions, large-diameter cysts may lead to cauda equina syndrome. Thoracic or cervical cysts compress the cord and result in a slowly progressive myelopathy.

Imaging Studies

The X-ray findings are those commensurate with age and spinal degeneration: degenerative disc disease, facet arthropathy, degenerative spondylolisthesis, and spur formation. Spinal CT may detect the cyst when its wall has calcified or when its cavity contains gas or blood due to a hemorrhage. In the latter case the cyst space will appear hyperdense in comparison to the spinal canal. Occasionally large cysts may erode the adjacent bone and become detectable on bone windows. Contrast CT may show some enhancement in the cyst's wall. MRI, the procedure of choice, will show an extradural lesion with smooth surfaces adjacent to the facet joint. T1-weighted images may show the cyst as hypointense, isointense, or hyperintense when it contains blood. T2-weighted images show a hyperintense lesion that, at times, may communicate with the facet joint. In contrast studies the cyst's walls may enhance and show its impact on the adjacent nerve roots (Figures 7-1A, 7-1B, and 7-1C).

The MRI examination helps rule out an extruded disc or a tumor as their T1 and T2 signal characteristics and response to contrast administration are different from those of a cyst. Unlike cysts, extruded discs are not hyperintense on T2-weighted images. Following contrast administration, however, the disc's periphery may enhance due to local scarring or inflammation. Tumors, typically, will become hyperintense to a greater degree after contrast administration.

Management

Following the diagnosis of a facet cyst it is worth trying conservative measures as the symptoms may spontaneously regress. Analgesic

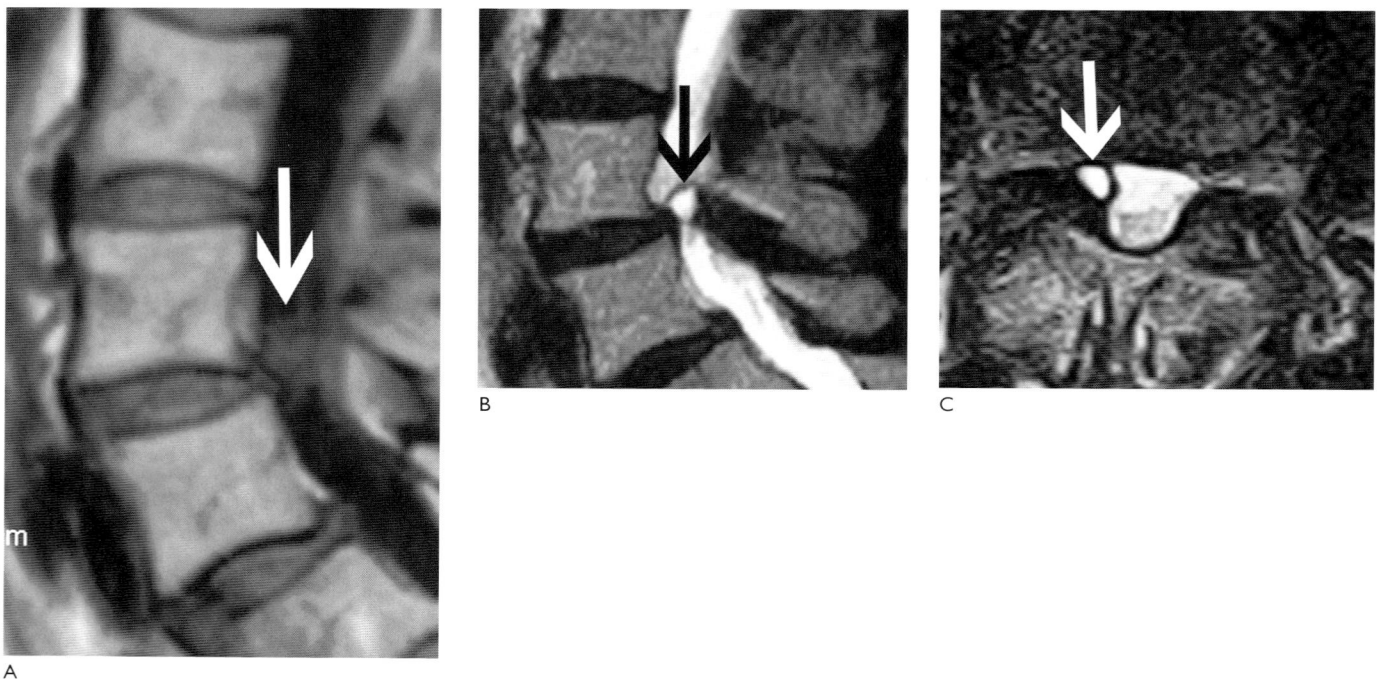

FIGURE 7-1

MRI of the lumbar spine. (A) In the sagittal T1-weighted MRI a lesion with signal intensity brighter than the CSF is seen filling the sagittal diameter of the spinal canal (arrow). (B) The lesions appear to be cystic and of high signal intensity (arrow) on the T2WI. (C) Axial T2WI MR of the same patient. A facet joint synovial cyst is seen within the right lateral recess bulging into the lateral recess and the intervertebral neural foramen. The proximity of the cyst to the facet joint is clearly demonstrated.

and anti-inflammatory medication may be tried first. If the symptoms persist the cyst can be drained percutaneously. A needle is introduced into the cyst under fluoroscopy or guided by CT scan. Following drainage of the cyst's contents steroids can be injected into the cyst's cavity. This procedure can bring about symptom relief lasting for weeks, months, or, at times, longer periods of time. If no relief is obtained or when the symptoms recur, surgery should be considered. Total cyst excision is performed in order to prevent cyst recurrence. Spinal stabilization should be performed in patients with local instability. Most patients do well postoperatively.

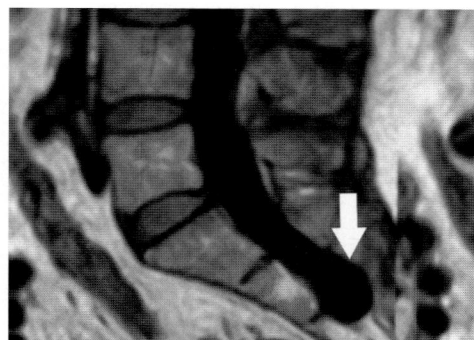

FIGURE 7-2
Sagittal T1WI showing a rounded sacral cyst having the same signal intensity as the CSF.

PERINEURAL CYST (TARLOV CYST)

Tarlov cysts are commonly seen in MRI studies of the lumbosacral spine. The cysts were described by Tarlov in 1938 and bear his name. In most instances the cysts are an incidental finding, have no clinical relevance, and are not responsible for the patient's symptoms. In a small number of patients, especially those with large cysts, symptoms such as back pain, radicular pain, and pelvic pain may be caused by the cysts.

Tarlov cysts are most frequently encountered in the sacral region, especially at the S2 and S3 levels (Figure 7-2). At times the cysts may occur in the lumbar region and less frequently in the thoracic region. The cysts usually develop at the junction of the dorsal root with the dorsal root ganglion in the space between the perineurium and the endoneurium. At times the nerve rootlets are embedded in the cyst's walls. It is postulated that the cysts are formed secondary to an inflammatory or degenerative process or local trauma. Not infrequently, multiple bilateral cysts resembling a cluster of grapes are formed. At times, the cysts attain a large diameter of several centimeters. Large cysts, especially those with a valve-like mechanism that may lead to gravitational fluid accumulation, may cause sacral ectasia, enlarge the neural foramen, and, at times, lead to a pathological fracture.

It is very difficult to decide what role, if any, the cyst plays in the patient's symptomatology. In most patients other coexisting pathology is the likely cause of the symptoms. Several small series of patients have been described where surgery dealing with other pathology, such as disc, facet arthropathy, or spinal stenosis, has been performed, while the cyst was left untouched. In many instances all the symptoms subsided.

Rarely, sacral, perineal, and radicular pain or compromised bladder and bowel function may be caused by large cysts. In the absence of other significant pathology, surgery should be considered. The cysts should be decompressed and their content aspirated. As nerve fibers are frequently embedded within the cyst's wall, it is not surprising that some patients can be left with neurological deficits following excision.

Imaging Studies

X-ray studies are usually negative and do not indicate the presence of the cysts. Occasionally, enlarged neural foraminae or thinned pedicles provide a clue to the presence of a space-occupying lesion. CT scans, especially bone windows, may show enlarged neural foraminae or sacral spinal canal. Soft tissue windows may show a mass with the same density as the CSF. The mass does not enhance with contrast. MRI studies easily detect the cysts and clearly show their size and location. The sagittal cuts will show a pea-sized or larger mass that is isointense with the CSF and is located at the end of the thecal sac in the sacral region. The cysts are usually hyperintense in T2-weighted images and remain so following fat suppression. Unlike metastatic disease or primary nerve root tumors, perineural cysts do not enhance with contrast (Figures 7-3A, 7-3B, and 7-3C).

ARACHNOID CYSTS

Acquired arachnoid cysts are usually found at the thoracic spine. These cysts result from CSF accumulation within a diverticulum of arachnoid membrane that communicates with the subarachnoid space. They develop post-traumatically, following an infection, or after surgery. The cysts may be large and extend over several vertebral levels. They may enlarge the spinal canal, thin out the facets, and at times

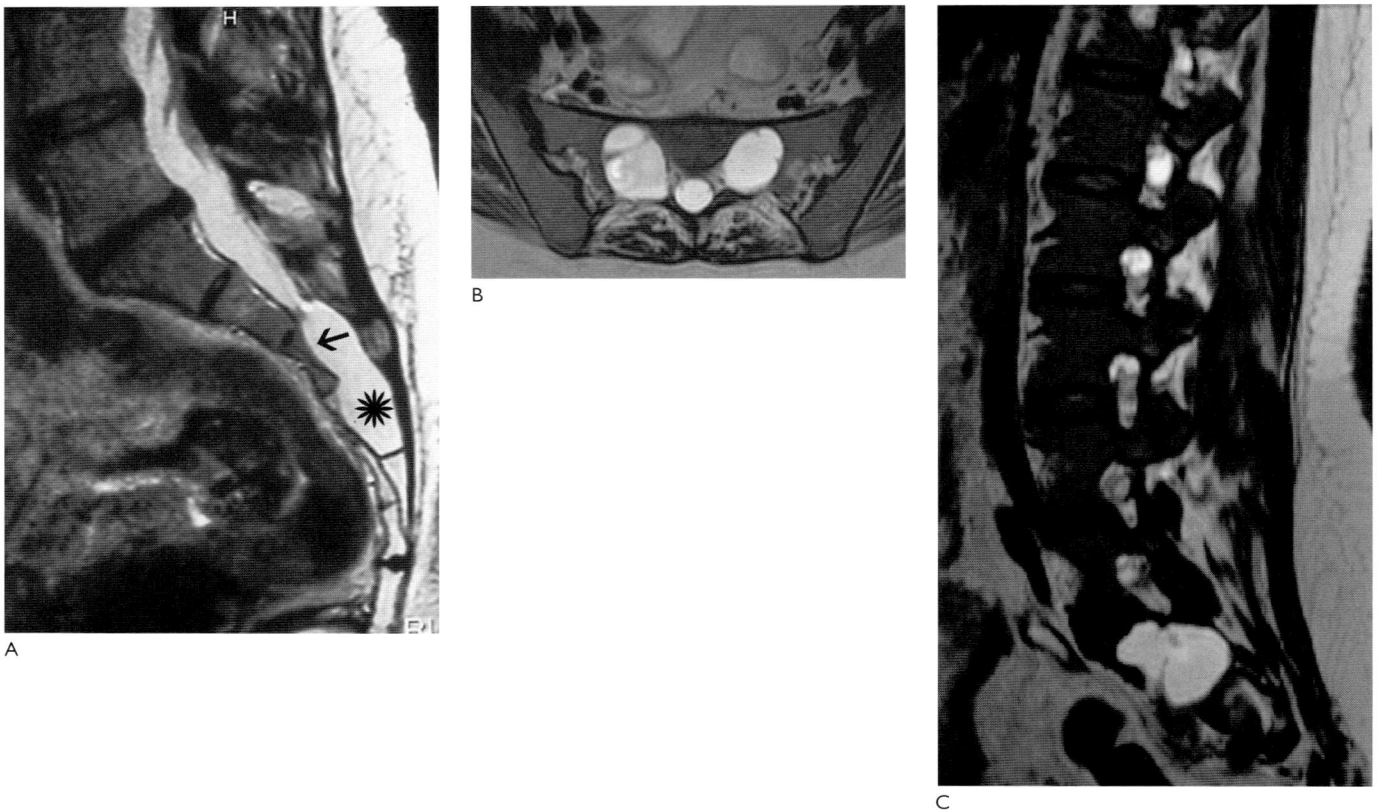

FIGURE 7-3
(A) Sagittal T2-weighted MRI showing a Tarlov cyst isointense to the CSF (star). Posterior scalloping of the sacrum is demonstrated (arrow). (B) Very large Tarlov cysts protruding laterally and anteriorly through the sacral foraminae and indenting the sacral allae. The cysts are isointense with the CSF in all sequences. The right cyst has a small area that is hyperintense and a hypointense strand that represents septations with the cyst's wall. (C) A parasagittal cut (T2WI) through the neural foraminae clearly shows the hyperintense cyst eroding the foraminal wall and extending beyond the sacral foramen.

may enlarge neural foraminae as well. The cysts may compress the spinal cord and lead to thinning and atrophy of this structure.

Clinical Presentation

As with perineural cysts, most patients with arachnoid cysts remain asymptomatic. If the cysts are large and affect the vertebrae the patients may present with fluctuating back pain and radicular pain that may be severe and is worse during straining or coughing. Spinal cord compression results in myelopathic symptoms: gait dysfunction, paraparesis, and sphincter involvement. In the latter cases the patients should be operated on promptly as undue delay may lead to compromised function.

Imaging Studies

The cyst may appear as a solitary, oval structure. At times, multiple cysts may be present. The density and signal characteristics of these cysts on CT and MRI studies are similar to those of perineural cysts.

Management

Complete excision of the cyst is the definitive treatment.

Bibliography

Banning CS, Thorell WE, Leibrock LG: Patient outcome after resection of lumbar juxtafacet cysts. Spine 26: 969–972, 2001.

Bassiouni H, Hunold A, Asgari S, Hubschen U, Konig HJ, Stolke D: Spinal intradural juxtamedullary cysts in the adult: Surgical management and outcome. Neurosurgery 55: 1352–1360, 2004.

Charest DR, Kenny BG: Radicular pain caused by synovial cyst: An underdiagnosed entity in the elderly? J Neurosurg 92: 57–60, 2000.

DePalma MJ, Strakowski JA, Mandelker EM, Zerick WR: An instance of an atypical intraspinal cyst presenting as S1 radiculopathy: A case report and brief review of pathophysiology. Arch Phys Med Rehabil 85: 1021–1025, 2004.

Doita M, Nishida K, Miura J, Takada T, Kurosaka M, Fujii M: Kinematic magnetic resonance imaging of a thoracic spinal extradural arachnoid cyst: An alternative suggestion for exacerbation of symptoms during straining. Spine 28: E229–E233, 2003.

Kaneko K, Inoiue Y: Haemorrhagic lumbar synovial cyst: A case of acute radiculopathy. J Bone Joint Surg Br 82: 583–584, 2000.

Khan AM, Synnot K, Cammisa FP, Girardi FP: Lumbar synovial cysts of the spine: An evaluation of surgical outcome. J Spinal Disord Tech 18: 127–131, 2005.

Langdown AJ, Grundy JRB, Birch NC: The clinical relevance of Tarlov cyst. J Spinal Disord Tech 18: 29–33, 2005.

Paulsen RD, Call RD, Murtagh FR: Prevalence and percutaneous drainage of cysts of the sacral nerve root sheath (Tarlov cysts). Am J Neuroradiol 15: 293–297, 1994.

Ross JS, Brant-Zawadzki M, Moore KR, Crim J, Chen MZ, Katman GL: Infections, pp. 2–13 in Ross JS, Brandt-Zawadzki M, Moore KR, Crim J, Chen MZ, Katman GL: Diagnostic imaging, vol IV: Spine. Amirsys, 2004.

Sabers SR, Ross SR, Grogg BE, Lauder TD: Procedure-based nonsurgical management of lumbar zygapophyseal joint cyst-induced radicular pain. Arch Phys Med Rehabil 86: 1767–1771, 2005.

Sabo RA, Tracey PT, Weinger JM: A series of 60 juxtafacet cysts: Clinical presentation, the role of spinal instability, and treatment. J Neurosurg 85: 560–565, 1996.

Shah R, Lutz G: Lumbar intraspinal synovial cysts: Conservative management and review of the world's literature. Spine J 3: 479–488, 2003.

Takeuchi A, Miyamoto K, Sugiyama S, Saitou M, Hosoe H, Shimizu K: Spinal arachnoid cysts associated with syringomyelia: Report of two cases and a review of the literature. J Spinal Disord Tech 16: 207–211, 2003.

Tarlov IM: Perineural cysts of the spinal root. Arch Neurol Psychiat 40: 1067–1074, 1938.

Tillich M, Trummer M, Lindbichler F, Flaschka G: Symptomatic intraspinal synovial cysts of the lumbar spine: Correlation of MR and surgical findings. Neuroradiology 43: 1070–1075, 2001.

Tunialan LM, Cawley CM, Barrow DL: Arachnoid cyst with associated arachnoiditis developing after subarachnoid hemorrhage: Case report. J Neurosurg 103: 1088–1091, 2005.

Voyadzis JM, Bhargava P, Henderson FC: Tarlov cysts: A study of 10 cases with review of the literature. J Neurosurg 95: 25–32, 2001.

SPONDYLOARTHROPATHY

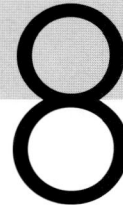

8

The term *spondyloarthropathy* refers to a cluster of interrelated seronegative chronic inflammatory diseases that affect the spine and the peripheral joints. Other systems, such as the ocular, gastrointestinal, cardiovascular, and cutaneous systems, are affected as well.

The point of attachment of ligaments and tendons to bone is known as the enthesis. In the spondyloarthropathies, structural changes occur throughout the skeleton, including the spine at the enthesis sites. Initially, bone resorption takes place, and subsequently excessive bone formation occurs. These structural changes at the enthesis sites have been called enthesopathy.

Many patients with spondyloarthropathy have a positive HLA-B27. The rheumatoid factor, however, remains negative in these diseases. Seronegative spondyloarthropathy is the term that is applied to this class of disorders, which includes ankylosing spondylitis, psoriatic arthropathy, Reiter's disease, inflammatory bowel arthropathy, and Behcet's disease.

CLINICAL PRESENTATION

Patients suffering from these diseases present with musculoskeletal complaints such as spinal stiffness, pain, and/or arthralgia. Typical of inflammatory diseases, the pain tends to improve with motion. Many patients complain predominantly of morning stiffness and pain that subside once they get going. When spinal symptoms appear in isolation in these diseases they are frequently interpreted as nonspecific, or erroneously attributed to degenerative disc disease. When the complaints persist and a thorough work-up is initiated, and as other systems become involved (e.g., psoriatic skin changes, ocular symptoms), the correct diagnosis is often made.

ANKYLOSING SPONDYLITIS

Ankylosing spondylitis (AS) usually presents in the second or third decade. It affects mostly males but occasionally is reported in females.

Clinical Presentation

Patients present with morning stiffness and persistent, sometimes progressive, axial pain. When the disease affects the major joints of the lower extremities (hips, knees), the patients will complain of pain in those regions as well.

Over time, enthesopathic changes appear and may, eventually, result in spine fusion. The fusion is caused by ossification of the anterior, posterior, and interspinous ligaments; the facet joints; and the discs. The spine ends up as a very rigid, solid structure known as bamboo spine (Figure 8-1). Lack of spinal motion interferes with the ability of the spine to withstand flexion and extension moments and brings about spinal osteoporosis. The spine becomes very fragile and as a result even simple, noncomplicated falls may lead to an unstable spinal fracture. In many instances the fracture occurs through the calcified discs (Figure 8-2). Because of this fragility, new-onset spinal pain should never be taken lightly in patients with AS. If X-rays of the painful region fail to detect an apparent fracture, bone scan and thin-slice CT or multislice CT with the multiplanar reconstructions may help reveal it at an early phase. Spine fractures are more common in the thoracic segments but may occur in the lumbar as well as the cervical regions.

In AS, the physical examination usually reveals decreased range of motion in the lumbar spine and the thoracic cage. The Schober test

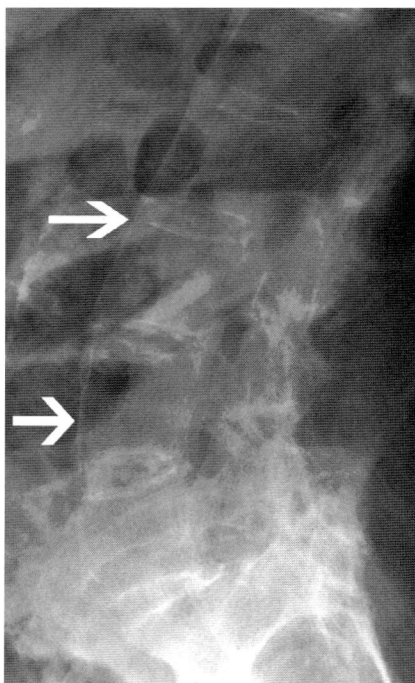

FIGURE 8-1
Lateral plain film of the lumbar spine showing a "bamboo spine." Ossification of the anterior longitudinal ligament is seen (arrows) bridging all the vertebral bodies across the discs. Note that the facet joints are fused as well.

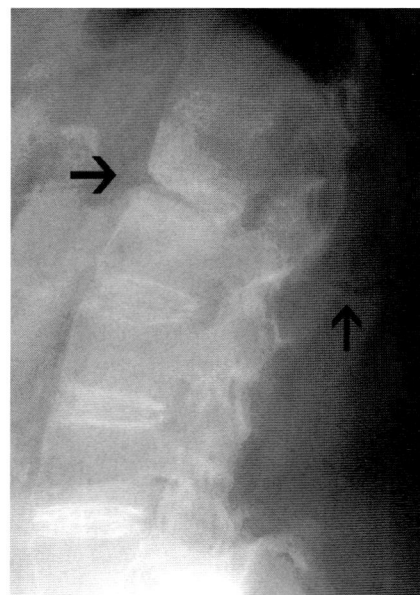

FIGURE 8-2
Lateral plain film of the lumbar spine in a patient with ankylosing spondylitis. Patient sustained a fracture through the disc following minor trauma. The fracture extends all the way back to involve the fused posterior elements (arrows). Courtesy Dr. N. Haramati.

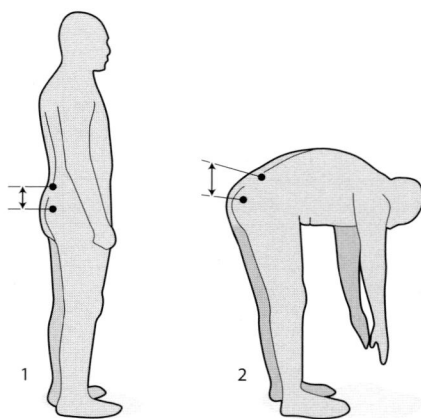

FIGURE 8-3
Schematic drawing of the Schober test. The test enables the physician to assess the mobility of the lumbar spine.

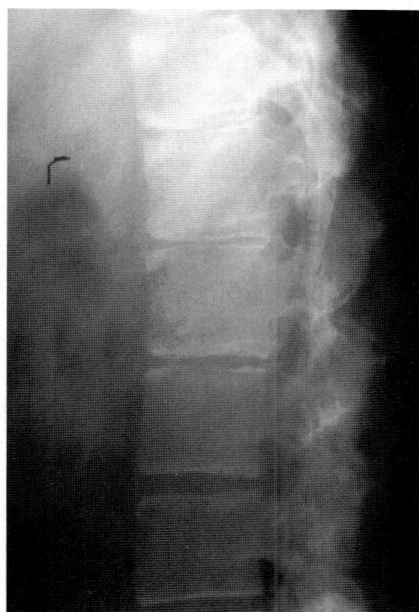

FIGURE 8-4
Lateral plain X-ray of the thoraco-lumbar spine. Straightening of the spinal column and loss of the normal lordosis are apparent. Squaring of the vertebral bodies with sclerosis at the vertebral corners is visible. Courtesy Dr. N. Haramati.

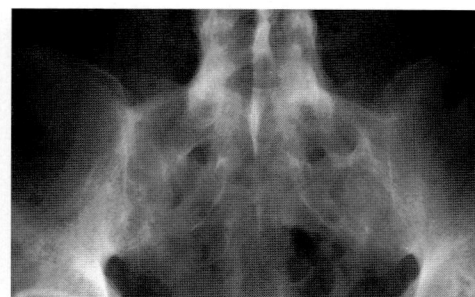

FIGURE 8-5
AP plain film of the lumbo-sacral region. Fusion of the sacroiliac joints and facet joints is seen. Note the calcification of the supraspinous ligament, which is bridging the spinous processes. Courtesy Dr. N. Haramati.

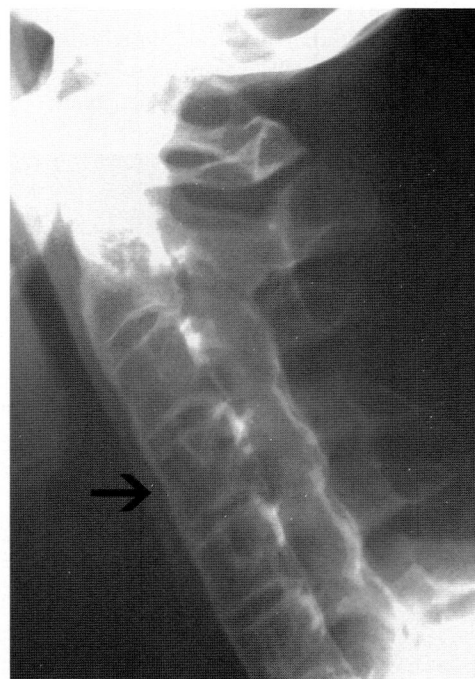

FIGURE 8-6
Cervical spine plain film in a patient with AS. Note the calcification of the anterior longitudinal (arrow) and posterior longitudinal ligaments, and fusion of the facet joints with preservation of the disc spaces. Courtesy Dr. N. Haramati.

may help detect decreased lumbar mobility. A mark is made on the skin overlying the low back region at two points while the patient is in the upright position. The lower point is placed between the dimples of Venus—at the level of the posterior superior iliac spines—and the more proximal point is placed ten centimeters cranially. The distance between the skin marks is measured again following forward bending. If the distance between the skin markings increases by more than five centimeters, it attests to normal lumbar motion (Figure 8-3). In patients with AS most of the forward bending would occur at the hip joints and the distance between the skin marks will increase only minimally, less than three centimeters.

Imaging Studies

Initially, enthesopathic changes, erosions followed by sclerosis, appear at the corners of the vertebral bodies and lead to squaring of the vertebrae. These changes can be easily detected on plain films (Figure 8-4). Erosions and whiskering appear in the sacroiliac joints and in the pubic region. These can be detected on CT and MRI and help reach a diagnosis at an early stage of the disease. Although CT excels in erosion detection and finding surface irregularities, the MRI may show signal changes (decreased on T1 and increased on T2) around these erosions and the corners of the vertebral bodies. Initially, widening of the sacroiliac joint space occurs and later on blurring of the sacroiliac joint margins will be seen. Over the course of months or years

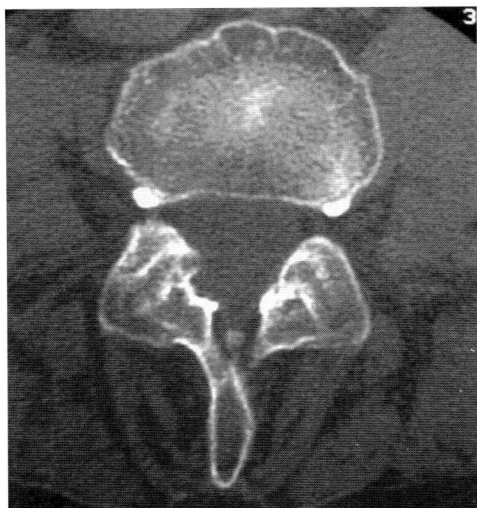

FIGURE 8-7
Axial CT showing fusion of both the facet joints. Note the calcification surrounding the disc periphery. Courtesy Dr. N. Haramati.

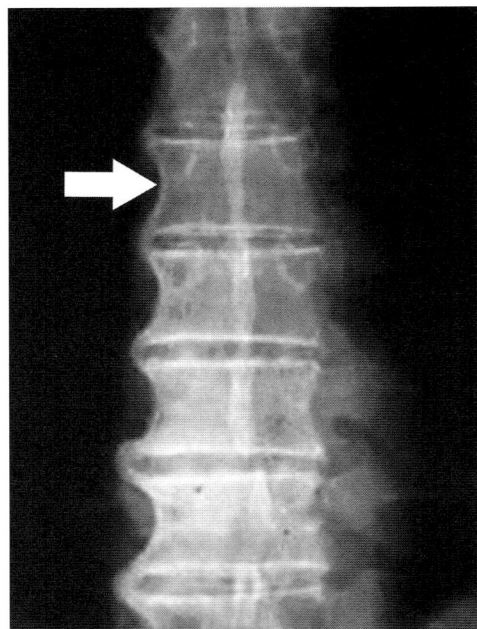

FIGURE 8-8
Plain AP film of the thoracic spine in a patient with DISH showing flowing osteophytes bridging the vertebral bodies on the right side. Note the absence of similar osteophytes on the left.

TABLE 8-1
Differences between AS and DISH

	Ankylosing Spondylitis	**Diffuse Idiopathic Skeletal Hyperostosis (DISH)**
Age	Second or third decade	Fifth to seventh decade
Gender	Mostly males	Both genders are affected
HLA-B27	Positive in over 90%	Negative
Sacroiliac joints	Involved, eventually ankylosed	Spared
Uveitis, aortitis, aortic insufficiency	Frequently present	Absent

the sacroiliac joints will fuse. Subsequently ossification of the vertebral bodies and the annulus pulposus leads to the formation of thin syndesmophytes. They form bridges between the vertebral bodies, eventually leading to spine fusion (Figures 8-5 and 8-6).

The facet joints become fused as well. The disc spaces may be preserved These features can be easily seen on a CT scan. It will show the sclerotic bone, calcified discs, syndesmophytes, and fused facet joints (Figure 8-7). The fused spine will appear hypointense on T1 as well as T2 weighted images, consistent with the abundant sclerotic bones. The calcifying discs may show increased signal intensity on T1 and T2 weighted images.

AS may be, at times, confused with diffuse idiopathic skeletal hyperostosis (DISH), a commonly seen benign condition (Figure 8-8).

Table 8-1 emphasizes some of the salient differences between these two conditions.

Management

The management of AS includes patient education, a lifelong exercise program, medications, and occasionally surgery. The patient should be referred for long-term physical therapy. Mobility preservation, muscle strengthening, fitness enhancement, and improvement in the sense of well-being are the main physical therapy goals. Stretching exercises, especially of the hip and knee flexors, are incorporated into the patient's daily routine in an attempt to prevent the development of flexion contractures. Every effort is made to preserve the upright posture and prevent the spine from fusing in kyphosis. General conditioning exercises combined with underwater aerobics may prove beneficial. Nonsteroidal anti-inflammatory drugs (NSAIDs) in full therapeutic doses should be tried first. Sulfasalazine, an effective and safe medication, can be prescribed at the early stages of the disease. It may be helpful in patients who do not respond to NSAIDs. In patients with severe, progressive disease methotrexate and cyclophosphamide should be prescribed. Tumor necrosis factor alpha inhibitors (etanercept, infliximab, or others) may be helpful in delaying disease progression and, according to some authors, should be prescribed early in the course of the disease.

PSORIATIC SPONDYLOARTHROPATHY

Psoriatic arthropathy usually involves the cervical spine and the upper extremities.

Clinical Presentation

Patients with psoriasis tend to develop erosive arthritis affecting the fingers, especially at the distal interphalangeal joints. Occasionally the arthritis is mutilating and leads to destruction of the interphalangeal joints. Shortened, telescoping fingers lead to "opera glass hand." Arthralgia in large joints and pain due to enthesopathy (heel cord pain, plantar fasciitis) are frequently seen. The disease commonly involves the skin and the nails.

Up to 30% of psoriatic patients develop spondyloarthropathy, especially of the cervical region. Many have unilateral or bilateral sacroiliitis as well. Not infrequently the spinal changes remain asymptomatic and are discovered only incidentally. This occurs more frequently in males. The spinal changes may be attributed to psoriasis only when cutaneous, nail, or joint changes consistent with the disease develop.

The spinal changes consist of multiple asymmetrical syndesmophytes that fuse adjacent vertebrae. A large region, mostly in the cervical spine, may be totally fused. The vertebral bodies as well as the facet joints may be fused. These changes are best seen on plain X-rays and CT scans and, in some cases, may be indistinguishable from those seen in AS.

ENTEROPATHIC ARTHRITIS AND POSTINFECTIOUS REACTIVE ARTHROPATHY

Up to 40% of patients with ulcerative colitis and Crohn's disease develop enteropathic arthritis and spondyloarthropathy that may include sacroiliac involvement. The findings in X-rays and CT and MRI scans may be similar or identical to those of AS.

The term "postinfectious reactive arthritis" refers to a peripheral, nonseptic arthritis that develops within a month of an infection somewhere else in the body. All the cultures that are obtained from the affected joints are negative. The arthropathy is usually limited to a small number of joints, develops acutely, and is asymmetric. Up to a third of these patients may develop recurrent or chronic arthropathy, sacroiliitis, and spondyloarthropathy that may resemble AS or psoriasis. Unlike AS, skip areas—spinal segments that are not affected—are seen, whereas in AS, especially in advanced cases, the whole spine is fused. Some of these patients are HLA-B27–positive. Quite commonly, patients present with an overlapping clinical picture and are diagnosed as having undifferentiated spondyloarthropathy.

Bibliography

Ahlstrom H, Feltelius N, Nyman R, Hallgren R: Magnetic resonance imaging of sacroiliac joint inflammation. Arthritis Rheum 33: 1763–1769, 1990.

Braun J, Bollow M, Sieper J: Radiologic diagnosis and pathology of the spondyloarthropathies. Rheum Dis Clin N Am 24: 697–735, 1998.

Curtis JR, Lander PH, Moreland LW: Swallowing difficulties from "DISH-phagia." J Rheumatol 31: 2526–2527, 2004.

Fast A, Shailesh P, Marin E: Spine fractures in ankylosing spondylitis. Arch Phys Med Rehabil 67: 595–597, 1986.

Grigoryan M, Roemer FW, Mohr A, Genant HK: Imaging in spondyloarthropathies. Curr Rheumatol Rep 6: 102–109, 2004.

Indar R, Jacob J, Aldam CH, Hussein AA: Dysphagia: An unusual orthopaedic cause. Hosp Med 66: 54–55, 2005.

Kahn MA: Update on spondyloarthropathies. Ann Intern Med 136: 896–907, 2002.

Laiho K, Kauppi M: The cervical spine in patients with psoriatic arthritis. Ann Rheum Dis 61: 650–652, 2002.

Oostveen JCM, Van de Laar MAFJ: Magnetic resonance imaging in rheumatic disorders of the spine and sacroiliac joints. Semin Arthritis Rheum 30: 52–69, 2000.

Queiro R, Belzunegui J, Gonzalez C, De DJ, Sarasqueta C, Torre JC, Figueroa M: Clinically asymptomatic axial disease in psoriatic spondyloarthropathy: A retrospective study. Clin Rheumatol 21: 10–13, 2002.

Resnick D, Shapiro RF, Wiesner KB, Niwayama G, Utsinger PD, Shaul SR: Diffuse idiopathic skeletal hyperostosis of Forestier and Rotes-Querol. Semin Arth Rheum 7: 153–187, 1978.

Scarpa R: Discovertebral erosions and destruction in psoriatic arthritis. J Rheumatol 27: 975–978, 2000.

Shaikh S: The spondyloarthropathies revisited. Semin Spine Surg 12: 74–86, 2000.

Sieper J, Rudwaleit M: How early should ankylosing spondylitis be treated with tumor necrosis factor blockers? Ann Rheum Dis 64: 61–64, 2005.

Sosner J, Fast A, Kahan B: Odontoid fracture and C1-2 subluxation in psoriatic cervical spondyloarthropathy. Spine 21: 519–521, 1996.

van Tubergen A, Hidding A: Spa and exercise treatment in ankylosing spondylitis: Fact or fancy. Best Pract Res Clin Rheumatol 16: 653–666, 2002.

Update on spondyloarthropathies. Ann Intern Med 136: 897–905, 2002.

Wittram C, Whitehouse GH, Williams JW, Bucknall RC: A comparison of MR and CT in suspected sacroiliitis. J Comput Assist Tomogr 20: 68–72, 1996.

Yu W, Feng F, Dion E, Yang H, Jiang M, Genant HK: Comparison of radiography, computed tomography and magnetic resonance imaging in the detection of sacroiliitis accompanying ankylosing spondylitis. Skeletal Radiol 27: 311–320, 1998.

RHEUMATOID ARTHRITIS

9

Rheumatoid arthritis (RA) is a chronic progressive systemic disorder affecting multiple synovial joints. Spine involvement, particularly at the craniocervical junction, usually occurs together with peripheral sites. The disease appears in the second to fourth decades and affects more women than men at a 3:1 ratio. The trigger for the disease is still unknown. It is believed to be an immune-mediated disease in which immune complexes are deposited in the synovial tissues. The inflamed synovial tissue, the pannus, contains giant cells, T and B lymphocytes, and plasma cells. As the pannus thickens and grows it invades adjacent structures, destroys the cartilage and bone, and leads to joint destruction, deformities, and instability. Eventually, fibrous or bony ankylosis may develop.

RA has a strong predilection to the cervical spine, especially but not exclusively to the C1-C2 region. The disease usually spares the thoracic, lumbar, and sacral regions. Up to 86% of RA patients develop cervical spine pathology, which may progress and lead to neurological involvement.

PATHOPHYSIOLOGY

The pathophysiology of RA in the cervical region is the same as that seen in the peripheral joints. Synovitis and pannus formation lead to bony erosions and ligamentous degradation, which may eventually result in instability that can lead to spinal cord and, occasionally, brain stem compression.

CLINICAL PRESENTATION

RA patients usually present with morning stiffness and pain affecting primarily the small joints of both hands and wrists. The metacarpal and proximal interphalangeal joints are the most frequently affected joints. Typical deformities in the hands and wrists develop over time. Rheumatoid nodules may appear around the posterior aspect of the elbows. Blood work-up may detect an elevated sedimentation rate and C-reactive protein, anemia, and a positive rheumatoid factor.

Patients with cervical spine involvement may be initially asymptomatic. As the disease progresses neck pain may appear. Suboccipital headaches aggravated by neck movements are common, and electrical-like sensation in the torso or extremities that is precipitated by neck flexion or extension may appear. This is frequently referred to as *L'hermitte's sign*. Some patients develop earache and occasionally facial pain due to compression or irritation of the sensory fibers of the greater auricular nerve or the spinal trigeminal nucleus. Neurological findings are less common than pain but may be present in up to one-third of the patients. Gait dysfunction (unstable gait, wide-based gait), decreased upper extremity dexterity and weakness, and sphincter dysfunction may develop due to cervical myelopathy.

Occasionally a clunking sensation appears during neck extension. This correlates with reduction of the subluxed atlanto-axial junction.

The physical examination of patients with cervical involvement should be thoroughly performed. Special attention should be devoted to the presence of upper motor neuron signs: upgoing toes, positive Hoffmann sign, clonus, and hyperreflexia. It should be emphasized that the presence of painful deformed peripheral joints and disuse muscle atrophy make the neurological assessment of the rheumatoid patient quite challenging.

ATLANTO-AXIAL SUBLUXATION

The dens is tightly bound to the first cervical vertebra via the transverse ligament (Figures 9-1A and 9-1B). Synovitis and pannus formation lead to dens erosions and structural deterioration and weakening of the stabilizing ligaments, the transverse and apical ligaments. At times, severe erosions lead to total disruption of these ligaments allowing atlanto-axial subluxation, especially during neck flexion. The subluxation results in posterior migration of the dens, reduction of the space available for the cord and may eventually end-up in cord compression. This occurs in almost half of the RA patients.

IMAGING STUDIES

The atlanto-axial region can be evaluated by X-ray, CT, and MRI examinations. Cervical spine X-rays should include AP, lateral, and open-

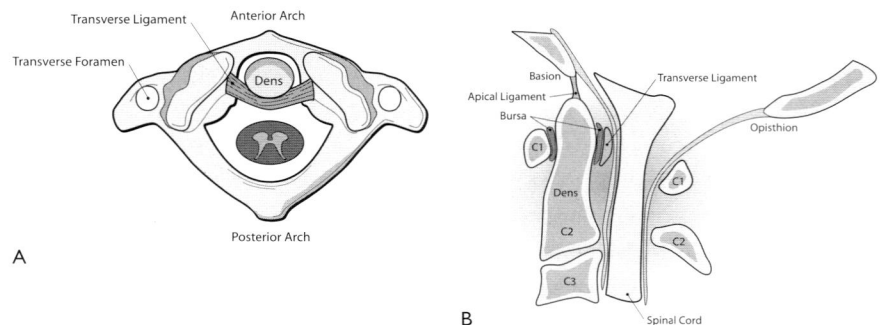

FIGURE 9-1
Schematic drawings of the C1-C2 region. (A) Note how the transverse ligament holds the odontoid process in close proximity to the anterior arch of the atlas. (B) Sagittal view.

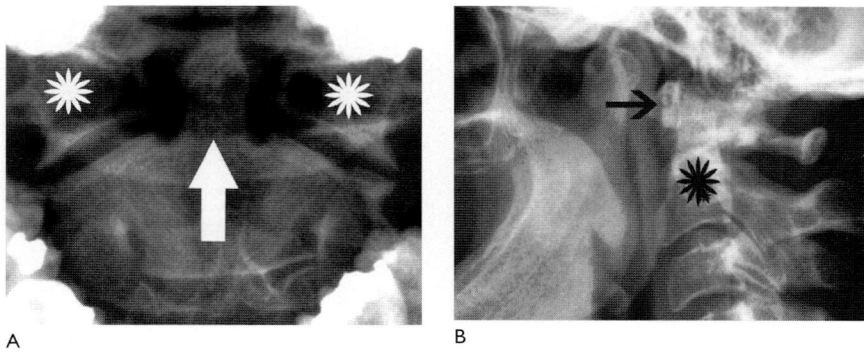

FIGURE 9-2

(A) Trans-oral X-ray of a normal atlanto-axial vertebrae showing the odontoid process of C2 (arrow) and the lateral masses of C1 (stars). Note that the lateral edges of the C1 lateral masses perfectly align with those of C2 vertebra. (B) Lateral view of the C1-C2 region. Note the close proximity of the dens (star) to the anterior arch of the atlas (arrow).

mouth views. In addition, upright (sitting, standing) lateral flexion and extension films should be obtained. Open-mouth view allows good visualization of the dens, provided that the mouth is widely opened so that the teeth do not obstruct the view (Figures 9-2A and 9-2B). Good quality lateral films allow direct measurement of the space between the posterior aspect of the anterior arch of the atlas and the anterior aspect of the dens, the anterior atlanto-dental interval (AADI). In healthy adults this space measures up to 3 mm, even during flexion. AADI of more than 3 mm points to the presence of instability. Intervals of 8 or 9 mm correlate with neurological compromise due to posterior migration of the dens and spinal cord compression. When the gap between the dens and the atlas does not reduce during extension it may attest to the presence of a pannus in front of the dens. Some authors emphasize the importance of the posterior atlanto-dental interval (PADI). Normally, the PADI measures 18 mm. PADI measuring less than 14 mm was found to be a reliable indicator for patients that are at high risk for cord compression and neurological compromise (Figures 9-3 and 9-4).

Single-slice CT scan at 1 mm cuts, or multislice helical CT with axial and coronal reformatted images, can provide invaluable information about the C1-C2 region (Figures 9-5A and 9-5B). It may help detect erosions in the dens that may otherwise be missed on plain films and may disclose cervical instability. Postcontrast CT studies can reliably detect inflammatory soft tissue proliferation (pannus) around the dens and may point to the presence of cord compression.

MRI, the study of choice, provides excellent information about the bones and the soft tissues (ligaments, brain stem, cord, and pannus) and allows a reliable assessment of this critical region. The pannus appears as low signal structure on T1-weighted images (T1WI). The signal on T2-weighted images (T2WI) reflects its vascularity and changes accordingly from low intensity with poorly vascularized, through a heterogeneous signal, to a high-intensity signal when highly vascularized. It enhances following contrast administration. The cord

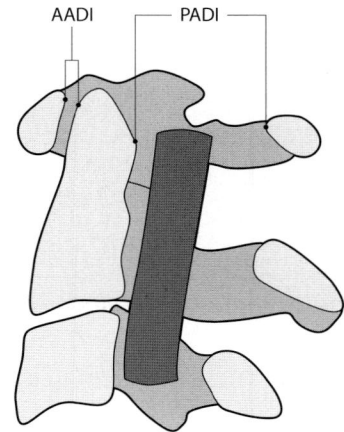

FIGURE 9-3

(A) Schematic drawing of the sagittal view of the C1-C2 vertebrae. Note the atlanto-axial interval, which is less than 3 mm in a healthy adult.

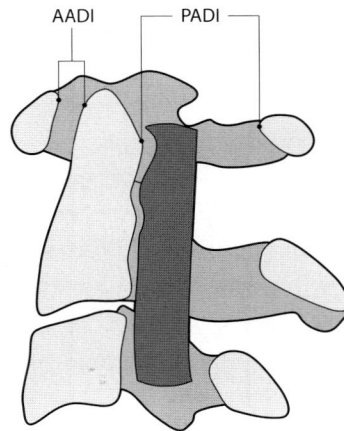

FIGURE 9-4

Schematic drawing showing posterior migration of the dens resulting in spinal cord impression. Note the enlarged atlanto-axial interval.

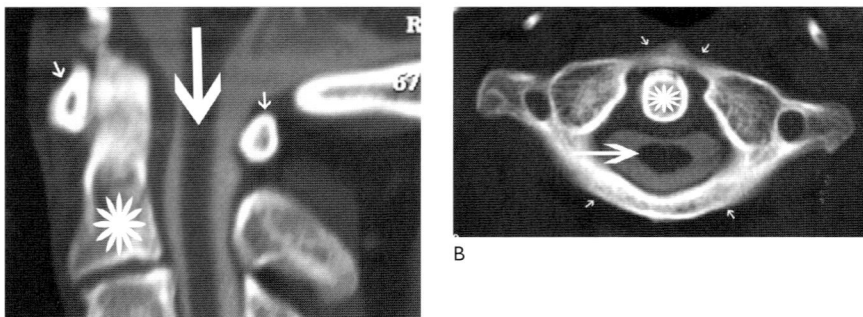

A

B

FIGURE 9-5
CT-myelography of the C1-C2 region. (A) Sagittal and (B) axial cuts. The spinal cord (large arrow) occupies about a third of the spinal canal diameter and the dens another third of the space (star). Note the anterior and posterior arches of the atlas (B, small arrows).

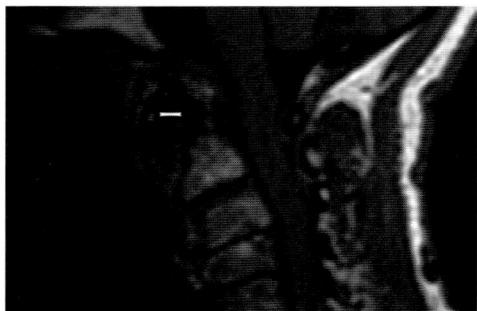

FIGURE 9-6
Sagittal T1WI MR showing increased atlanto-dental space. The spinal cord is pushed against the posterior arch of C1.

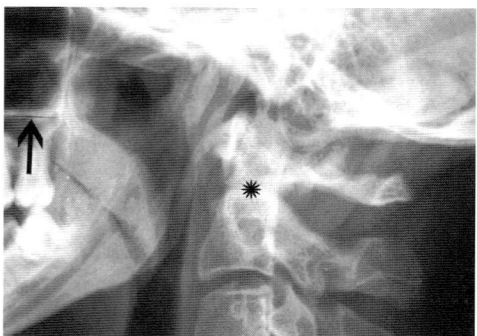

FIGURE 9-7
Lateral plain film of the cranio-cervical junction from the occiput to C3 level. Arrow points toward the hard palate. The dens (star) is in close proximity to the anterior arch of C1.

signal and its shape and diameter help determine the course of action: continuous observation versus surgical intervention. Increased cord signal intensity on T2WI is a poor prognostic indicator for neurological recovery as it may represent irreversible cord damage such as gliosis and myelomalacia. Severe cord atrophy also represents chronic nonreversible changes that may tip the balance against surgical intervention. The recently introduced open MRI in which images can be obtained in flexion is important in demonstrating the amount of instability and showing abnormalities that may not seem so impressive in the neutral position (Figure 9-6).

BASILAR INVAGINATION

Basilar invagination, also known as cranial settling or superior migration of the dens, is less common than C1-C2 instability but far more dangerous. It occurs in up to 38% of rheumatoid patients. This complication is brought about by destruction of the occiput-C1 and C1-C2 joints by the proliferating pannus. The dens migrates superiorly and can compress the brain stem at the foramen magnum level. Because the brain stem contains critical autonomic centers, pressure on these structures can lead to labile blood pressure, arrhythmias, and even sudden death. Patients with established cord compression and neurological deficits have a poor potential for recovery and high surgical morbidity. Early identification and referral for surgery are therefore critical and may preserve the functional status and prevent impending disastrous neurological deterioration.

RADIOLOGICAL ASSESSMENT

Several methods have been developed to identify basilar invagination on cervical spine plain films. All the methods require recognition of certain basic, simple, and important landmarks on lateral films: the basion (ventral border of the foramen magnum), opisthion (dorsal border of the foramen magnum), hard palate, atlas, C2 pedicles, and the tip of the odontoid process (Figure 9-7). The following methods are quite simple and helpful. This is not a complete list of all the methods that are listed in the literature.

Chamberlain line: a line drawn from the posterior edge of the hard palate to the opisthion (Figure 9-8). Normally, the tip of the dens should not protrude more than 3 mm above this line.

McRae line: a line drawn from the basion to the opisthion (across the foramen magnum) (Figure 9-8). Normally, the tip of the odontoid should be below this line.

Wackenheim line: a line drawn along the superior surface of the clivus (Figure 9-9). Normally, the tip of the odontoid should not be posterior to this projected line.

McGregor line: a line drawn from the postero-superior aspect of the hard palate to the most caudal point of the occipital curve (Figure 9-10). Normally, the tip of the odontoid should not protrude more than 4.5 mm above this line.

Clark stations: the odontoid process is divided into three equal parts in the sagittal plane (Figure 9-10). Normally the anterior ring of the atlas should be level with the upper third. If it is level with the middle or lower third basilar invagination exists.

Unfortunately, none of these methods in isolation has been found to be totally reliable. None reaches sensitivity above 90% or specificity over 80%. The methods with the least false negative results were found to be the Wackenheim line and the Clark stations.

When basilar invagination is suspected MRI studies should be obtained. Special attention should be paid to the brain stem, spinal cord, and the cervico-medullary angle. The latter normally ranges between 135 and 175 degrees. Cranial settling and peridental pannus formation may decrease this angle and correlate well with the presence of myelopathy and neurological changes.

SUBAXIAL SUBLUXATION

Subaxial subluxation is a term pointing to instability below the C1-C2 region. It is less common than C1-C2 instability and tends to develop later in the course of the disease.

This deformity results from facet joints destruction and deterioration of the stabilizing ligaments. Subaxial subluxation may develop in a single level or at multiple cervical levels and may lead to stepladder or staircase deformity. It usually develops at the C2-C3 or C3-C4 levels and may lead to spinal cord compression and myelopathy (Figure 9-11).

Imaging Studies

The staircase deformity can be easily spotted on X-rays in lateral views of the cervical spine (Figure 9-12). The deformity is also clearly

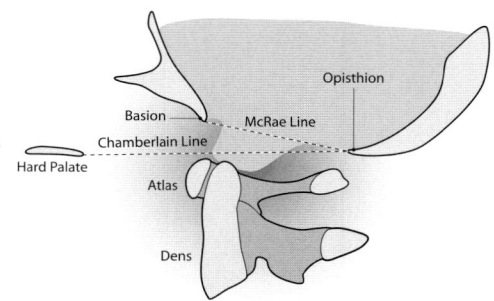
FIGURE 9-8
McRae line: a line drawn from the basion to the opisthion (across the foramen magnum).

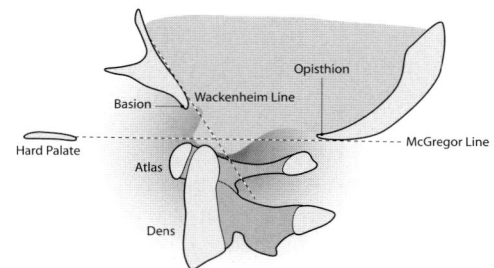
FIGURE 9-9
Wackenheim line: a line drawn along the superior surface of the clivus.

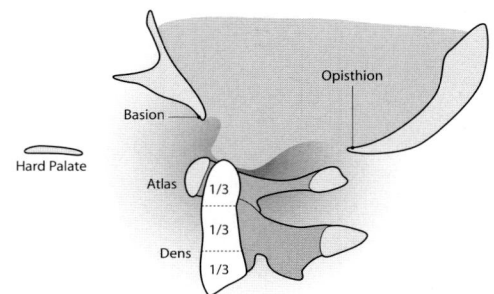
FIGURE 9-10
Clark stations: the odontoid process is divided into three equal parts in the sagittal plane.

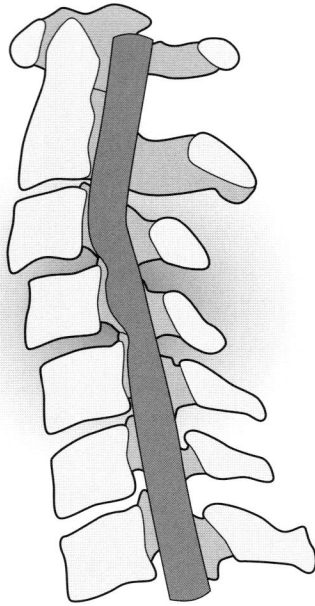

FIGURE 9-11
Schematic drawing showing subaxial subluxation at C3-C4 and C4-C5 with cord compression.

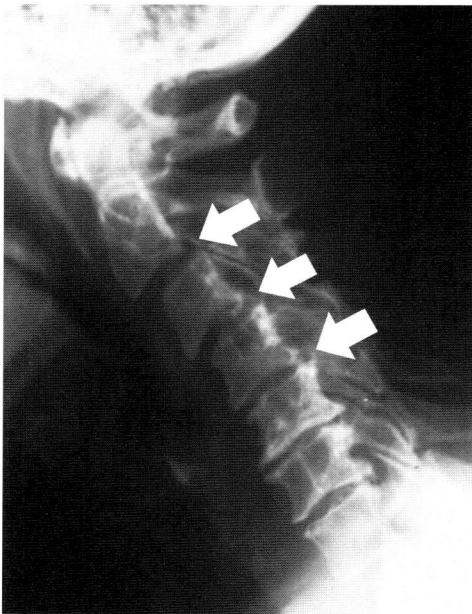

FIGURE 9-12
Lateral plain film of the cervical spine showing subaxial instability from C2-C3 through C4-C5 (arrows).

seen on sagittal images in CT as well as in MRI studies. The latter can disclose cord compression and show signal changes within the cord substance.

Management

The challenges posed by the cervical spine in rheumatoid patients are complex and require vast knowledge and expertise. In the last two decades the medical management of RA has changed with the rather early administration of disease-modifying agents. Early utilization of drugs such as sulfasalazine, methotrexate, or leflunomide is expected to suppress synovial pathology and postpone or reduce irreversible bony structural changes. It is hoped that earlier administration of these agents will eventually result in decreased cervical spine involvement in RA patients.

Nonmyelopathic patients can benefit from conservative care: education (cervical anatomy, pathophysiology), activity modification (staying away from contact sports, avoiding activities that require acute neck flexion), isometric neck exercises (emphasizing strengthening of upper cervical extensors), and custom-made cervical collars can all help patients with atlanto-axial instability at least in the early stages of the disease.

There is still, however, no well-accepted approach to the neurologically intact rheumatoid patient who has radiologically proven atlanto-axial instability. Because the natural history of the disease has not been completely elucidated, the timing of surgical intervention remains controversial. Should the surgeon wait for the development of long tract signs, or should the patients be operated on prophylactically?

Recent research suggests that prophylactic posterior fusion may be superior to conservative care, and can decrease the morbidity and the mortality and improve the quality of life of patients with RA.

Patients with C1-C2 instability and a PADI of less than 14 mm, cervico-medullary angle smaller than 135 degrees (normal angle is between 135 and 175 degrees), and atlanto-axial impaction where the dens has migrated more than 5 mm above the McGregor line should be referred for neurosurgical consultation without delay.

Bibliography

Boden SD, Dodge LD, Bholman HH, Rechtine GR: Rheumatoid arthritis of the cervical spine. J Bone Joint Surg Am 75: 1282–1297, 1993.

Breedveld FC, Algra PR, Vielvoye CJ, Cats A: Magnetic resonance imaging in the evaluation of patients with rheumatoid arthritis and subluxations of the cervical spine. Arthritis Rheum 30: 624–629, 1987.

Castro S, Verstraete K, Mielants H, Vanderstraeten G, de Reuck J, Veys EM: Cervical spine involvement in rheumatoid arthritis: A clinical , neurological and radiological evaluation. Clin Exp Rheumatol 12: 369–374, 1994.

Chang J, Kavanaugh A: Novel therapies for rheumatoid arthritis. Pathophysiol 12: 217–225, 2005.

Dreyer SJ, Boden SD: Natural history of rheumatoid arthritis of the cervical spine. Clin Orthop 366: 98–106, 1999.

Einig M, Higer HP, Meairs S, Faust-Tinnefeldt G, Kapp H: Magnetic resonance imaging of the craniocervical junction in rheumatoid arthritis: Value, limitations, indications. Skeletal Radiol 19: 341–346, 1990.

Fujiwara K, Owaki H, Fujimoto M, Yonenobu K, Ochi T: A long-term follow-up study of cervical lesions in rheumatoid arthritis. J Spinal Disord 13: 519–526, 2000.

Fujiwara K, Yonenobu K, Ochi T: Natural history of upper cervical lesions in rheumatoid arthritis. J Spinal Disord 10: 275–281, 1997.

Grauer JN, Tingstad EM, Rand N, Christie MJ, Hilibrand AS: Predictors of paralysis in the rheumatoid cervical spine in patients undergoing total joint arthroplasty. J Bone Joint Surg Am 86: 1420–1424, 2004.

Hamilton JD, Gordon MM, McInnes IB, Johnston RA, Madhok R, Capell HA: Improved medical and surgical management of cervical spine disease in patients with rheumatoid arthritis over 10 years. Ann Rheum Dis 59: 439–447, 2000.

Hermann KG, Bollow M: Magnetic resonance imaging of the axial skeleton in rheumatoid disease. Best Pract Res Clin Rheumatol 18: 881–907, 2004.

Heywood AWB, Learmonth ID, Thomas M: Cervical spine instability in rheumatoid arthritis. J Bone Joint Surg Br 70: 702–707, 1988.

Kauppi M, Leppanen L, Heikkila S, Lahtinen T, Kautianinen H: Active conservative treatment of atlantoaxial subluxation in rheumatoid arthritis. Br J Rheumatol 37: 417–420, 1998.

Kim DH, Hilibrand AS: Rheumatoid arthritis in the cervical spine. Am Acad Orthop Surg 13: 463–474, 2005.

Kudo H, Iwano K: Surgical treatment of subaxial cervical myelopathy in rheumatoid arthritis. J Bone Joint Surg Br 73: 474–480, 1991.

Lee SJA, Kavanaugh A: Pharmacological treatment of established rheumatoid arthritis. Best Pract Res Clin Rheumatol 17: 811–829, 2003.

Maeda T, Saito T, Harimaya K, Shuto T, Iwamoto Y: Atlantoaxial instability in neck retraction and protrusion positions in patients with rheumatoid arthritis. Spine 29: 757–762, 2004.

Nguyen HV, Ludwig SC, Silber J, Gelb DE, Anderson PA, Frank L, Vaccaro AR: Contemporary concepts review. Rheumatoid arthritis of the cervical spine. Spine J 4: 329–334, 2004.

Oda T, Fujiwara K, Yonenobu K, Azuma B, Ochi T: Natural course of cervical spine lesions in rheumatoid arthritis. Spine 20: 1128–1135, 1995.

Oostveen JCM, Van de Laar MAFJ: Magnetic resonance imaging in rheumatic disorders of the spine and sacroiliac joints. Semin Arthritis Rheum 30: 52–69, 2000.

Puttlitz CM, Goel VK, Clark CR, Traynelis VC, Scifert JL, Grosland NM: Biomechanical rationale for the pathology of rheumatoid arthritis in the craniovertebral junction. Spine 25: 1607–1616, 2000.

Ragab AA: Surgical exposures of the cervical spine. Contemp Spine Surg 5: 43–47, 2004.

Redlund-Johnell I, Pettersson H: Radiographic measurements of the cranio-vertebral region. Designed for evaluation of abnormalities in rheumatoid arthritis. Acta Radiol Diag 25: 23–28, 1984.

Reiter MF, Boden SD: Inflammatory disorders of the cervical spine. Spine 23: 2755–2766, 1998.

Riew KD, Hilibrand AS, Palumbo MA, Sethi N, Bohlman HH: Diagnosing basilar invagination in the rheumatoid patient. The reliability of radiographic criteria. J Bone Joint Surg Am 83: 194–200, 2001.

Shen FH, Samartzis D, Jenis LG, An HS: Rheumatoid arthritis: evaluation and surgical management of the cervical spine. Spine J 4: 689–700, 2004.

Tanaka N, Sakahashi H, Ishima T, Takahashi H, Ishii S: Results after 24 years of prophylactic surgery for rheumatoid atlantoaxial subluxation. J Bone Joint Surg Br 87: 955–958, 2005.

METABOLIC BONE DISEASE

10

OSTEOPOROSIS

Osteoporosis is commonly seen in postmenopausal Caucasian women. However, it is found in women of all racial groups including black women. The disease does not spare males in the late stages of life; they too may be affected by *senile osteoporosis*. Osteoporosis may be caused by endocrinopathies, nutritional deficiencies, drugs (long-term steroid therapy), or immobilization. Smoking is a well-recognized risk factor for osteoporosis.

Osteoporosis may be akin to a "silent thief." As it evolves, the patient has no symptoms and is not aware of the developing disease. Routine blood work-up including sedimentation rate, complete blood count, creatinine, calcium, phosphorus, uric acid, liver function tests, thyroid stimulating hormone, parathyroid hormone, alkaline phosphatase, and serum vitamin D levels remain normal throughout. Frequently the disease is diagnosed late when the patient sustains a spontaneous vertebral fracture or breaks a long bone following minimal trauma. Fractures tend to occur in the vertebral bodies, proximal hip, distal radius, and proximal humerus. Vertebral fractures are a major source of morbidity and affect the quality of life of many patients. There are approximately 700,000 new vertebral fractures each year in the United States. These fractures may be incidentally discovered in films obtained for other reasons and are frequently missed by inexperienced physicians.

Clinical Presentation

Severe axial pain may develop following a trivial trauma, or spontaneously after nontraumatic events such as coughing or sneezing. The pain increases with movements and disappears with complete rest. The pain may prevent the patient from ambulating. Tenderness to percussion over the fractured vertebra is apparent. In many instances the pain is addressed with the proper medications but no work-up is offered, and the patient is left undiagnosed. This "benign neglect" results in

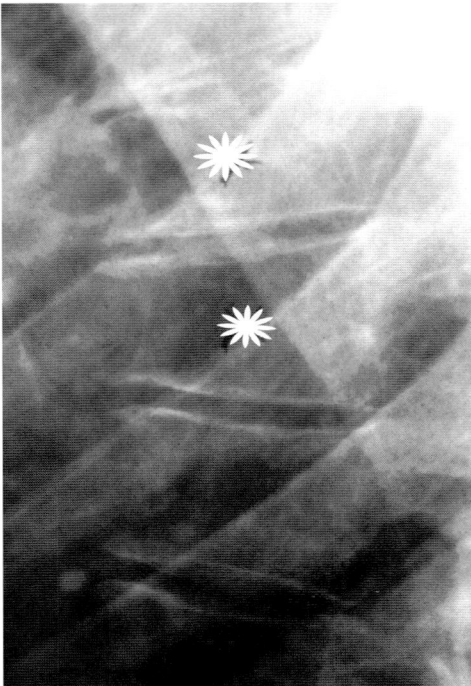

FIGURE 10-1
Lateral plain film of the dorsal spine showing two mild compression fractures (stars). Note that the vertebrae look washed out.

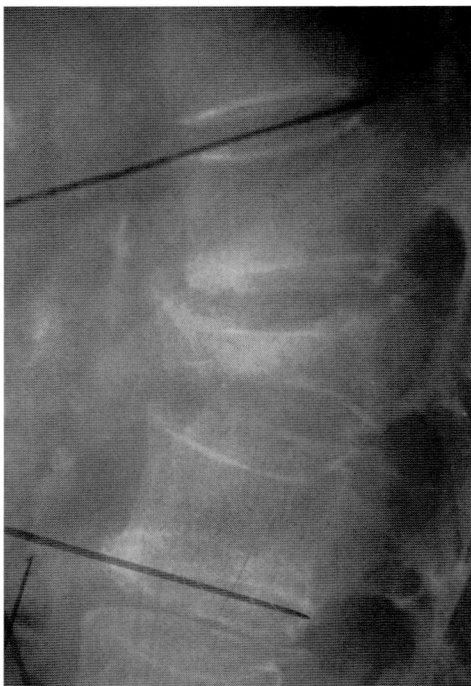

FIGURE 10-2
Severe osteoporotic fracture. Lateral X-ray showing that both the superior and inferior endplates have been affected leading to a kyphotic deformity.

disease progression. Over the course of time, patients develop additional fractures that may result in kyphotic deformities leading, in a significant percentage of patients, to chronic persistent back pain and, at times, to neurological complications and pulmonary dysfunction.

When osteoporosis or vertebral fractures are detected, systemic diseases such as hematological malignancies (multiple myeloma or metastatic disease) should be excluded. The work-up should include sedimentation rate, complete blood count, serum calcium, phosphorus, uric acid, serum and urine protein electrophoresis, and liver function tests. Osteoporosis work-up should also include blood levels of 25-hydroxyvitamin D, parathyroid hormone, osteocalcin (a bone formation marker), and 24-hour urine calcium excretion.

Imaging Studies

Bone density studies using dual photon X-ray absorptiometry (DEXA) can confirm the presence of osteoporosis and quantify its severity.

Plain films are not sensitive and remain normal in the early stages of osteoporosis. Up to 50–70% of bone loss can occur before osteoporosis is detectable on plain films. The main features of spinal osteoporosis are cortical bone thinning and resorption of bone trabeculae expressed on plain X-rays as decreased bone density. The bones appear more radiolucent; they look washed out or darker on plain films. Thinning of the cortical bone can be easily identified on CT images, while trabecular bone resorption brings about a lower density due to the changed relation of bone/bone marrow quantities.

The hallmark of osteoporotic vertebral fracture is loss of vertebral body height. This can be best viewed on lateral spine films. When the vertebral body loses 20% or more of its height, a vertebral fracture is present. These fractures occur when the axial load exceeds the osteoporotic vertebral body strength.

Thorough inspection of plain films may increase the diagnostic yield. Special attention should be devoted to the shape of neighboring vertebral bodies. Mild endplate deformities and lack of endplate parallelism may point to a fracture at a rather early stage (Figure 10-1).

A wedge fracture or anterior compression fracture occurs when height is lost at the anterior portion of the vertebral body while the posterior vertebral wall and the neural arch remain intact. These fractures are very common in osteoporotic individuals, are found in the thoracic as well as the lumbar region, and result from axial loading in flexion. Frequently, only the superior endplate is affected. At times, both, the superior and the inferior endplates are involved (Figure 10-2). These fractures have been considered stable and were not addressed appropriately in the past. Recently it has been observed that osteoporotic fractures in which the anterior wall of the vertebra "swells" or "projects" forward have a tendency to collapse due to involvement of both the anterior and the middle vertebral columns. When the anterior as well as the posterior walls of the vertebral body are affected, the fracture is termed a *burst fracture*. Burst fractures are clinically significant because they may be associated with a retropulsed fragment—a bone fragment that is pushed posteriorly into the spinal canal—leading to neurological compromise (Figures 10-3 and 10-4). When height is lost in the middle of the vertebral body leaving the periphery more or less intact, a biconcave-shaped vertebra is seen (Figure 10-5).

Schmorl's nodes, which represent intravertebral disc herniation through the endplate region, may be misread and erroneously interpreted as vertebral fracture. They can occur at the superior as well as the inferior endplate, and over time may be surrounded by a sclerotic bony rim. Schmorl's nodes are most frequently found in the lower thoracic and upper lumbar vertebrae. Commonly they are an incidental finding with no clinical significance (Figure 10-6).

CT and MRI studies provide invaluable assistance in determining a vertebral fracture's age and in establishing its etiology: osteoporotic or pathological. Establishing the fracture's age is important as it enables the clinician to determine whether the symptoms are related to the fracture or not. Furthermore, it provides some guidelines for treatment, such as vertebroplasty or kyphoplasty. The age of the fracture cannot be accurately determined by radiographs only. MRI is the best available modality to determine the fracture's age. The presence of bone marrow edema around the fracture site is a good indication that the fracture is acute. On T1-weighted images (T1WI) the edematous

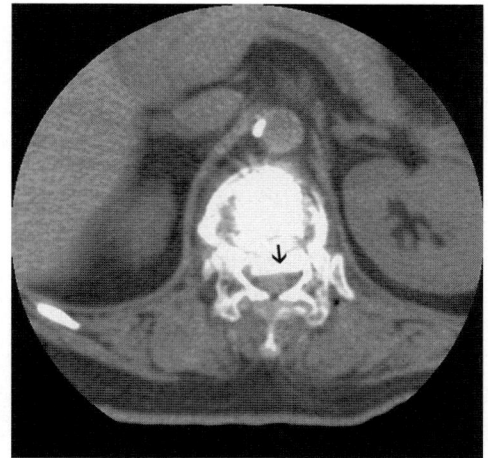

FIGURE 10-3
Axial CT showing a burst fracture with a retropulsed segment into the spinal canal (arrow). The posterior vertebral wall (middle column) has been fractured, and a large bony segment is compromising the spinal canal.

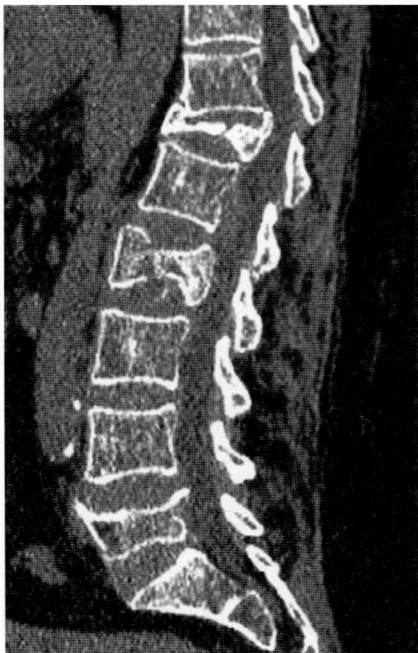

FIGURE 10-4
Sagittal reformatted CT scan showing a severely osteoporotic spine with fractures at T11, L2, and L5. Both the T11 and L2 fractures have a retropulsed segment that narrows the spinal canal.

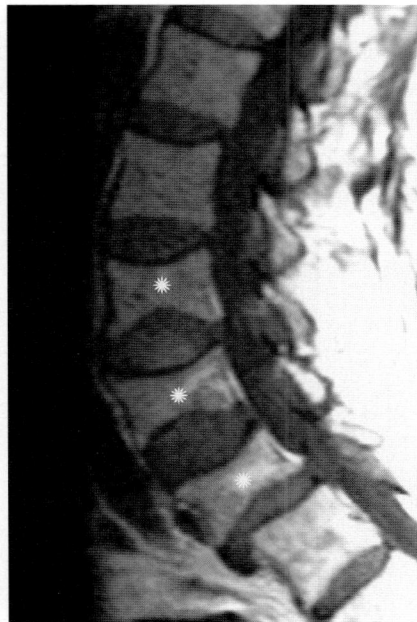

FIGURE 10-5
Sagittal T1WI MR showing an osteoporotic spine with three biconcave vertebrae (stars). Courtesy Dr. N. Haramati.

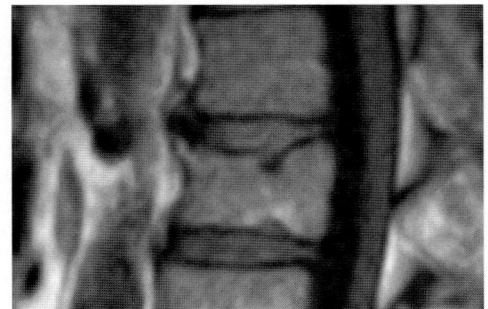

FIGURE 10-6
Sagittal T1WI MR showing Schmorl's nodes in the superior and inferior vertebral endplates. The vertebra itself looks somewhat compressed.

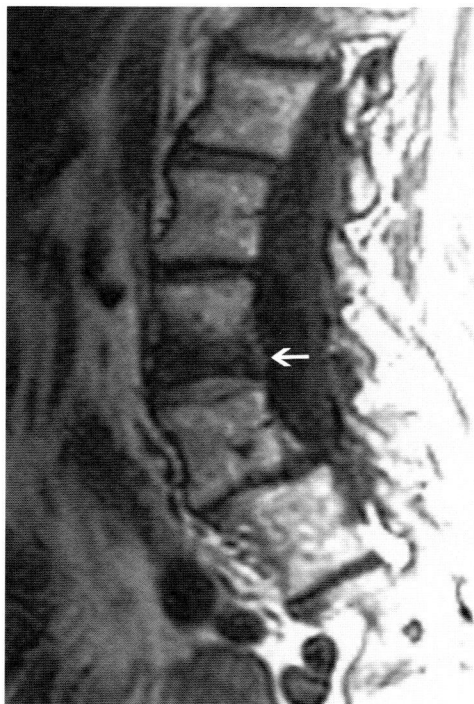

FIGURE 10-7
Sagittal T1WI of the lumbar spine in a 70-year-old female following a fall. X-rays were negative. Due to the severe pain an MRI was obtained. A large area of decreased signal is seen in the lower half of the L2 vertebra.

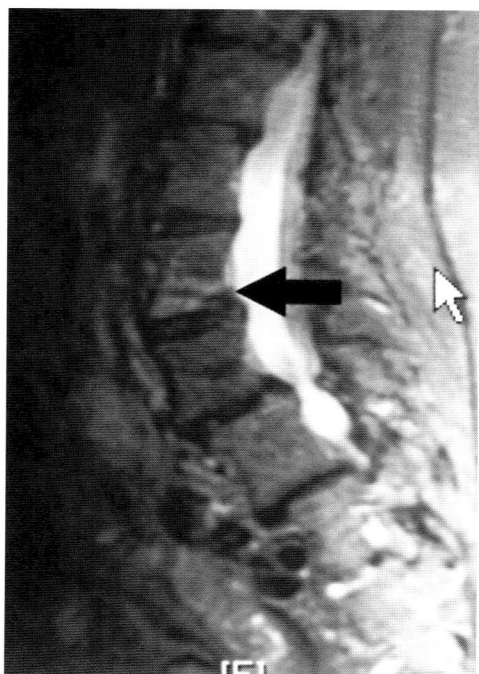

FIGURE 10-8
T2WI in the same patient as Figure 10-7. A hyperintense area is clearly seen. In the center of that area a line of decreased signal—the fracture itself—is visible (black arrow).

area will appear hypointense, whereas on T2-weighted images (T2WI) that same region will appear hyperintense. This area will remain hyperintense following fat suppression sequences. Over time, as the edema subsides, the hyperintense signal will disappear. When the fracture heals the region may remain hypointense or isointense with the rest of the vertebral body when the bone marrow fat has been restored (Figures 10-7 and 10-8).

Some patients with vertebral compression fractures, especially those around the thoraco-lumbar region, develop a cleft within the compressed vertebra. The cleft is usually located in the anterior-superior portion of the vertebral body, just beneath the superior endplate, and may contain air or fluid. Over time the margins of the cleft may calcify and become apparent on spinal radiographs, mostly in lateral views. It has been proposed that the clefts represent an unhealed, mobile and unstable compression fractures. The propensity of clefts to develop in the thoraco-lumbar region may be explained by the fact that this region withstands great dynamic loads that lead to vertebral instability and compromise fracture healing. It is now believed that Kummell disease, delayed post-traumatic avascular necrosis of the vertebral body, is similar in nature to clefted thoraco-lumbar compression fractures.

Sagittal reformatted CT images may help identify mild compressions by showing endplate depression and irregularity in the vertebral contour. CT can easily show violation of the posterior vertebral body wall in cases of burst fractures (Figures 10-9 and 10-10).

In patients with pathological compression fracture CT can detect even small lesions, which can then be biopsied under fluoroscopy or under CT guidance. MRI with contrast will help rule out metastatic disease, as the signal of the adjacent vertebral bodies will typically appear homogenous when the vertebral bodies are normal and heterogeneous when they are infiltrated by cancer.

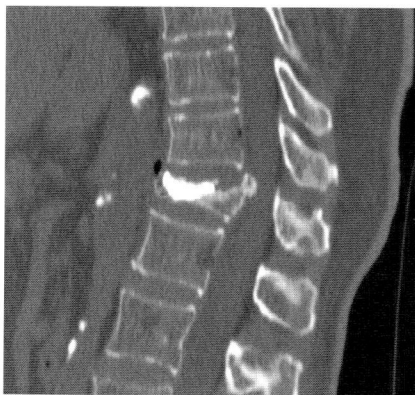

FIGURE 10-9
Reformatted sagittal CT showing the results of vertebroplasty in an osteoporotic patient with a burst fracture. Although the patient's kyphosis did not change, her pain significantly subsided.

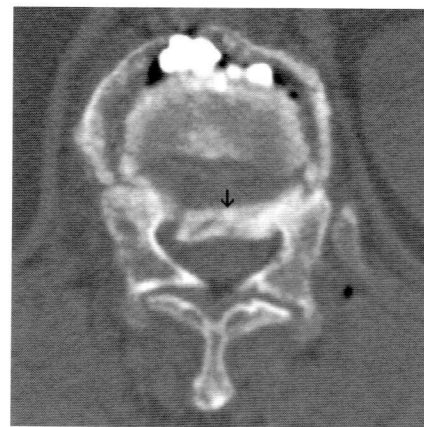

FIGURE 10-10
Axial CT showing a large retropulsed segment (arrow) that narrows the AP diameter of the spinal canal (same patient as in Figure 10-9).

TABLE 10-1
MRI Differences between Pathological and Benign Compression Fractures

	MRI Characteristics of Pathological Compression Fractures	**MRI Characteristics of Benign Compression Fractures**
Posterior body wall	May be convex or disrupted	Usually normal
T1, T2 signals of posterior elements	Frequently abnormal	Normal
Epidural or paraspinal soft tissue infiltration	May be present	Mostly absent
Adjacent vertebral bodies appearance on MRI	Abnormal signals may be observed: T1 decreased, T2 increased	Normal signal characteristics throughout

Management

Past management of compression fractures included analgesic or narcotic medications and immobilization, initially in bed and subsequently in a rigid brace. Patients with refractory pain were frequently managed by prolonged bed rest, which negatively affected the bones as it increased bone breakdown.

Osteoporosis management requires lifestyle changes. Smoking and drinking should be curtailed while fitness and strengthening exercises are advocated. The fractures should be initially immobilized with a proper-fitting brace in order to prevent further collapse. When the pain subsides, high-intensity resistance training exercises should be prescribed. Upper extremity, lower extremity, and spinal extensor muscles should be engaged. It has been shown that the severity of the thoracic kyphosis may be influenced by back extensor strength and that strong back extensors may ameliorate or prevent spinal deformity even in the presence of decreased bone density. These exercises should be combined with general conditioning and fitness exercises.

The introduction of vertebroplasty and kyphoplasty has allowed early painless mobilization in many patients. In both procedures, polymethylmethacrylate, a form of cement that sets quickly in an exothermic reaction, is injected percutaneously into the fractured vertebral body. The difference between the two procedures is that in kyphoplasty a balloon is introduced into the vertebral body and is then inflated. The inflated balloon restores some of the vertebral height prior to the introduction of cement and thus has the ability to decrease or prevent altogether the development of a kyphotic deformity. Following extraction of the balloon, cement is injected into the space it created (Figures 10-11 and 10-12). Better results can be obtained when vertebroplasty and kyphoplasty are performed rather early, preferably in the first 2–3 weeks of fracture occurrence. When these procedures are delayed, the crushed vertebrae heal in situ and the treatment results may not be as effective. These procedures are less effective in vertebrae that have lost over 70% of their height. The major advantages of these

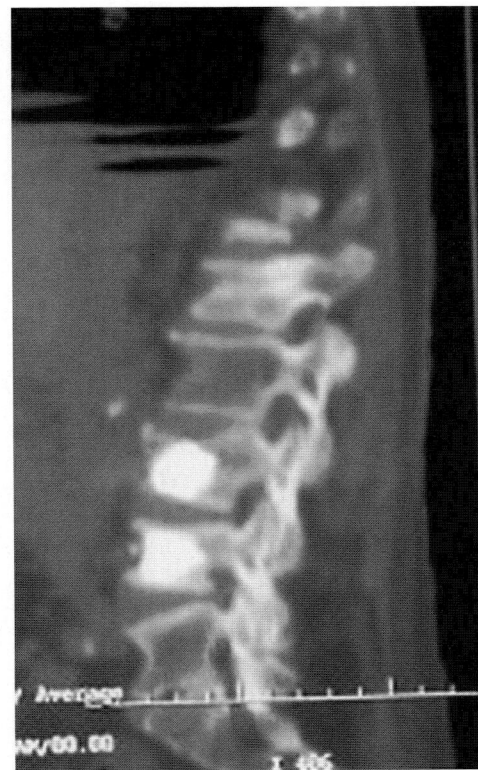

FIGURE 10-11
Reformatted sagittal CT of the lumbar spine in an osteoporotic woman. The patient underwent kyphoplasty in L3 and L4 vertebrae. Courtesy Dr. A. Brook.

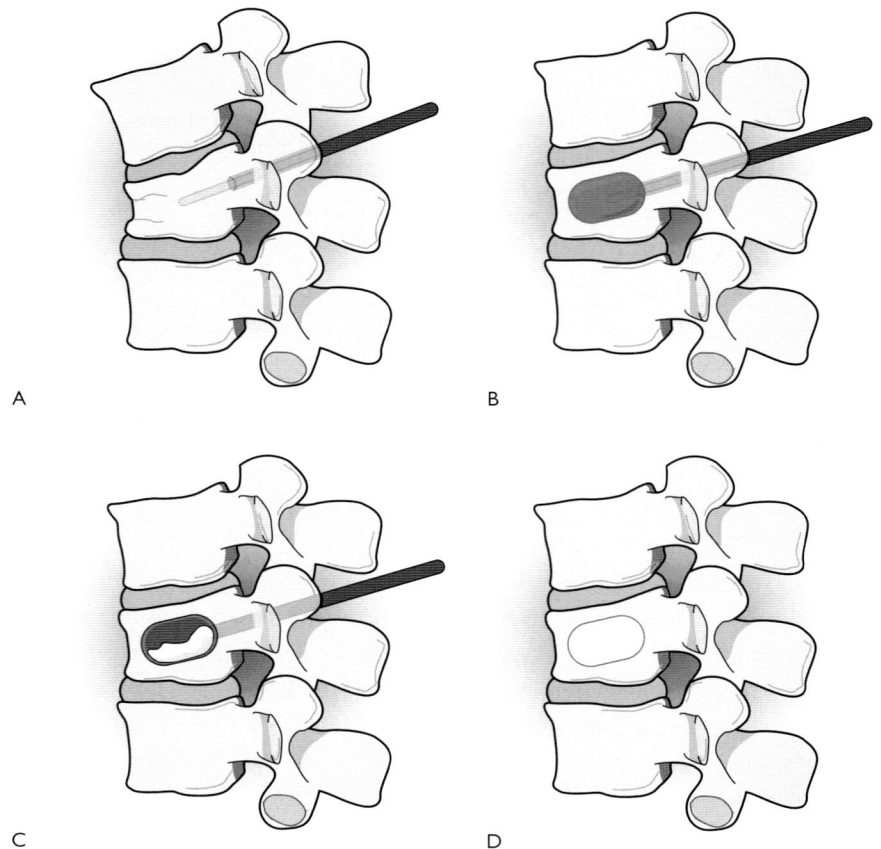

FIGURE 10-12
Schematic representation of kyphoplasty. (A) Introduction of a balloon into the vertebral body cavity. (B) The inflated balloon decreases the amount of compression. (C) Cement is introduced into the space that was created by the balloon. (D) The vertebra as it appears after withdrawal of the balloon and completion of cement filling.

procedures are that they provide immediate, sometimes dramatic, pain relief; enhance vertebral body strength; and, in the case of kyphoplasty, increase vertebral body height and reduce the kyphotic deformity. It has been suggested that the heat, generated while the cement is setting, destroys the nerve fibers that innervate the vertebral cortex and thus explains the immediate pain relief.

Balance exercises combined with tai chi exercises should be prescribed in an effort to improve the patient's stability and prevent future falls. Daily calcium (1,000–1,200 mg) and vitamin D (400–800 IU) supplementation is recommended. Adequate, well-balanced nutrition is of utmost importance, especially in the elderly, whose absorption of key nutrients declines.

Subcutaneous injections of Teriparatide (Forteo) can be tried as a first line of treatment. Forteo, a recombinant human parathyroid hormone, promotes bone formation and can be administered daily by subcutaneous injection into the thigh or abdominal wall. The injections (20 mcg) are administered daily for a period of up to 18 months. Increased bone density by up to 12% can be expected within a year.

At the termination of Forteo injections, in order to maintain the gain in bone density, antiresorptive medications can be administered. The bisphosphonate drugs (Alendronate, Risedronate, and others) are well tolerated antiresorptive drugs that can be taken once a week. These drugs inhibit osteoclast-mediated bone resorption and thus tip the balance toward bone buildup. Ibandronate (Boniva), a recently introduced bisphosphonate, is administered orally once a month.

Patients who cannot tolerate or do not respond to these drugs should try estrogen receptor modulators (Raloxifene), or Calcitonin. The latter medication also has analgesic effects. Bone density studies should be obtained every 12–18 months in order to confirm response to treatment.

SACRAL INSUFFICIENCY FRACTURES

Sacral insufficiency fractures are relatively uncommon. When they occur, however, they are frequently missed. They develop in osteoporotic individuals, mostly slim elderly women, frequently without any preceding trauma or following a fall. Occasionally, bilateral fractures in the allae of the sacrum are encountered. At times, in addition to the sacral fractures the patients sustain pelvic rim fractures, especially in the pubic rami region.

Clinical Presentation

The usual presenting symptom is severe pain that is located in the low back region or proximal buttock. The pain interferes with the patient's ability to ambulate. The neurological examination remains normal. The straight-leg raising test remains negative but the patient may experience increased pain when the lower extremity is manipulated.

Imaging Studies

Plain films often do not reveal the fracture because the area is commonly obscured by bowel shadows. When the plain films are negative, bone scan and/or pelvic CT or MRI may help in establishing the diagnosis. The bone scan may show increased uptake at the fracture site (Figure 10-13). CT scan can easily detect cortical defects and may show the fracture lines, which are usually found adjacent to but not involving the sacroiliac joints. In older fractures the CT will show sclerotic bands adjacent to the sacroiliac joints (Figure 10-14). MRI can establish the correct diagnosis and help rule out metastatic disease. It will detect bony edema at the fracture site, which will appear as a hypointense region on T1WI and hyperintense on T2WI. Fat suppression may further help define the extent of the edematous area (Figure 10-15).

Management

Patients with sacral insufficiency fractures should be kept ambulatory when possible. Pain management is critical in the early stages.

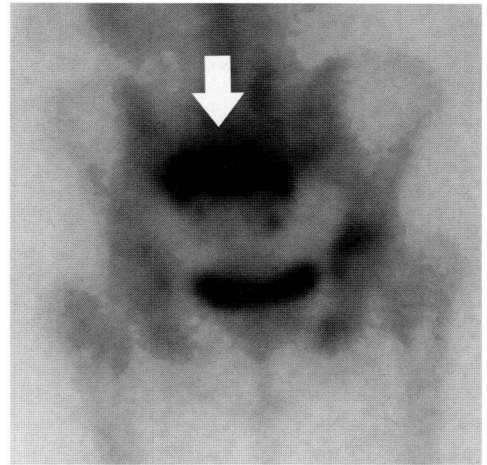

FIGURE 10-13
Bone scan of a 75-year-old woman who developed severe "back" pain with gait dysfunction. A large area of increased uptake is seen in the sacrum. Courtesy Dr. A. Brook.

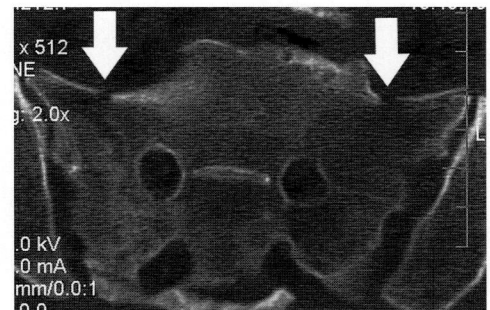

FIGURE 10-14
Coronal reformatted CT of the sacrum. Bilateral cortical defects in the sacral ala are seen (arrows). On the right side the fracture line can be identified. Courtesy Dr. A. Brook.

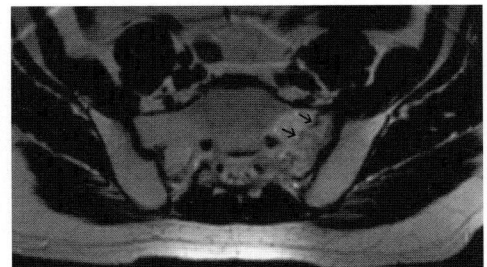

FIGURE 10-15
T2WI of the sacrum. A linear area of hypointensity (fracture) is seen in the left sacral region (arrows). Courtesy Dr. A. Brook.

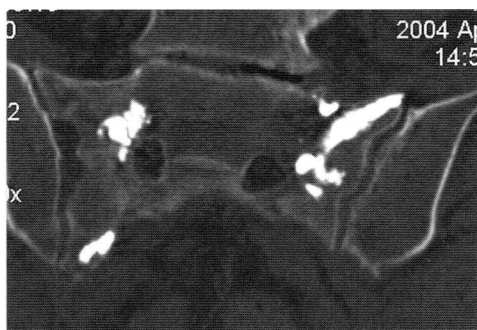

FIGURE 10-16
Coronal view CT of the sacrum after cement injection into bilateral sacral insufficiency fractures. Patient was able to ambulate with significantly less pain following the injections. Courtesy Dr. A. Brook.

The patients should be provided with a walker for protected weight bearing. This should be discarded and switched to a cane within 3–4 weeks. The fractured area can be injected with a small amount of cement in a *sacroplasty* procedure in order to stabilize the fracture, reduce the pain, and promote ambulation (Figure 10-16). The prognosis in these patients is favorable. Most patients become asymptomatic within 4–6 weeks.

OSTEOMALACIA

Osteomalacia (OM) is a metabolic bone disease resulting from defective mineralization of bone that leads to the accumulation of unmineralized osteoid matrix. The disease most frequently affects elderly housebound sedentary people who are not exposed to sunlight and consume a diet deficient in vitamin D. OM is caused by biochemical disturbances of the calcium-phosphate metabolism, which may be caused by intestinal malabsorption, senile hypovitaminosis D, hypophosphatemia, chronic renal insufficiency, or various drugs that are used long term, including anticonvulsants, bisphosphonates, and nonabsorbable antacids. A high degree of awareness of this disease is required in order to include it in the differential diagnosis. The classical biochemical changes of OM consist of low calcium, low phosphorus, and an elevated bone-specific alkaline phosphatase. In many elderly patients, however, the values of these substances may remain normal. The presence of the disease can be confirmed with a bone biopsy. The serum 25-hydroxyvitamin D and 1,25-dihydroxyvitamin D (calcitriol) may be decreased, and the parathyroid hormone may be elevated. The following paragraphs deal with OM due to hypovitaminosis D.

Clinical Presentation

Quite often OM is identified rather late because it presents with vague nonspecific complaints that simulate other common conditions such as fibromyalgia, polymyalgia rheumatica, polymyositis, osteoporosis, and metastatic diseases.

The presenting symptoms include three p's: pain, polyarthralgia, and proximal muscle weakness. Most patients present with pain of insidious onset. The pain may be progressive and involve the spine, rib cage, pelvis, and the limb girdles. Several areas may be painful and tender simultaneously, thus simulating fibromyalgia and other systemic diseases. Many patients complain of bilateral joint pain and diffuse muscle aches. Polyarthralgia with synovitis of the hands and feet may develop. Myopathy can result in proximal muscle weakness, especially of antigravity muscles such as the quadriceps. The weakness gradually evolves and brings about functional deficits. Initially the patients complain of fatigue. Later on they develop difficulties getting up from the seated position, stair climbing, and maintaining their balance, and they eventually suffer falls. In longstanding untreated patients bony deformities such as kyphosis, scoliosis, bowed legs, and protrusio acetabuli may develop.

Imaging Studies

Plain films may show diffuse demineralization with blurring of the bony trabeculae. Lucent sites appear in cortical bones, attesting to osteoid accumulation. These sites are oriented at a right angle to the cortex and are called *pseudofractures* or *Looser's zones*. Pseudofractures are not common. They may be seen in the pelvis, especially at the pubic rami and the bones of the extremities. Quite often they appear bilaterally and symmetrically. Calcified enthesopathies, fuzzy sacroiliac joints, and subchondral bone resorption of the symphysis pubis may be encountered as well. Occasionally sacral insufficiency fractures may occur. Their appearance on CT and MRI is not different from osteoporotic fractures (Figures 10-17 and 10-18).

Management

Large doses of vitamin D or its derivatives (calcitriol or alfacalcidol) can reverse the symptoms over time. Vitamin D–deficient patients should receive 2,000–3,000 IU of vitamin D per day for several months. Alternatively they may be treated with intramuscular injections of ergocalciferol, 50,000–100,000 IU per week for 1 month followed by one injection per month for the next five months. Daily calcium supplementation should be provided until the OM has resolved.

Vitamin D supplementation, however, can increase calcium and phosphate serum levels by enhancing intestinal absorption of these elements. Regular renal monitoring is important because progressive kidney calcification—*nephrocalcinosis*—may develop.

Bibliography

Berry JL, Davies M, Mee AP: Vitamin D metabolism, rickets, and osteomalacia. Semin Musculoskelet Radiol 6: 173–182, 2002.

Bhalla S, Reinus WR: The linear intravertebral vacuum: A sign of benign vertebral collapse. Am J Roentgenol 170: 1563–1569, 1998.

Blake SP, Connors AM: Sacral insufficiency fracture. Br J Radiol 77: 891–896, 2004.

Brook AL, Mirsky DM, Bello JA: Computerized tomography guided sacroplasty: A practical treatment for sacral insufficiency fracture. Case report. Spine 30: E450–E454, 2005.

Cooper KL, Beabout JW, Swee RG: Insufficiency fractures of the sacrum. Radiology 156: 15–20, 1985.

Cuenod CA, Laredo JD, Chevret S, Hamze B, Naouri JF, Chapeau X, Bondeville JM, Tubiana JM: Acute vertebral collapse due to osteoporosis or malignancy: Appearance on unenhanced and gadolinium-enhanced MR images. Radiology 199: 541–549, 1996.

Dublin AB, Hartman J, Latchaw RE, Hald JK, Reid MH: The vertebral body fracture in osteoporosis: Restoration of height using percutaneous vertebroplasty. Am J Neuroradiol 26: 489–492, 2005.

Flicker L, MacInnis RJ, Stein MS, Scherer SC, Mead KE, Nowson CA, Thomas J, Lowndes C, Hopper JL, Wark JD: Should older people in residential care receive vitamin D to prevent falls? Results of a randomized trial. J Am Geriatr Soc 53: 1881–1888, 2005.

Glerup H, Mikkelsen K, Poulsen L, Hass E, Overbeck S, Andersen h, Charles P, Eriksen EF: Hypovitaminosis D myopathy without biochemical signs of osteomalacic bone involvement. Calcif Tissue Int 66: 419–424, 2000.

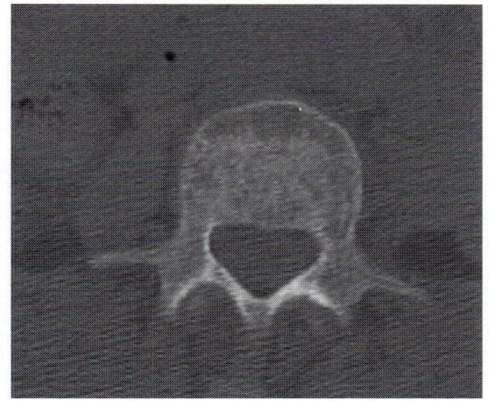

FIGURE 10-17
Axial CT image of a lumbar vertebra in a patient with severe osteomalacia. Note the paucity of bony trabeculae creating large "holes" within the cancellous bone, especially in the anterior portion of the vertebral body. Courtesy Dr. N. Haramati.

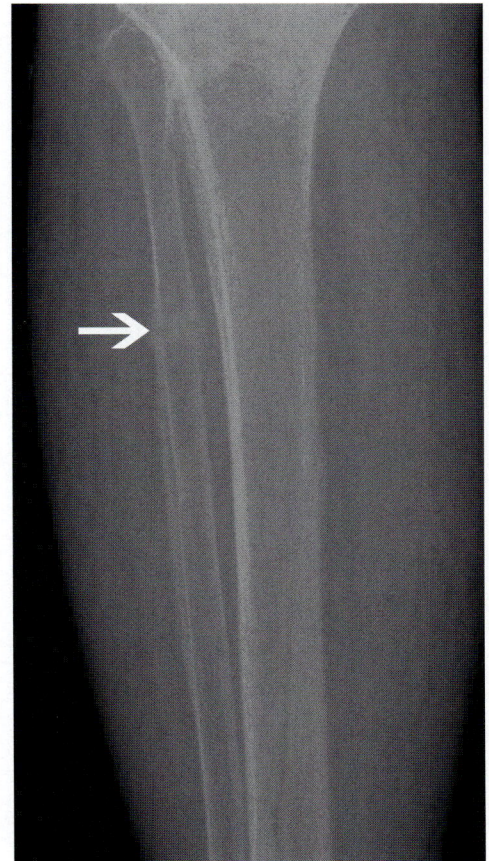

FIGURE 10-18
Plain X-ray of the leg in a patient with osteomalacia. A looser zone is clearly seen in the upper third of the fibula. Courtesy Dr. N. Haramati.

Hadjipavlou AG, Tzermiadianos MN, Katonis PG, Szpalski M: Percutaneous vertebroplasty and balloon kyphoplasty for the treatment of osteoporotic vertebral compression fractures and osteolytic tumors. J Bone Joint Surg Br 87: 1595–1604, 2005.

Iqbal MM: Osteoporosis: Epidemiology, diagnosis, and treatment. South Med J 93: 2–18, 2000.

Jevtic V: Imaging of renal osteodystrophy. Eur J Radiol 46: 85–95, 2003.

Kanberoglu K, Kantarci F, Cebi D, Yilmaz MH, Kurugoglu S, Bilici A, Koyuncu H: Magnetic resonance imaging in osteomalacic insufficiency fractures of the pelvis. Clin Radiol 60: 105–111, 2005.

Kelman A, Lane NE: The management of secondary osteoporosis. Best Pract Res Clin Rheumatol 19: 1021–1037, 2005.

Kobayashi K, Shimoyama K, Nakamura K, Murata K: Percutaneous vertebroplasty immediately relieves pain of osteoporotic vertebral compression fractures and prevents prolonged immobilization of patients. Eur J Radiol 15: 360–367, 2005.

Lenchik L, Rogers LF, Delmas PD, Genant HK: Diagnosis of osteoporotic vertebral fractures: Importance of recognition and description by radiologists. Am J Radiol 183: 949–958, 2004.

Lyman D: Undiagnosed vitamin D deficiency in the hospitalized patient. Am Fam Physician 71: 299–304, 2005.

Maddalozzo GF, Snow CM: High intensity resistance training: Effects on bone in older men and women. Calcif Tissue Int 66: 399–404, 2000.

McKiernan F, Faciszewski T: Intravertebral clefts in osteoporotic vertebral compression fractures. Arthritis Rheum 48: 1414–1419, 2003.

Newhouse KE, El-Khoury GY, Buckwalter JA: Occult sacral fractures in osteopenic patients. J Bone Joint Surg Am 74: 1472–1477, 1992.

Oostveen JCM, Van de Laar MAFJ: Magnetic resonance imaging in rheumatic disorders of the spine and sacroiliac joints. Semin Arthritis Rheum 30: 52–69, 2000.

Orr RD: Treatment of osteoporotic vertebral compression fractures with vertebral augmentation: Vertebroplasty and kyphoplasty. Contemp Spine Surg 5: 27–32, 2004.

Osterhouse MD, Kettner NW: Delayed posttraumatic vertebral collapse with intravertebral vacuum cleft. J Manipulative Physiol Ther 25: 270–275, 2002.

Plotnikoff GA, Quigley JM: Prevalence of severe hypovitaminosis D in patients with persistent, nonspecific musculoskeletal pain. Mayo Clin Proc 78: 1463–1470, 2003.

Rao RD, Singrakhia MD: Current concepts review: Painful osteoporotic vertebral fractures. Pathogenesis, evaluation, and roles of vertebroplasty and kyphoplasty in its management. J Bone Joint Surg Am 85: 2010–2022, 2003.

Reginato AJ, Falasca GF, Pappu R, McKingth B, Agha A: Musculoskeletal manifestations of Osteomalacia: Report of 26 cases and literature review. Semin Arthritis Rheum 28: 287–304, 1999.

Richardson JP: Vitamin D deficiency: The once and present epidemic. Am Fam Physician 71: 241–242, 2005.

Soubrier M, Dubost JJ, Boisgard S, Sauvezie B, Gaillard P, Michel JL, Ristori JM: Insufficiency fracture. A survey of 60 cases and review of the literature. Joint Bone Spine 70: 209–218, 2003.

Sugita M, Watanabe N, Mikami Y, Hase H, Kubo T: Classification of vertebral compression fractures in the osteoporotic spine. J Spinal Disord Tech 18: 376–381, 2005.

Theodorou DJ: The intravertebral vacuum cleft sign. Radiol 221: 787–788, 2001.

Thomas MK, Demay MB: Vitamin D deficiency and disorders of Vitamin D metabolism. Endocrinol Metab Clin N Am 29: 611–627, 2000.

Togawa D, Lieberman IH, Bauer TW, Reinhardt MK, Kayanja MM: Histological evaluation of biopsies obtained from vertebral compression fractures: Unsuspected myeloma and osteomalacia. Spine 30: 781–786, 2005.

Vaccaro AR, Kim DH, Brodke DS, Harris M, Chapman J, Schildhauer T, Routt C, Sasso RC: Diagnosis and management of sacral spine fractures. J Bone Joint Surg Am 86: 166–175, 2004.

White PH: Osteopenic disorders of the spine. Semin Spine Surg 2: 121–129, 1990.

NEOPLASTIC DISEASES

11

Neoplastic diseases of the spine may be classified according to their location in the spine: *extradural*, *intradural*, or *intramedullary*. Their clinical presentation is usually related to their location. They may progress slowly and gradually or, at times, develop rapidly, especially in malignant and aggressive neoplasms. This chapter does not deal with all the existing tumors. Only the more common ones will be discussed.

EXTRADURAL TUMORS

Extradural tumors comprise about 60% of all spinal tumors. They may be either *primary*, that is, originating in the spine, or *metastatic*; either *benign*, such as, osteoid osteoma or hemangiomas, or *malignant and aggressive*, such as, chordoma; and either *osteolytic*, that is, leading to bone destruction and breakdown, such as multiple myeloma, or *osteoblastic*, that is, bone-forming tumors, such as in the case of metastases from prostate cancer. Spinal metastases are the most common extradural tumors as the spine is frequently affected by metastatic disease. Unlike spinal infections, which often invade and destroy the intervertebral discs, spine tumors almost never involve these structures.

Clinical Presentation

The most common clinical manifestation of spine tumors is axial pain. It may or may not be accompanied by radicular pain. Frequently the pain has an insidious onset, does not subside with rest, and, with time, may increase. When the first manifestation of a tumor is due to a pathological fracture the patient will present with severe pain of sudden onset. At times, the pain may be mechanical in nature (aggravated by weight bearing or movement and improved by rest), thus simulating other benign conditions. Frequently nocturnal pain is a dominant feature. Radicular pain and neurological symptoms may appear over the course of weeks and months, depending on the tumor aggressiveness and its location. Because many tumors are diagnosed relatively late, motor and sensory changes may already be present at the time of diagnosis and provide important information toward tumor localization. Chronic unremitting axial or radicular pain, nocturnal pain, weight loss, iron deficiency anemia, or progressive neurological loss can all be caused by a spine tumor and should trigger an aggressive and thorough diagnostic work-up. Early diagnosis and intervention are critical as patients with cord compression who are ambulatory when diagnosed have a much better prospect for ambulation following therapeutic interventions than those who are already paraplegic at the time of diagnosis.

SPINAL METASTASES

Skeletal metastases are 25 times more common than primary bone tumors. Spinal metastases are common because they tend to develop in hematopoietic active bone marrow, which is predominantly located in the adult spine. Most spinal metastases are found in the thoracic and lumbar regions. They are frequently disseminated via the blood-hematogenous spread. Both venous dissemination and arterial dissemination may occur. Batson's plexus of valveless veins, a major source of spinal metastases, connects with venous plexuses inside the spinal canal. Pressure difference in these veins directs tumor cells from the pelvis (prostate) into the lumbar or thoracic vertebral bodies. The tumors may also get to the spine by direct dissemination or through the lymphatic system. They frequently invade the vertebral bodies or the pedicles. Metastases can also grow along nervous tissue and thus enter the epidural space inside the spinal canal. The most common sources of vertebral metastases are the *b*reast, *l*ungs, *t*hyroid, *k*idney, and *p*rostate. An easy way to remember these organs is by bringing to mind the "classical" NY sandwich: *b*acon, *l*ettuce, and *t*omatoes with a *k*osher *p*ickle.

As the metastatic lesions grow, they destroy the vertebral body, penetrate through cortical bone, invade the spinal canal, and compromise the neural elements. Cord compression and neurological deficits may also occur when vertebral bodies collapse due to compromised structural integrity.

Imaging Studies

X-rays are the less sensitive diagnostic tool for spinal metastases detection. Vertebral bodies can loose upwards of 50% of their density before it becomes detectable in plain films. The vertebral bodies may appear heterogeneous or motley on plain films. This appearance is not specific and can be found in osteoporosis as well. The vertebral bodies' shape, texture, and cortices should be critically observed. Special attention should be paid to the posterior vertebral body wall. The presence of a lytic (darker) or blastic (whiter) vertebral body may give away the presence of metastases. In some patients with metastatic prostate cancer the vertebral bodies may seem completely white (Figures 11-1A and 11-1B). The pedicles should be critically inspected. They are

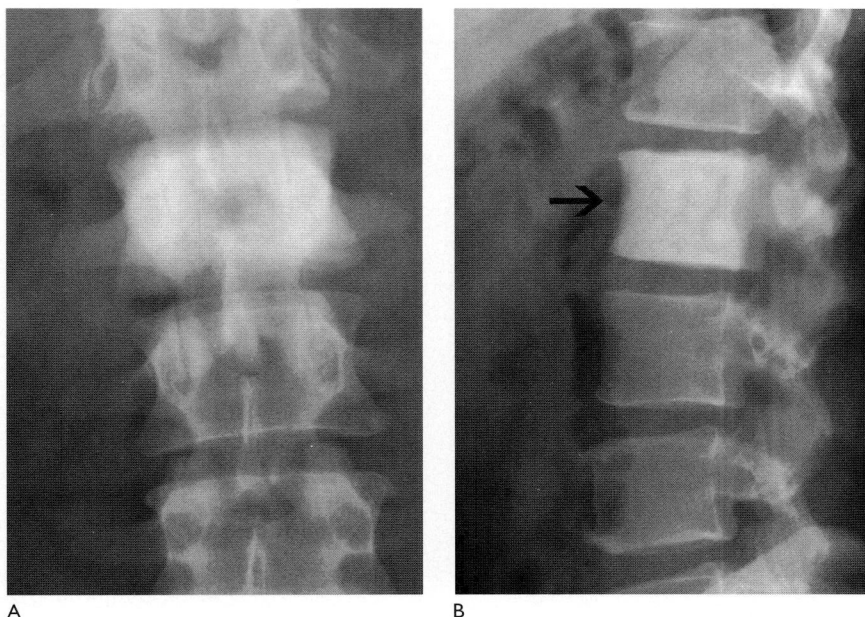

A
B

FIGURE 11-1
Plain films in (A) AP and (B) lateral view showing an ivory vertebra. Courtesy Dr. N. Haramati.

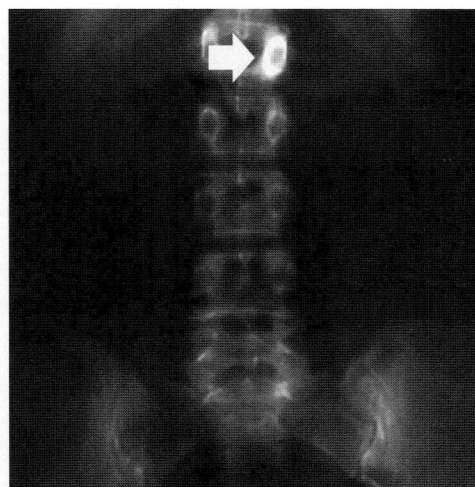

FIGURE 11-2
Plain film in AP view of the lumbar spine showing a sclerosed left pedicle at L2.

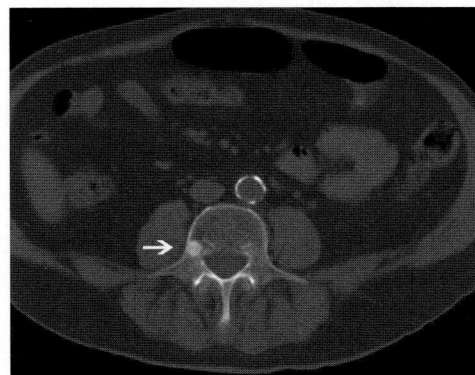

FIGURE 11-3
Axial CT slice through the L2 vertebral body showing a sclerosed right pedicle. The lesion was difficult to identify on plain films.

well seen in posteroanterior views and can be screened rather quickly. Absence, erosion, or sclerosis of a pedicle may indicate the presence of a bone metastase at that location (Figure 11-2).

Bone scanning is an efficient and cheap tool to detect cancer at an early stage. It has a high sensitivity with lower specificity but may remain falsely negative in patients with lytic lesions such as multiple myeloma.

High-resolution CT is very helpful in detecting small bony lesions. Axial CT allows accurate depiction of bony details without being hampered by overlap bones as is the case with plain films (Figure 11-3). Sagittal and coronal reconstructions of multislice CT help in determining the integrity and the stability of the affected vertebral bodies, and are highly recommended when a search for bony metastases is conducted (Figure 11-4). The diagnostic yield can be further enhanced by the administration of contrast material, because it can differentiate innocent fatty infiltration or hemngioma from metastatic soft tissue within the vertebrae as well as facilitate the detection of epidural and, at times, intradural tumor extension. Recently the combination of CT and positron emission tomography (CT-PET) has become available. It might add a powerful diagnostic tool for bony metastases in the workup of the oncological patient.

MRI is an excellent diagnostic modality for tumor detection, especially of bone marrow metastases, and it is the most sensitive modality compared with other imaging techniques. It might detect tiny lesions that may have otherwise been overlooked by nuclear imaging or by CT. MRI provides important information about the vertebrae as well as the soft tissues. It helps detect epidural tumor extension and, following contrast administration, it may show leptomeningeal spread.

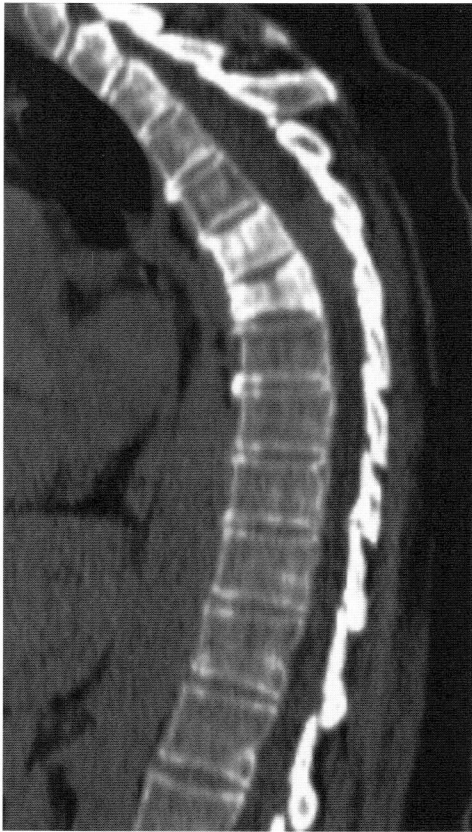

FIGURE 11-4
Sagittal reconstruction of a CT study discloses two consecutive sclerotic vertebrae due to osteoblastic breast metastasis. The body of the lower vertebra is significantly compressed, whereas the body of the one above is affected to a lesser extent.

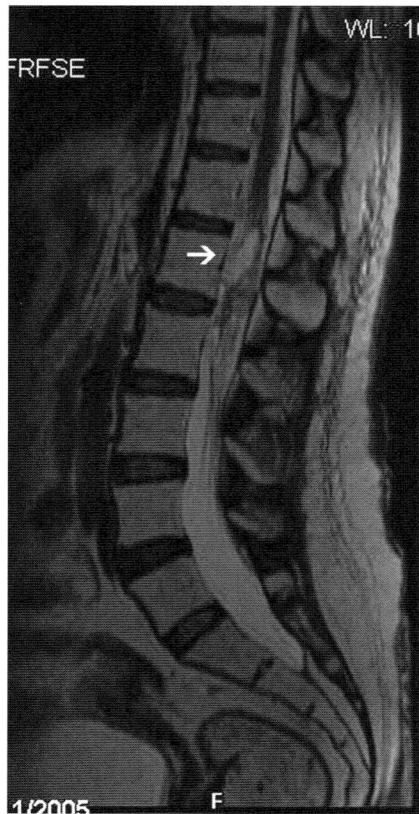

FIGURE 11-5
Sagittal T2WI of the lumbar spine showing a high-intensity tumor opposite the L1 vertebral body. The tumor is engulfing the distal cord.

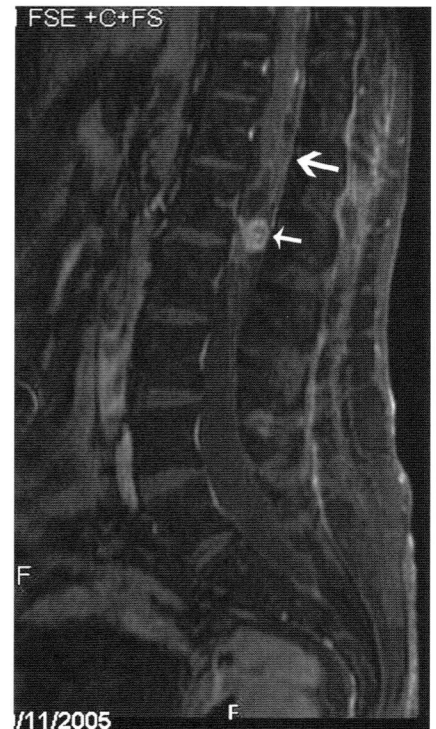

FIGURE 11-6
Sagittal T1WI following gadolinium administration and with fat suppression demonstrating enhancement along the cauda equina roots (larger arrow) in a patient with leptomeningeal metastatic disease. Larger metastases are visible at the L1-L2 junction (smaller arrow).

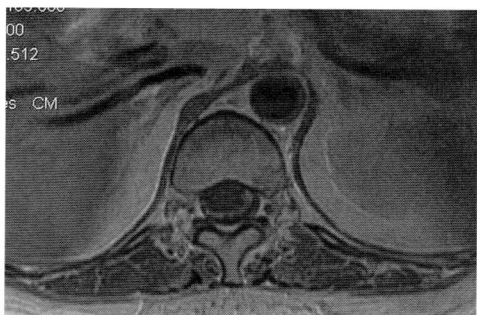

FIGURE 11-7
Axial T1WI with fat suppression and contrast showing enhancement in the periphery of the thecal sac due to leptomeningeal spread.

This is commonly seen in the lumbosacral spine when cancer cells, directed by gravity, cling to and coat the nerve roots and the cauda equina (Figures 11-5, 11-6, and 11-7). Blastic tumors appear hypointense on T1- and T2-weighted images (T1WI and T2WI). Extensively involved vertebral bodies may seem darker than the adjacent discs on T1WI. Hypointense sclerotic bone metastases may appear somewhat brighter then the normal bone following contrast administration, especially when a fat suppression sequence is utilized.

The signal characteristics of lytic metastases are similar to those of blastic metastases on T1WI: hypointense compared with uninvolved, normal bone marrow. Following contrast administration, the involved vertebral segments will enhance usually and will become more conspicuous when fat suppression is applied (Figure 11-8). T2WI will show either hypointense or hyperintense segments or a combination of both; they have a heterogeneous appearance. Occasionally, areas of hyperintensity surrounding a region that is hypointense—the *target sign*—can be seen. Extensive infiltration may weaken the vertebral body and lead to vertebral collapse with retropulsed segments that may compromise the neural elements. This can be clearly captured on both sagittal and axial T1WI and T2WI (Figure 11-9).

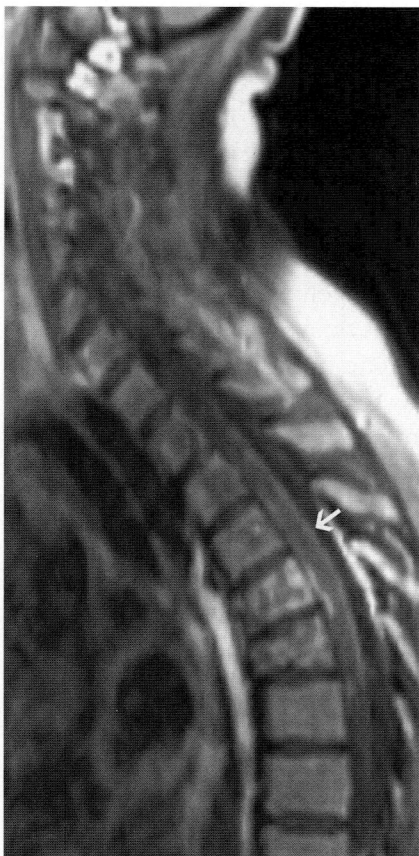

FIGURE 11-8
Sagittal T1WI with contrast showing enhancement of the involved vertebrae. A pathological fracture can be seen involving two of the motley-appearing vertebrae. There is also leptomeningeal enhancement enveloping the cord (arrow).

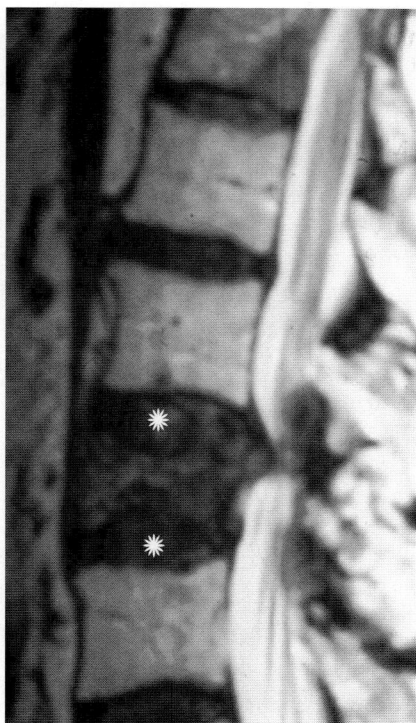

FIGURE 11-9
Pathological fracture of a metastatic vertebra with retropulsed segment encroaching into the spinal canal causing cord compression. The adjacent discs are marked by stars.

Management

Decompression and stabilization are required in patients with unstable fractures and neurological involvement. Osteolytic tumors may be managed with vertebroplasty enabling early pain-free mobilization. At times, radiation therapy may bring about pain relief.

MULTIPLE MYELOMA

Multiple myeloma is a systemic malignant disease. It is the most common primary tumor of bone. In its initial stages, marrow infiltration with plasma cells and increased bone resorption result in radiological appearance identical to that seen in osteoporosis. The disease leads to anemia, increased sedimentation rate, hypercalcemia, accumulation of paraprotein in the serum, and Bence-Jones protein in the urine. The diagnosis can be confirmed by finding abnormal serum and urine electrophoresis. Bone marrow biopsy establishes the diagnosis by demonstrating abundance (over 10%) of malignant plasma cells.

Clinical Presentation

Multiple myeloma is more common in males and usually presents in the fifth or sixth decades. Most patients present with pain. Initially the pain may be mechanical in nature, increasing on weight bearing and disappearing with rest. Soon afterward, the pain intensifies, becomes permanent, and may disturb the patient's sleep. At times, sudden, severe axial pain develops due to a pathological fracture. Vague symptoms such as fatigue, generalized weakness, and weight loss accompany the pain. The disease affects the vertebral bodies as well as the posterior elements. The thoracic and lumbar spine regions are the most commonly affected areas. At times a solitary lytic-multicystic bone lesion is found presenting a solitary myeloma or "plasmacytoma."

Imaging Studies

Bone scan may remain negative in the presence of bone marrow infiltration and the absence of fractures. CT may detect lytic lesions, especially in the trabecular bone of the vertebral bodies even in the presence of normal-looking plain films (Figures 11-10A, 11-10B, and 11-10C). Lytic lesions may involve cortical bone as well. About 1% of the lesions may be sclerotic. Spiral or multidetector CT may be able to provide detailed information on osseous involvement. In advanced stages the CT will show destruction of vertebral bodies and the presence of compression fractures with tumor extending beyond the vertebral boundaries (Figure 11-11).

MRI is the best screening test in multiple myeloma patients who appear to have normal plain films or diffuse osteoporosis. In the initial stages of the disease, however, up to 50% of patients with proven bone marrow infiltration may have a normal-looking MRI.

Three patterns of marrow involvement by the disease are known. The most common type consists of focal, well-demarcated low-signal-intensity lesions on T1WI and high intensity on T2WI. Post-contrast

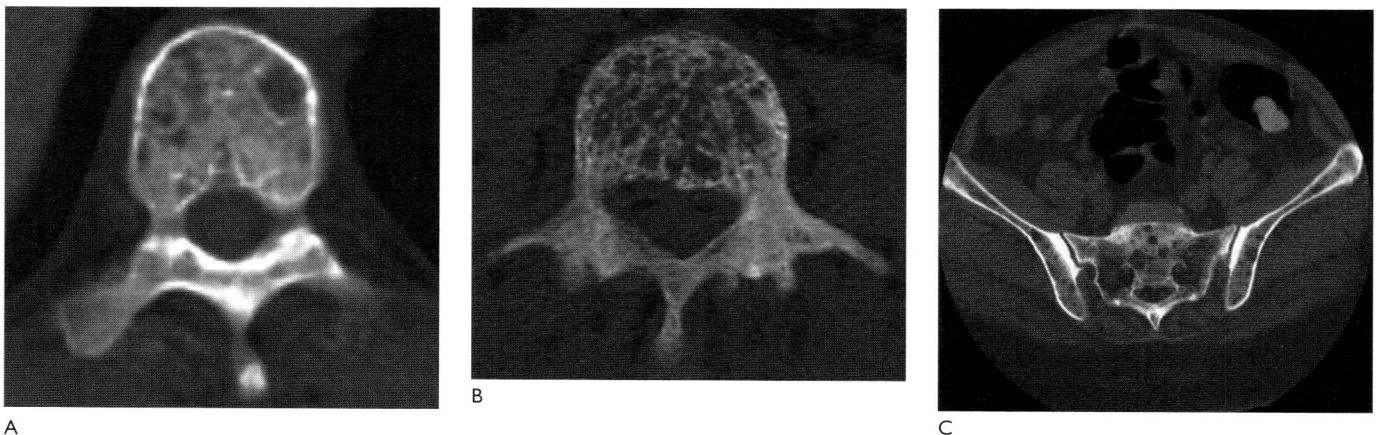

A

B

C

FIGURE 11-10
(A, B) Axial CT scans through a thoracic vertebra showing multiple lytic lesions within the vertebral body and posterior elements. (C) Extensive involvement of the pelvic bones in the same patient. Courtesy Dr. A. Brook.

T1WI will show marked enhancement and facilitate the diagnosis. The second type is that of tiny foci with similar signal characteristics to the larger lesions. The third type is that of diffuse bone marrow involvement. T1WI in these patients will show a homogenously decreased signal throughout the bone marrow that can be easily overlooked. The obtained signal may be similar to that of the intervertebral discs or even of lower intensity. T2WI in these patients will show a diffuse increased signal, and there may be diffuse enhancement following contrast administration (Figures 11-12A and 11-12B).

Management

Multiple myeloma is an aggressive disease with a high mortality rate. High-dose chemotherapy, total body radiation, and bone marrow or stem cell transplantation can extend survival in some patients. Vertebroplasty and kyphoplasty may help preserve vertebral height, decrease pain, and enhance function.

CHORDOMA

Spinal chordomas are relatively rare, slow-growing, low-grade malignant tumors. The peak incidence is in the fifth and sixth decades.

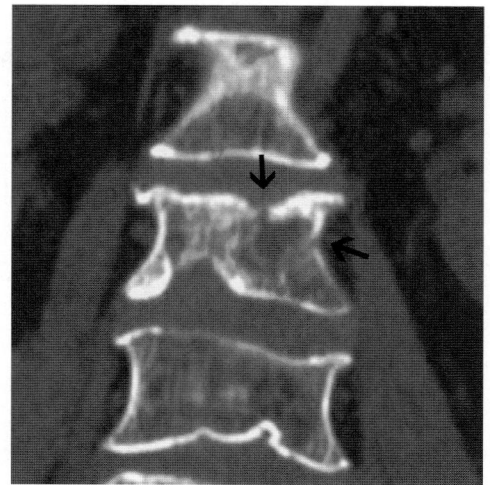

FIGURE 11-11
Coronal reconstruction of the lumbar spine showing punched out lesions in the vertebral bodies and fractured cortical bone in the vertebral body (arrows).

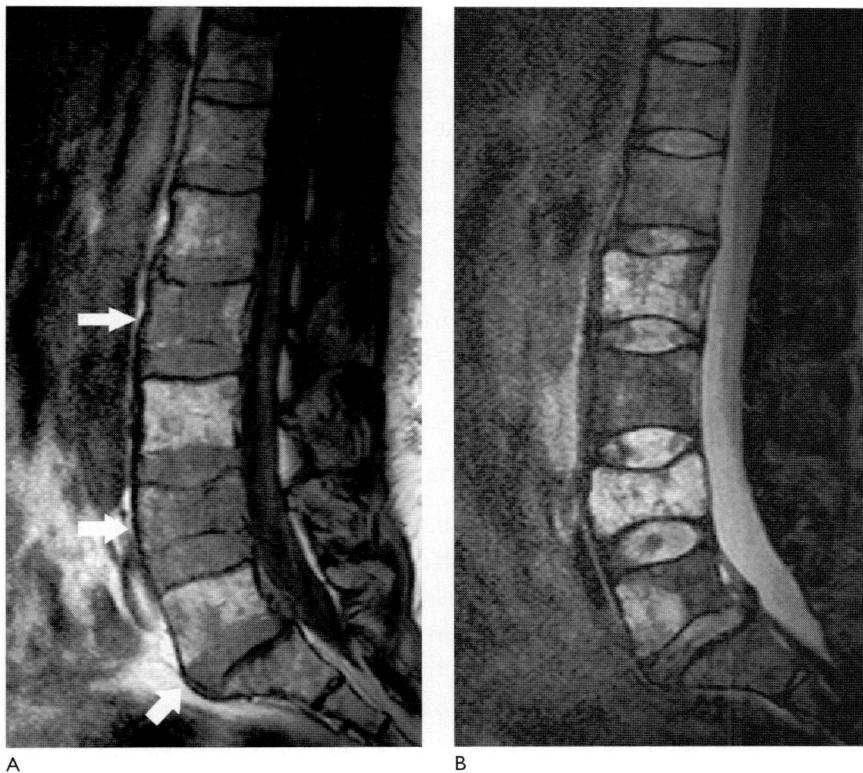

A   B

FIGURE 11-12
(A) Sagittal T1WI and (B) T2WI with fat suppression MRI of the lumbar spine in a myeloma patient. Note that the affected vertebrae (L2, L4, and L5) have a decreased signal on T1- and an increased signal on T2WI. When a vertebra is partially involved, as the L2 and L5 are in this case, the signal appears heterogeneous. Courtesy Dr. T. Miller.

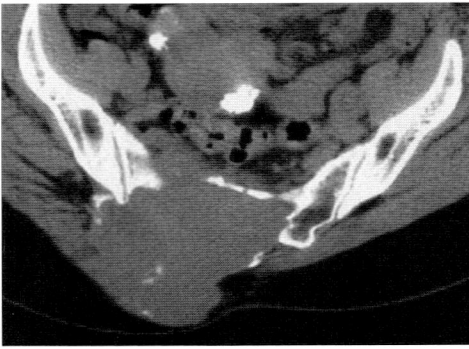

FIGURE 11-13

Pelvic CT showing an extensive destructive lytic lesion that involves the sacral bone and invades the right sacroiliac joint. The mass bulges anteriorly into the pelvis and posteriorly into the subcutaneous fatty tissue. Note some amorphous intratumoral calcifications. Courtesy Dr. D. Lerer.

Males are affected twice as often as females. About half of spinal chordomas affect the sacrum, a third the clivus area, and the rest are found in other regions of the spine, with a predilection for C2. The tumor originates from remnants of the notochord. This is a locally aggressive tumor that slowly infiltrates and destroys cancellous bone. The mean duration of symptoms is 11 months before the diagnosis is established.

Clinical Presentation

Most patients present with back pain, radicular pain, lower extremity weakness, and bladder, bowel, or sexual dysfunction.

Imaging Studies

Plain films may reveal a destructive sacral lesion or clivus mass, which may be lucent with some amorphous calcification. The mass can destroy the bone and invade adjacent structures. Quite often the sacral tumor penetrates into the epidural space and/or the paravertebral tissues. On CT, the tumor mass appears hypodense to the adjacent normal tissue and enhances mildly or moderately following contrast administration (Figure 11-13). MRI is the procedure of choice in establishing the size of the tumor and its extent. Most chordomas appear heterogeneous on MRI. They tend to be isointense on T1WI with foci of high signal intensity, and hyperintense on T2WI. Low signal septations may appear on T2WI. Postcontrast enhancement may vary from mild (blush) to intense enhancement (Figures 11-14A, 11-14B, and 11-14C). T2WI with fat saturation may help delineate the extension of the tumor into the adjacent soft tissues. Frequently the tumor appears lobulated.

Management

Early diagnosis combined with radical en bloc resection and, at times, radiation improves disease-free intervals and enhances quality of life.

VERTEBRAL HEMANGIOMA

The prevalence of vertebral hemangiomas increases with age, peaking in the fourth through sixth decades. This is the most common benign spinal tumor; it may be present in up to 10% of all spinal MRI studies. It occurs most frequently in the thoracic spine, less frequently in the lumbar region, and rarely in the cervical region. Commonly, multiple hemangiomas may be seen affecting several vertebrae. Ninety percent of hemangiomas develop within the vertebral bodies. The rest are found in the posterior elements.

Clinical Presentation

Most hemangiomas are asymptomatic and do not harbor any risk. They may be seen on images obtained in the process of patient evaluation and do not require any clinical response. Symptomatic hem-

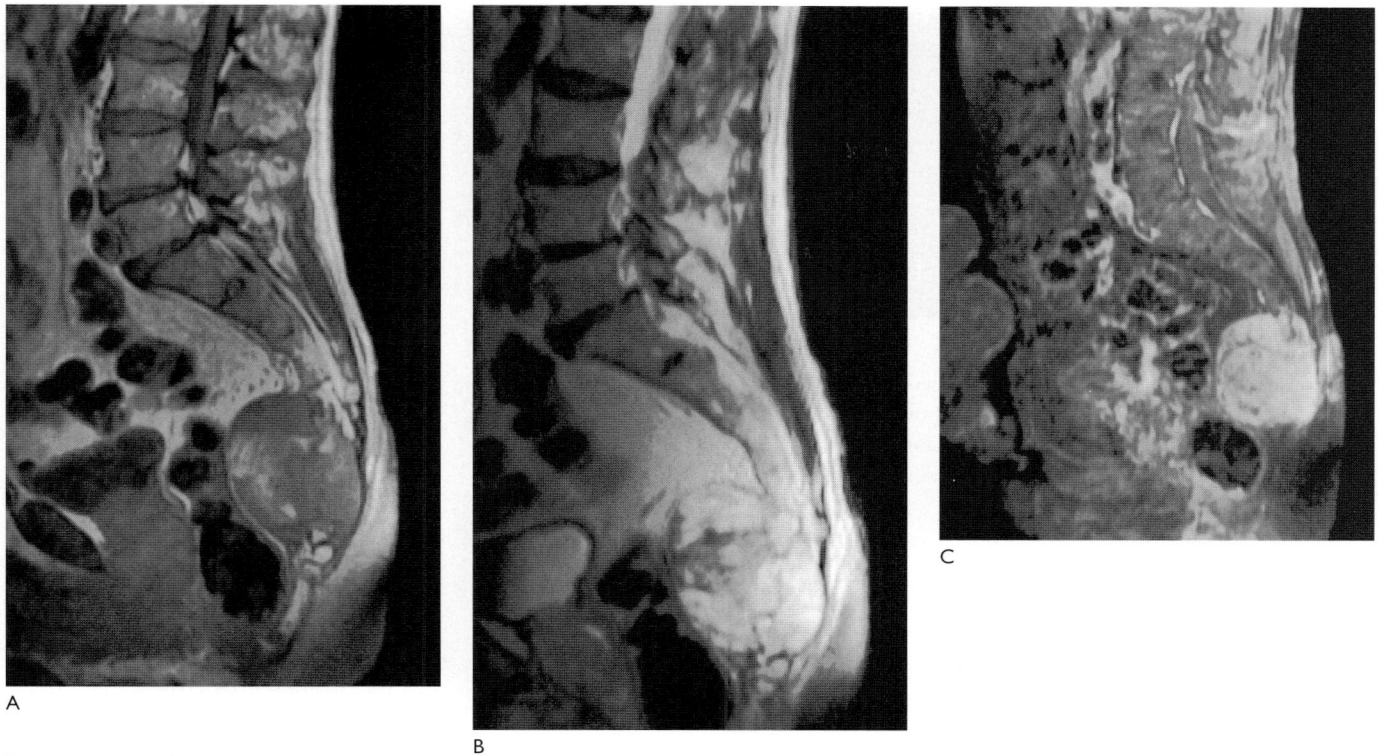

FIGURE 11-14

(A) Sagittal T1WI, (B) T2WI, and (C) postcontrast T1WI of a large chordoma. A very large tumor is demonstrated. The tumor has grown anteriorly into the pelvis from the lowermost edge of the sacrum, involving the coccyx and pushing the rectum forward. It is heterogeneous but mostly hypointense on T1WI (with some areas of increased signal) (A), and iso- to hyperintense on T2 with septations of low intensity. Following contrast administration it enhances and is easily depicted with fat suppression (C).

angiomas tend to occur in the lower thoracic spine. The more aggressive ones grow beyond the vertebral body boundaries and may compress the spinal cord or the exiting nerve roots. As they grow within the vertebral body they may compromise its structural integrity to the point of collapse. Patients with aggressive hemangiomas present with axial pain and tenderness. Only a minority develop slowly progressive radicular symptoms or myelopathic signs. Rarely, rapid-onset, progressive neurological compromise is seen. The symptoms may be caused by epidural expansion of the tumor, expansion of the vertebral body in response to tumor expansion, sudden bleeding, or vertebral body collapse.

Imaging Studies

Plain films reveal either parallel linear streaks or "honeycomb" appearance or vertical striation within the vertebrae (Figure 11-15). CT easily detects these lesions. The affected vertebra will show a "polka dot" appearance on axial cuts. Thickened trabeculae are surrounded with hypodense fatty tissue (Figure 11-16). Aggressive hemangiomas may extend beyond the vertebral body, penetrate into the spinal canal, and compress the spinal cord. In these cases MRI will better demonstrate the extent of soft tissue involvement. Benign hemangiomas usually appear hyperintense on both T1WI and T2WI (FSE) when there is a great amount of fatty tissue within the tumor. They may enhance

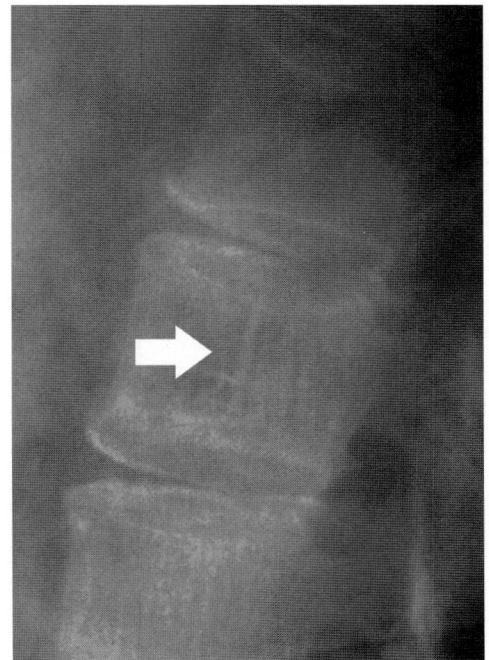

FIGURE 11-15

A lateral plain film showing thickened, vertically oriented trabeculae within the vertebral body (arrow). This appearance is characteristic of a hemangioma.

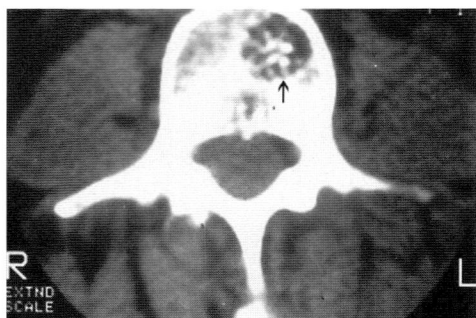

FIGURE 11-16
An axial CT showing a well-circumscribed, hypodense round lesion within the vertebral body with a "spotted" appearance of sparse thickened trabeculae surrounded by hypodense fat, typical for hemangioma (arrow).

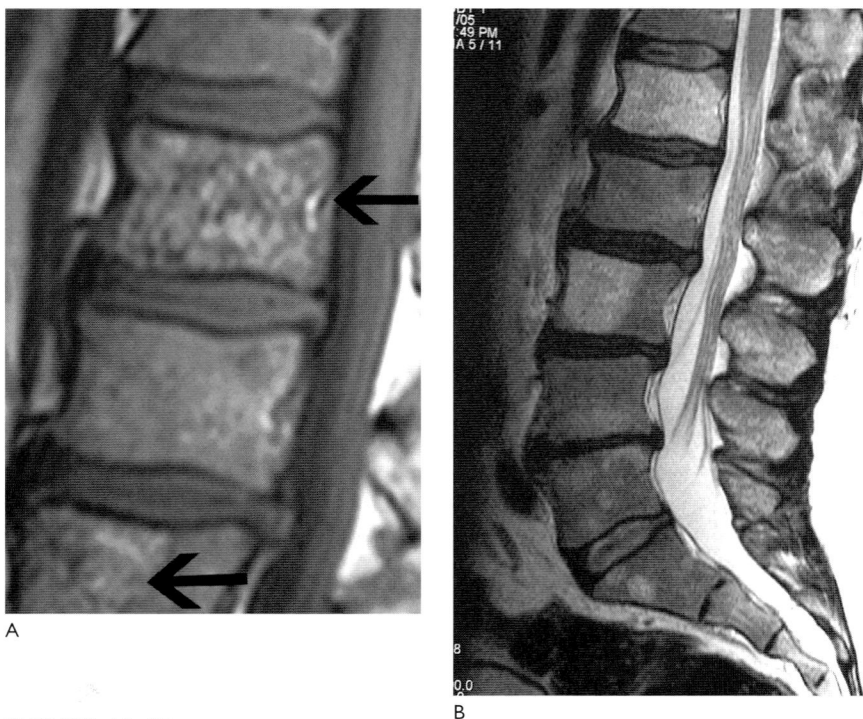

A

B

FIGURE 11-17
Sagittal MRI of hemangiomas. (A) On T1WI both lesions have a mildly increased signal. (B) On T2WI they are clearly hyperintense.

following contrast administration (Figures 11-17A and 11-17B). The rare aggressive hemangiomas have no fatty tissue and are usually isointense or hypointense and may mimic metastases or primary vertebral lesions such as plasmacytoma.

Management

The management of hemangiomas depends on whether they cause only pain or compromise the neural elements. In patients complaining of pain other causes that may explain the patient's symptoms should be explored. Symptomatic hemangioma can be treated by radiation. Aggressive hemangiomas that invade the epidural space or jeopardize the structural integrity of the vertebral body should be excised.

OSTEOID OSTEOMA

Osteoid osteoma is a benign tumor found in young males in the second decade of life. Typically, the tumor is located in the posterior elements—the pedicles or the laminae. Most of these tumors are found in the lumbar region and, less frequently, in the cervical region.

Clinical Presentation

Patients complain of unrelenting axial pain that is worse at night. The pain responds well to aspirin and NSAIDS. Antalgic scoliosis may be observed on physical examination.

Imaging Studies

Plain films and CT can show a round, lucent nidus (core) surrounded by sclerotic bone. The tumor appears "hot" on bone scan (Figure 11-18).

On MRI, the tumor will appear hypointense on T1WI. On T2WI the nidus may appear hyperintense, and the surrounding sclerotic bone will appear hypointense. Postcontrast, the nidus will enhance.

Management

Patients with unrelenting symptoms should be operated on. Total excision offers permanent cure.

OSTEOBLASTOMA

Osteoblastoma appears histologically similar to osteoid osteoma, and the difference between them is determined by their size: Osteoblastomas tend to be larger than osteoid osteoma, extending over 1.5 cm. They have a tendency to expand. Osteoblastoma has a greater predilection for the spine than osteoid osteoma and occurs more commonly in the cervical region. At times, the tumor may appear in other locations throughout the spine.

Clinical Presentation

Patients present with axial pain and antalgic scoliosis.

Imaging Studies

Imaging will demonstrate the expansile lesion, which may penetrate through the bone and expand into the soft tissue (Figure 11-19). The imaging characteristics of osteoblastoma are quite variable.

INTRADURAL EXTRAMEDULLARY TUMORS: MENINGIOMA

Meningioma is a slow-growing benign tumor commonly found in females. The most common location for spinal meningiomas is the thoracic spine. Less frequently these tumors may be detected in the cervical region. The tumors are often attached to the dura, the nerve roots, or spinal cord.

Clinical Presentation

Meningiomas usually present in the fifth or sixth decades, mostly in women. Patients may present with progressive gait dysfunction due to myelopathy, sensory changes, back pain, and, less frequently, sphincter dysfunction. Physical examination may detect long tract signs, mainly hyperreflexia. Occasionally weakness in the lower extremities is documented.

Imaging Studies

Plain films may show the tumor only when it is heavily calcified. Meningiomas can be easily overlooked on CT scan when they are

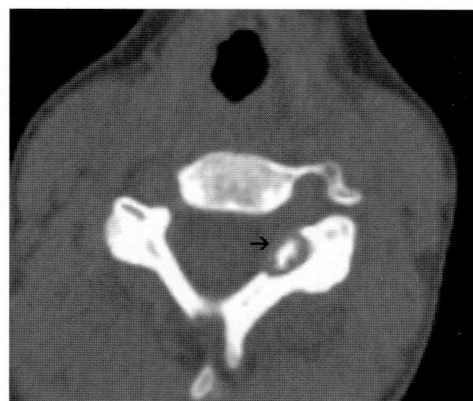

A

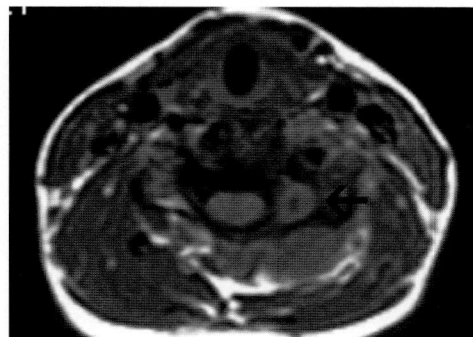

B

FIGURE 11-18
(A) Axial CT cut through the fourth cervical vertebra shows an osteoid osteoma at the larminar–pedicle junction. It has a sclerotic nidus. (B) Axial T1WI showing a well-demarcated lesion (arrow). Note the somewhat thickened sclerotic lamina and facet and soft tissue mass behind the affected lamina.

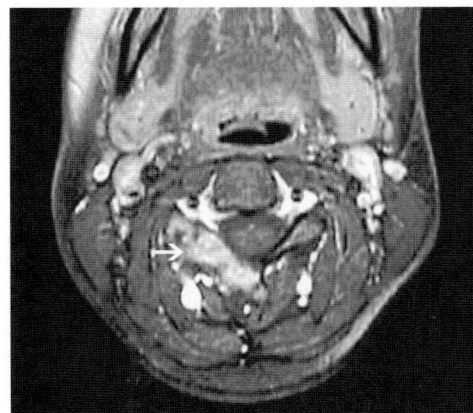

FIGURE 11-19
Osteoblastoma. The lesion expands the right lamina (arrow). T1WI with gadolinium and fat suppression.

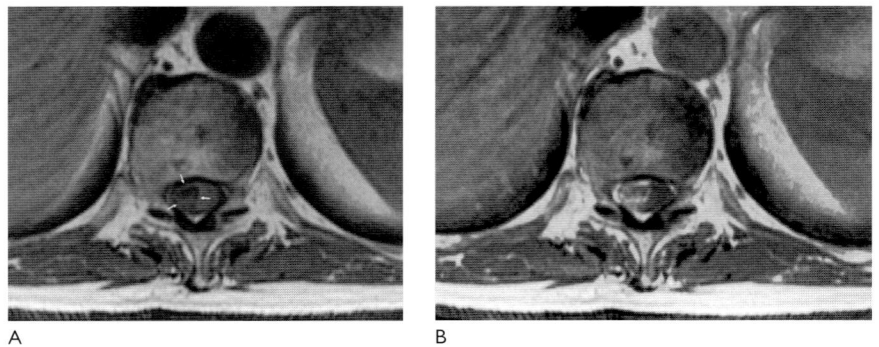

FIGURE 11-20
(A) A large meningioma shown in axial T1WI. The tumor is occupying most of the spinal canal and compressing the spinal cord (star). (B) The tumor enhanced following contrast administration. Courtesy Dr. E. Ashkenazi.

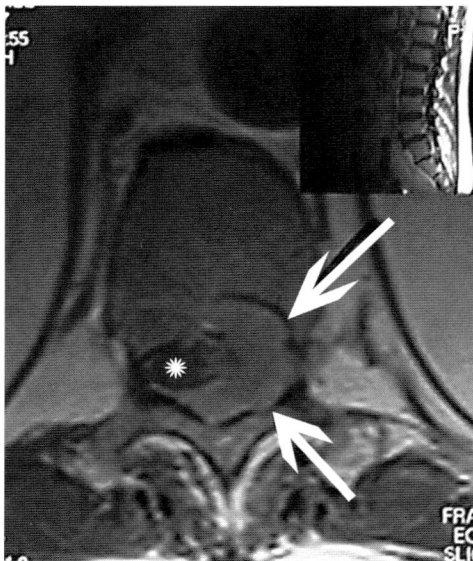

FIGURE 11-21
Axial T1WI showing a right-side calcified intra-dural meningioma (arrows) of low intensity at the T12 level.

isodense to the spinal cord. They can be more easily detected when calcified as they appear hyperdense to the cord or following intrave-nous contrast administration when they usually enhance. Most spinal meningiomas are located posterolaterally within the spinal canal. The tumor may be heavily calcified and as such will appear as a hyperdense mass. On MRI most spinal meningiomas are isointense to the spi-nal cord on T1WI and T2WI. Heavily calcified tumors will remain hypointense in most sequences (Figures 11-20A and 11-20B). The tumors will prominently enhance (if they are not heavily calcified) fol-lowing contrast material administration (Figure 11-21).

Management

Most patients do well following tumor excision and have a good functional outcome.

NERVE SHEATH TUMORS: SCHWANNOMAS

Schwannomas, also known as neurinomas or neurilemmomas, are benign nerve sheath tumors. These are slow-growing solitary tumors that affect both genders equally and may appear throughout the spine, although they have a stronger predilection for the thoracic and lumbar regions. The tumors are usually attached to the posterior sensory roots.

Clinical Presentation

The most common presentation is with gradually increasing radicular pain, numbness, and paraesthesia. The pain may increase with movements. Presentation usually occurs in the third to sixth decades. The neurological examination usually remains normal.

Imaging Studies

On plain films findings are secondary to an existing mass and may appear as a thinned pedicle, an enlarged neural foramen, or posterior vertebral erosion. On CT a well-defined mass isodense with the cord and roots with occasional cystic changes might be demonstrated. Bone ero-sions and remodeling such as scalloping of the vertebral bodies are readily depicted. On MRI nerve root sheath tumors are typically isointense or hypointense to the cord on T1WI and hyperintense on T2WI. Intense enhancement that might be homogenous or heterogeneous appears following contrast administration. At times, a target sign appearance is encountered on T2WI with a low-intensity center and a high-signal rim. Cystic tumors may appear heterogeneous (Figure 11-22).

NEUROFIBROMA/SCHWANNOMA

Neurofibromas may appear as solitary tumors or, in patients with neurofibromatosis, as multiple tumors affecting spinal nerve roots at multiple levels.

Imaging Studies

The appearance of neurofibromas on imaging studies may have the same characteristics as that of schwannomas: they may be isodense to the spinal cord on CT and enhance after contrast administration. On MRI they are usually isointense on T1WI and, at times, a target sign may appear with central hypointensity surrounded by a hyperintense peripheral rim. These tumors may enhance homogeneously following contrast administration (Figure 11-23). They may grow to a large size and bring about bone remodeling resulting in thinning of the pedicles, enlarged neural foraminae, and scalloped vertebral bodies.

INTRAMEDULLARY TUMORS

Ependymoma is the most common intramedullary tumor. Myxopapillary ependymoma is a slow-growing glioma that is mostly found at the conus medullaris, filum terminale, and cauda equina regions (Figure 11-24). In patients over 50 years of age ependymomas tend to develop in the thoracic region. Astrocytoma tends to affect children and young adults. Infrequently, other intramedullary tumors such as lipoma, metastasis, or hemangioblastoma are encountered.

Clinical Presentation

Intramedullary gliomas usually become symptomatic in the third and fourth decades and are most often seen in the upper thoracic and cervical regions. They usually present with slow-onset myelopathy. Ependymomas tend to occur in the fourth and fifth decades, affect both genders, and in over 50% of cases are located in the thoracic spine. The initial presentation may include dysesthesia and pain and may be followed by gait dysfunction, weakness, atrophy, and myelopathic symptoms. Because these tumors are slow-growing they tend to be diagnosed late and by that time cause significant morbidity.

Imaging Studies

Plain films in patients with longstanding intramedullary lesions such as ependymomas may show enlarged spinal canal with increased

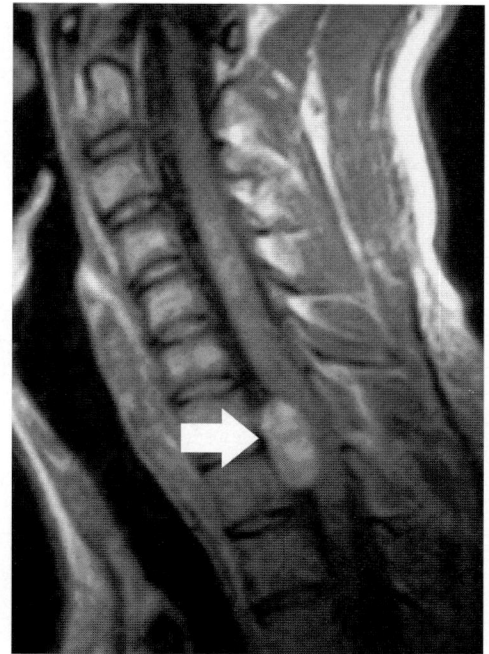

FIGURE 11-22
Sagittal T1WI with contrast demonstrates a large hyperintense tumor that pushes on the cord and deforms it. Courtesy Dr. J. Houten.

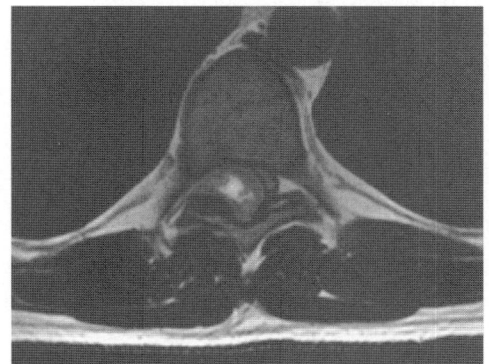

FIGURE 11-23
Axial T2WI clearly demonstrating a schwannoma.

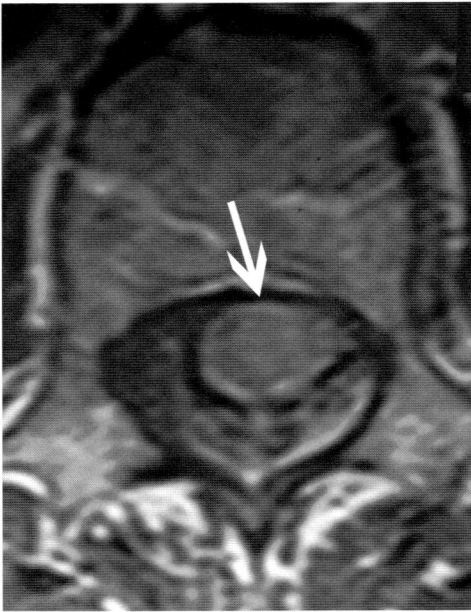

FIGURE 11-24
A large myxopapillary ependymoma in the cauda region. On T1WI the tumor has almost the same intensity as the cord, which is compressed and pushed backward. Courtesy Dr. E. Ashkenazi.

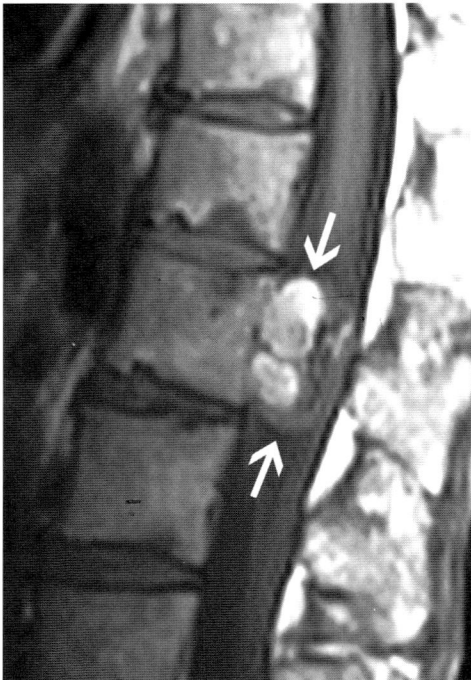

FIGURE 11-25
Sagittal T1WI with contrast showing a large, lobulated, strongly hyperintense ependymoma. Courtesy Dr. J. Houten.

interpedicular distance, scalloping of the posterior vertebral bodies, and at times widened foraminae and eroded pedicles. CT discloses the enlarged spinal canal and might depict an isodense intradural mass that might enhance following contrast administration. On MRI, an isointense mass on T1WI that appears hyperintense to the cord on T2WI and intensely enhances following contrast administration can be seen (Figure 11-25).

Plain films in astrocytomas may be negative. Occasionally canal expansion may be noticed. On CT images cord thickening is noted, with possible mild enhancement following contrast administration. MRI will clearly demonstrate the dilated cord, which may appear on T1WI hypointense or isointense to the cerebrospinal fluid. Occasionally hypointense cysts may be spotted on T1WI within the mass. The mass will appear hyperintense on T2WI and will further enhance following contrast administration. Occasionally cysts and syrinx may be observed in MRI studies.

Management

Microsurgery with tumor debulking may offer some hope for functional improvement. In patients with high-grade tumors, postoperative radiotherapy is indicated.

Bibliography

Barba D, Marshall LF: Intradural tumors. Semin Spine Surg 2: 228–242, 1990.

Baur-Melnyk A: Bone marrow imaging in MRI. Eur J Radiol 55: 1, 2005.

Byrne TN: Spinal cord compression from epidural metastases. N Engl J Med 327: 614–619, 1992.

Celli P, Trillo G, Ferrante L: Extrathecal intraradicular nerve sheath tumor. J Neurosurg Spine 3: 1–11, 2005.

Cohen-Gadol AA, Zikel OM, Koch CA, Scheithauer BW, Krauss WE: Spinal meningiomas in patients younger than 50 years of age: a 21 year experience. J Neurosurg Spine 98 (3 suppl.): 258–263, 2003.

Crist BD, Lenke LG, Lewis S: Osteoid osteoma of the lumbar spine. A case report highlighting a novel reconstruction technique. J Bone Joint Surg Am 87: 414–418, 2005.

DiChiro G, Doppman IL, Dwyer AJ, Patronas NJ, Knop RH, Bairamian D, Vermess M, Oldfield EH: Tumors and arterio-venous malformations of the spinal cord. Assessment using MR. Radiology 156: 689–697, 1985.

Fox MW, Onofrio BM: The natural history and management of symptomatic and asymptomatic vertebral hemangiomas. J Neurosurg 78: 36–45, 1993.

Gezen F, Kahraman S, Canakci Z, Beduk A: Review of 36 cases of spinal cord meningiomas. Spine 25: 727–731, 2000.

Gitelis S, Wilkins R, Conrad EU: Benign bone tumors. J Bone Joint Surg Am 77: 1756–1782, 1995.

Hadjipavlou AG, Tzermiadianos MN, Katonis PG, Szpalski M: Percutaneous vertebroplasty and balloon kyphoplasty for the treatment of osteoporotic vertebral compression fractures and osteolytic tumors. J Bone Joint Surg Br 87: 1595–1604, 2005.

Harrington KD: Current concepts review: Metastatic disease of the spine. J Bone Joint Surg Am 68: 1110–1115, 1986.

Klimo P, Schmidt MH: Surgical management of spinal metastases. Oncologist 9: 188–196, 2004.

Lecouvet FE, Vande Berg BC, Malghem J, Maldague BE: Magnetic resonance and computed tomography imaging in multiple myeloma. Semin Musculoskelet Radiol 5: 43–55, 2001.

McCormick PC, Stein BM: Intramedullary tumors in adults. Neurosurg Clin N Am 1: 609–630, 1990.

McLain RF, Weinstein JN: Tumors of the spine. Semin Spine Surg 2: 157–180, 1990.

Nobauer I, Uffmann M: Differential diagnosis of focal and diffuse neoplastic diseases of bone marrow in MRI. Eur J Radiol 55: 2–32, 2005.

Oeppen RS, Tung K: Case report. Retrograde venous invasion causing vertebral metastases in renal cell carcinoma. Br J Radiol 74: 759–761, 2001.

Oliverio PJ, Davis BT: Imaging of malignant and benign lesions of the vertebral column. Semin Spine Surg 12: 2–16, 2000.

Park SW, Lee JH, Ehara S, Park YB, Sung SO, Choi JA, Joo YE: Single shot fast spine echo diffusion-weighted MR imaging of the spine: Is it useful in differentiating malignant metastatic tumor infiltration from benign fracture edema? Clin Imaging 28: 102–108, 2004.

Portenoy RK, Lipton RB, Foley KM: Back pain in the cancer patient: An algorithm for evaluation and management. Neurology 37: 134–138, 1987.

Ross JS, Brant-Zawadzki M, Moore KR, Crim J, Chen MZ, Katman GL: Neoplasms, pp. 2–127 in Ross JS, Brandt-Zawadzki M, Moore KR, Crim J, Chen MZ, Katman GL: Diagnostic imaging: Spine, vol. IV. Amirsys, 2004.

Schiff D, O'Neill BP, Suman VJ: Spinal epidural metastasis as the initial manifestation of malignancy: Clinical features and diagnostic approach. Neurology 49: 452–456, 1997.

Shrivastava RK, Epstein FJ, Perin NI, Post KD, Jallo GI: Intramedullary spinal cord tumors in patients older than 50 years of age: Management and outcome analysis. J Neurosurg Spine 2: 249–255, 2005.

Sung MS, Lee GK, Kang HS, Kwon ST, Park JG, Suh JS, Cho GH, Lee SM, Chung MH, Resnick D: Sacrococcygeal chordoma: MR imaging in 30 patients. Skeletal Radiol 34: 87–94, 2005.

Templin CR, Stambough JB, Stambough JL: Acute spinal cord compression caused by vertebral hemangioma. Spine J 4: 595–600, 2004.

Tolli TC, Cammisa FP, Lane JM: Metastatic disease of the spine. Semin Spine Surg 2: 181–196, 1990.

Van Goethem JWM, Van den Hauwe L, Ozsarlak O, De Schepper AMA, Parizel PM: Spinal tumors. Eur J Radiol 50: 159–176, 2004.

Welch WC: Tumors of the cauda equina. Semin Spine Surg 12: 117–127, 2000.

York JE, Kaczaraj A, Abi-Said D, Fuller GN, Skibber JM, Janjan NA, Gokaslan ZL: Sacral chordoma: 40-year experience at a major cancer center. Neurosurgery 44: 74–79, 1999.

Yuh WT, Quets JP, Lee HJ, Simonson TM, Michalson LS, Nguyen PT, Sato Y, Mayr NA, Berbaum KS: Anatomic distribution of metastases in the vertebral body and modes of hematogenous spread. Spine 21: 2243–2250, 1996.

PAGET'S DISEASE (OSTEITIS DEFORMANS)

12

Paget's disease (PD), also known as osteitis deformans, was initially described by Dr. James Paget in 1877 and bears his name. PD usually appears in the sixth through eighth decades, rarely under age 40, and is frequently incidentally discovered when patients take radiological tests for other reasons. The disease is commonly seen in Caucasian people of European descent and is more common in males. Up to 10% of Caucasians over 70 years old may be affected by PD. The disorder is rarely seen in people of Asian and African descent.

The etiology of Paget's disease (PD) is still unclear. Genetic factors and slow viruses have been implicated but there is still no conclusive evidence for either cause. Several studies have reported an increased level of interleukin-6, which induces osteoclast formation in PD. In the last two decades it has been observed that the incidence of PD and the severity of the illness in newly diagnosed patients are both decreasing.

PD is a chronic disorder characterized by increased osteoclast activity leading to bone resorption and, alongside it, increased osteoblastic activity resulting in the production of disordered, irregular new bone. The disease activity level can be monitored by following the bone isoenzyme of alkaline phosphatase.

CLINICAL PRESENTATION

In spite of the fact that the spine is the second most common area affected by PD the majority of patients with PD remain totally asymptomatic. Some patients present with axial pain, which may be constant and does get better with rest. The pain may be ill-localized and of dull, boring character. Occasionally it may have a mechanical nature and increase on weight bearing.

Other patients may present with facet arthropathy or spinal stenosis. In the former group, as pagetic bone is formed next to the facet joint, it frequently leads to the development of osteoarthritis in that joint. This leads to pain that increases on weight bearing, may radiate to the buttock (never below the knee), and can be unilateral or bilateral. In the latter group, new bone formation leads to spinal stenosis, resulting in neurogenic claudication, radicular pain, and, at times, cauda equina syndrome or frank myelopathy. Acute back pain may develop when a fracture occurs in the pagetic bone.

The disease most commonly involves the pelvis, axial skeleton, and both femurs. When the skull is affected hearing loss may develop. A small fraction of patients (<1%) are at risk of developing sarcomatous transformation.

IMAGING STUDIES

PD is often incidentally diagnosed in plain radiographs that were obtained for other reasons. The radiological hallmarks of PD include coarse trabeculae, thickened cortical bones, lytic areas (osteoporosis circumscripta) interspersed with dense sclerotic bone, and bony deformities. In typical cases sclerosis may occur in the vertebral margins resulting in "picture frame" vertebrae (Figures 12-1A and 12-1B). Rarely, diffuse, intense sclerosis of the entire vertebral body results in an "ivory" vertebra, which frequently looks like metastatic disease (prostate, breast, lymphoma). After prolonged periods of bone resorption and bone formation the affected bones thicken, enlarge, and, at times, deform. The adjacent soft tissues, however, remain normal. Bone scan should be obtained in order to establish the distribution of the disease.

CT and MRI studies should be obtained whenever coexisting pathology, malignant transformation, or other complications such as fracture, spinal stenosis, or myelopathy are suspected.

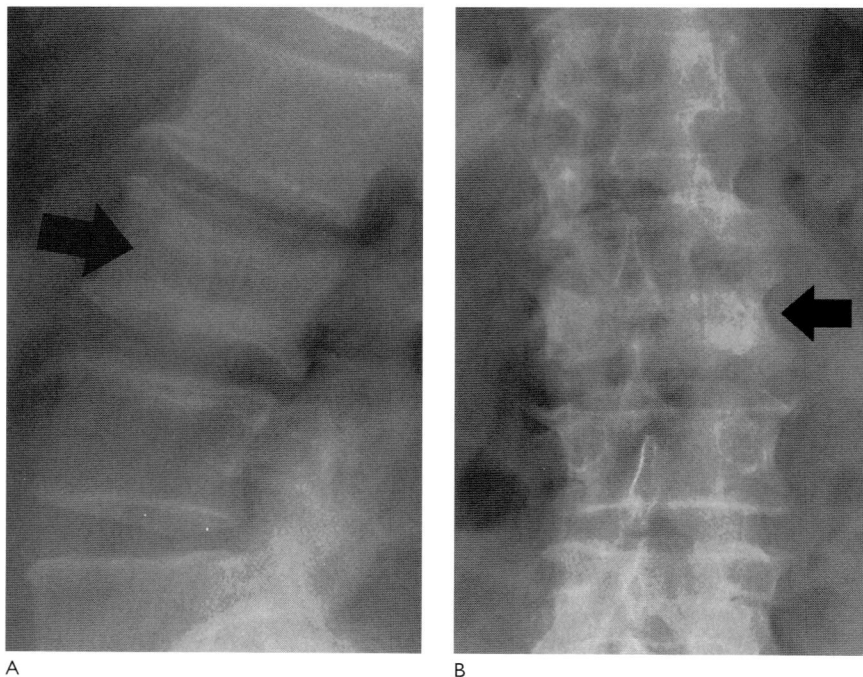

FIGURE 12-1

A 65-year-old male with back pain. (A) Lateral plain film and (B) AP view showing "picture frame" vertebra (arrow). Courtesy Dr. H. Dorfman.

CT of the involved vertebra will reveal coarse trabeculae interspersed with lytic areas and thickened sclerotic cortex (Figure 12-2). Contrast administration will enhance the bone marrow in locations with active disease. CT will also easily point to the presence of central canal or foraminal narrowing.

MRI is the procedure of choice whenever malignancy is concerned as it allows good visualization of the bone marrow and the adjacent soft tissues.

Uncomplicated PD may be overlooked on MRI studies because the coarse trabeculae do not generate a signal and, commonly, the bone marrow remains unremarkable even in the presence of active PD. Vertebral enlargement, focal areas of low signal on T1WI and T2WI (sclerotic bone) with increased bone marrow fat may be the only clear findings (Figures 12-3 and 12-4). Occasionally, areas of high signal intensity on T2WI are seen. These areas represent immature connective tissue with dilated vessels. Following contrast administration there may be a mild increase in signal intensity.

Normal-looking bone marrow, lack of cortical destruction, and normal-looking adjacent soft tissues may be the only features that differentiate PD from malignancies or bone infection on MRI. When in doubt, plain radiographs and CT of the suspicious region should be obtained. At times, bone biopsy is required to settle the issue of malignant transformation.

MANAGEMENT

Asymptomatic patients with normal biochemical studies do not require any intervention and can be clinically followed. Patients with

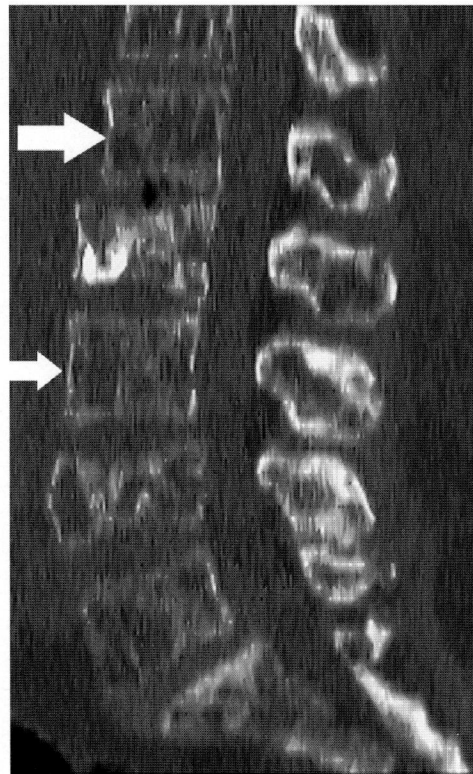

FIGURE 12-2
Sagittal reformatted CT showing thickened trabeculae within the vertebral bodies (arrows). Courtesy Dr. H. Dorfman.

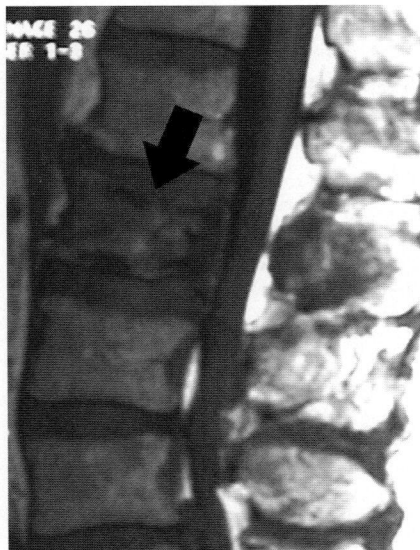

FIGURE 12-3
Sagittal T1WI MR showing a pagetic vertebra. The affected vertebra is hypointense (arrow) due to bony sclerosis. The adjacent vertebrae have a normal signal. Courtesy Dr. H. Dorfman.

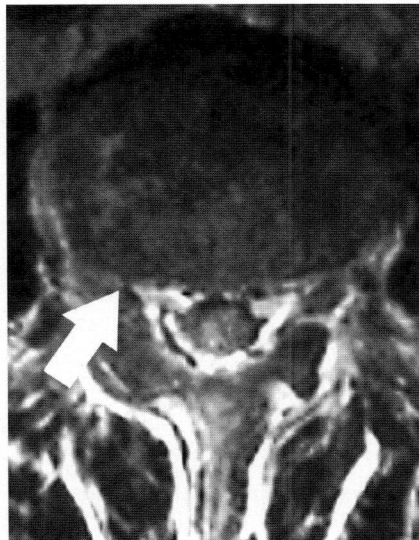

FIGURE 12-4
Axial T1WI MR of a pagetic vertebra. Note the decreased signal intensity and the thickened trabeculae (arrow). Courtesy Dr. H. Dorfman.

bone pain or symptomatic spinal stenosis should be started on anti-pagetic therapy. Several classes of drugs are presently available for the treatment of Paget's disease. The bisphosphonates have been used for quite some time with positive results. These drugs can eliminate symptoms and suppress disease activity for an extended period of time. Alendronate (Fosamax) and Risedronate (Actonel) can be given orally. The former should be administered weekly for a period of three to six months (70 mg/qweek), whereas the latter, the more effective of the two, should be administered daily (30 mg/qd) for a period of two months. Pamidronate, a more potent biphosphonate, can be intravenously administered. Sixty milligrams are mixed in saline and given over a few hours for two to three consecutive days. This drug, which may bring a rather dramatic clinical improvement, is reserved for patients with extensive PD.

Patients who do not tolerate these medications can be started on calcitonin, mithramycin, or gallium nitrate.

In severe symptomatic spinal stenosis that does not respond to medical treatment, and in cases in which cauda equina syndrome develops, surgery should be performed

Bibliography

Altman RD: Musculoskeletal manifestation of Paget's disease of bone. Arthritis Rheum 23: 1121–1127, 1980.

Altman RD: The spine in Paget's disease of bone. Semin Spine Surg 2: 130–135, 1990.

Brown JP, Chines AA, Myers WR, Eusebio RA, Ritter-Hrncirik C, Hayes CW: Improvement of pagetic bone lesions with risedronate treatment: A radiologic study. Bone 26: 263–267, 2000.

Chapman GK: The diagnosis of Paget's disease of bone. Aust N Z J Surg 62: 24–32, 1992.

Chen JR, Richard SCR, Wallach S, Avramides A, Flores A: Neurologic disturbances in Paget's disease of bone: Response to calcitonin. Neurology 29: 448–457, 1979.

Cherian RA, Haddaway MJ, Davie MWJ, MCCall IW, Cassar-Pullicino VN: Effect of Paget's disease of bone on areal lumbar spine bone mineral density measured by DXA, and density of cortical and trabecular bone measured by quantitative CT. Br J Radiol 73: 720–726, 2000.

Gagel RF, Logan C, Melette LE: Treatment of Paget's disease of bone with salmon calcitonin nasal spray. J Am Geriatr Soc 30: 1010–1014, 1988.

Hadjipavlou AG, Gaitanis IN, Katonis PG, Lander P: Paget's disease of the spine and its management. Eur Spine J 10: 370–384, 2001.

Hadjipavlou AG, Lander P: Paget's disease of the spine. J Bone Joint Surg Am 73: 1376–1381, 1991.

Jattiot F, Goupille P, Azais I, Roulot B, Alcalay M, Jeannou J, Bontoux D, Valat JP: Fourteen cases of sarcomatous degeneration in Paget's disease. J Rheumatol 26: 150–155, 1999.

Kaufman GA, Sundaram M, McDonald DJ: Magnetic resonance imaging in symptomatic Paget's disease. Skeletal Radiol 20: 413–418, 1991.

Lombardi A: Treatment of Paget's disease of bone with alendronate. Bone 24 (5 suppl.): 59–61, 1999.

Lyles KW, Siris ES, Singer FR, Meunier PJ: A clinical approach to diagnosis and management of Paget's disease of bone. J Bone Miner Res 16: 1379–1387, 2001.

Oostveen JCM, Van de Laar MAFJ: Magnetic resonance imaging in rheumatic disorders of the spine and sacroiliac joints. Semin Arthritis Rheum 30: 52–69, 2000.

Roberts MC, Kressel MD, Zlatkin MB, Dalinka MK: Paget disease: MR imaging findings. Radiology 173: 341–345, 1989.

Rousiere M, Michou L, Cornelis F, Orcel P: Paget's disease of bone. Best Pract Res Clin Rheumatol 17: 1019–1041, 2003.

Saifuddin A, Hassan A: Paget's disease of the spine: Unusual features and complications. Clin Radiol 58: 102–111, 2003.

Schajowicz F, Araujo SE, Berestein M: Sarcoma complicating Paget's disease of bone: A clinico-pathology study of 62 cases. J Bone Joint Surg Br 65: 299–307, 1983.

Tiegs RD, Lohse CM, Wollan PC, Melton LJ: Long-term trends in the incidence of Paget's disease of bone. Bone 27: 423–427, 2000.

Vande Berg BC, Malghem J, Lecouvet FE, Maldague B: Magnetic resonance appearance of uncomplicated Paget's disease of bone. Semin Musculoskelet Radiol 5: 69–77, 2001.

Walsh JP: Paget's disease of bone. Med J Aust 181: 262–265, 2004.

Walsh JP, Ward LC, Stewart GO, Will RK, Criddle RA, Prince RL, Stuckey BG, Dhaliwall SS, Bhagat CI, Retallack RW, Kent GN, Drury PJ, Vasikaran S, Gutteridge DH: A randomized clinical trial comparing oral alendronate and intravenous pamidronate for the treatment of Paget's disease of bone. Bone 34: 747–754, 2004.

Whitehouse RW: Paget's disease of bone. Semin Musculoskelet Radiol 6: 313–322, 2002.

Whitten CR, Saifuddin A: MRI of Paget's disease of bone. Clin Radiol 58: 763–769, 2003.

Zlatkin MB, Lander PH, Hadjipavlou AG, Levine JS: Paget disease of the spine. CT with clinical correlation. Radiology 160: 155–159, 1986.

VASCULAR DISORDERS

13

VASCULAR ANATOMY

This chapter's discussion of vascular disorders affecting the spine will begin with a brief overview of vascular anatomy of the spine. Three disorders will then be discussed: anterior spinal artery syndrome, spinal epidural hematoma, and malformations.

Arterial System

The spinal cord receives arterial blood from two systems: the longitudinal and the horizontal. The longitudinal system is made up of a single anterior spinal artery and a pair of posterior spinal arteries. The anterior spinal artery supplies the anterior two-thirds of the cord, which includes the pyramidal and the spinothalamic tracts. It descends from the foramen magnum to the filum terminale and is located in the midline. The artery is supplied along its course by multiple feeders. The central artery, a branch of the anterior spinal artery, runs through the anterior median sulcus, enters the cord, and provides blood to the gray matter and the adjacent white matter. The posterior one-third of the cord, which includes the posterior horns and the dorsal columns, is supplied by the paired posterior spinal arteries. These are located on the dorsal surface of the cord medial to the dorsal roots and connect with pial arterial branches that run around the cord to provide blood to the posterior horns and the white matter in the circumference of the cord. The latter arteries are also supplied by the anterior spinal artery.

Intramedullary branches that penetrate the spinal cord emanate from the anterior spinal artery and its branch, the central artery. These intramedullary branches are end arteries—terminal arteries that do not anastomose and end in watershed zones. This explains the high prevalence of spinal cord infarcts seen in areas supplied by the anterior spinal artery. The arteries emanating from the two posterior spinal arteries interconnect through multiple anastomoses and are, therefore, less vulnerable to ischemia.

The horizontal system consists of anterior and posterior radicular arteries. These arteries are formed by the nervomedullary arteries and reinforce the anterior and posterior spinal arteries. The blood supply to the nervomedullary arteries originates in arteries branching mainly off the vertebral, ascending cervical, intercostals, lumbar, and internal iliac arteries. The mid-thoracic region is sparingly supplied by radicular arteries. The largest artery in this region is the artery of Adamkiewycz, also called arteria radicularis magna or the great radicular artery. It is usually found in the thoraco-lumbar region, between T9 and L2 on the left side and supplies arterial blood to the distal thoracic cord and the conus medullaris. It travels into the spine along with the nerve root through the intervertebral foramen on its way to the anterior spinal artery. The artery may be inadvertently punctured during transforaminal injections resulting, unfortunately, in permanent cord damage due to cord infarction.

The anterior spinal artery communicates with the posterior spinal arteries in the conus region and forms an "arterial basket" that supplies arterial blood to the filum terminale.

Venous System

The venous drainage of the spinal cord occurs through two systems: an intrinsic venous system and an extrinsic venous system. The intrinsic system includes the anterior median and radial groups. Blood from the anterior one-third of the cord drains into the anterior median spinal vein. The radial veins channel blood into the coronal plexus of veins. They drain the periphery of the cord.

The extrinsic system transports venous blood into medullary veins that course with the nerve roots.

ANTERIOR SPINAL ARTERY SYNDROME

Anterior spinal artery syndrome occurs in middle-aged and elderly patients and affects both genders equally. Patients with hypertension and diabetes, two diseases that increase atherosclerosis, are more susceptible to spinal cord infarction. The syndrome may also develop in patients with dissecting abdominal aortic aneurysm, following aneurysm repair; in patients with coagulopathies, vasculitis, or hypotension; or during transforaminal steroid injection when the artery of Adamkiewicz is inadvertently penetrated.

Clinical Presentation

The symptoms of cord infarction have a sudden onset. Sharp low back pain develops and is followed, within a short period of time, by flaccid paraplegia and sphincter dysfunction. The physical examination will detect complete paraplegia with incomplete sensory deficits: loss of pain and temperature sensation in the involved segments with preservation of light touch. The neurological deficits remain permanent due to irreversible cord damage.

Imaging Studies

Plain radiography and CT are not helpful in this condition. They may detect, however, a calcified aortic aneurysm. T1-weighted images (T1WI) may remain normal early on. T2-weighted images (T2WI) will detect increased cord signal due to spinal cord edema. The gray matter or the entire section of the involved cord will become hyperintense. There may be some enhancement following contrast administration. This develops several days following cord infarction and lasts for several weeks (Figure 13-1). Eventually, cord atrophy will be observed. Angiography will detect anterior spinal artery thrombosis.

The prognosis is dire as the changes in the spinal cord are irreversible.

Management

Once the diagnosis is established, the patients should be anticoagulated and referred to a spinal cord injury unit for further care.

SPINAL EPIDURAL HEMATOMA

Spinal epidural hematoma (SEH) appears mostly in the fifth through the eighth decades and is reported more frequently in adult males. Although it is a rare condition, physicians should be aware of it. Unless promptly diagnosed and treated it results in severe, irreversible neurological sequelae. SEH develops when an epidural vein bleeds and a hematoma forms. The condition has been reported in patients with clotting disorders, in anticoagulated patients, during pregnancy, in patients with vascular malformations, and following simple trauma, interventional procedures, and multilevel spinal surgery. The hematoma forms in the epidural space and, when large enough, may compress the spinal cord. It may occur anywhere in the spine but tends to develop more in the C5-to-T2 region. In patients over 40 years of age the low thoracic and lumbar regions tend to be affected as well.

In most cases the hematoma forms on the dorsal-lateral surface of the cord and covers several spinal segments.

Clinical Presentation

The clinical presentation is rather dramatic. Patients may develop sudden, severe stabbing axial pain with a radicular component. Neurological deficits appear within a short period of time. Sensory loss and weakness may progress to paraparesis or quadriparesis, depending on the hematoma location. Lumbar hematoma may initially simulate a herniated disc, but within a short period of time more nerve roots may be affected and the symptoms spread bilaterally.

Imaging Studies

Plain films remain normal and are not helpful. CT may show a high-density epidural mass that is usually situated posterolaterally. MRI is the diagnostic procedure of choice. The sagittal views provide

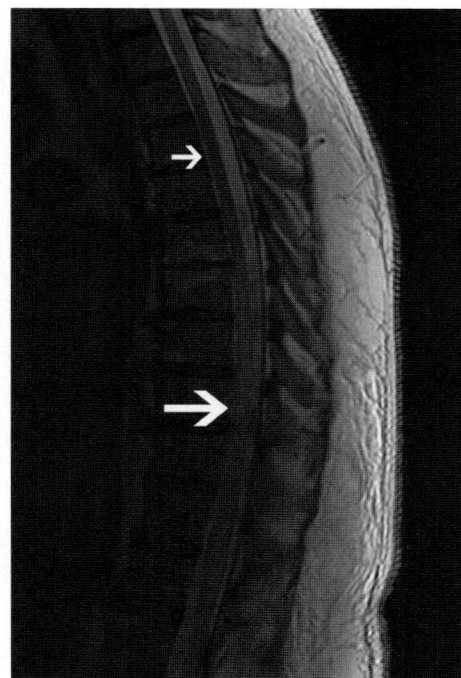

FIGURE 13-1
Sagittal T2WI of a 52-year-old male who, following bypass surgery, developed acute paraplegia. The upper thoracic cord has a normal cord signal and appearance. The lower part of the cord displays an increased signal, is swollen, and is less well defined than the proximal cord. Courtesy Dr. J. Houten.

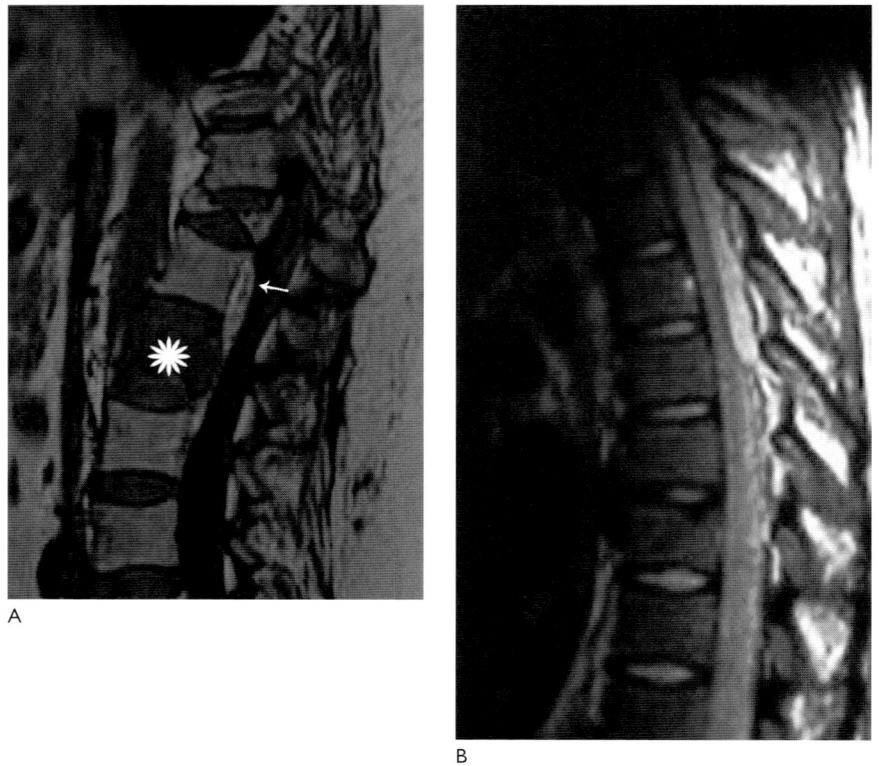

FIGURE 13-2

Sagittal T1WI MR. (A) A burst fracture (star) with a fragment displaced posteriorly into the spinal canal. Just behind and above the fractured vertebra a hyperintense mass with a hypointense core is found. (B) In another patient a hyperintense mass is seen posterior to the thoracic cord.

information about the extent of the hematoma, whereas the axial cuts provide information relative to cord compression. T1WI will show a mass with variable intensity. In patients with subacute or chronic hematoma the mass will appear hyperintense. Rapid-sequence T2WI provide excellent contrast. Unclotted blood has a high intensity, whereas clotted blood has low signal intensity (Figures 13-2A, 13-2B, 13-3A, 13-3B, and 13-3C). Contrast administration may show peripheral enhancement due to dural hyperermia and help rule out a tumor. If vascular malformation is suspected angiography should be performed.

Management

Prompt surgical hematoma evacuation may bring about good clinical recovery. Patients with severe, complete neurological loss prior to surgery have a less favorable prognosis.

MALFORMATIONS

Vascular malformations are frequently overlooked, uncommon lesions consisting of direct communications between spinal cord arteries and veins.

Several different classifications of spinal arteriovenous malformations (AVM) exist. A simple, fairly well accepted classification recognizes four types of AVM.

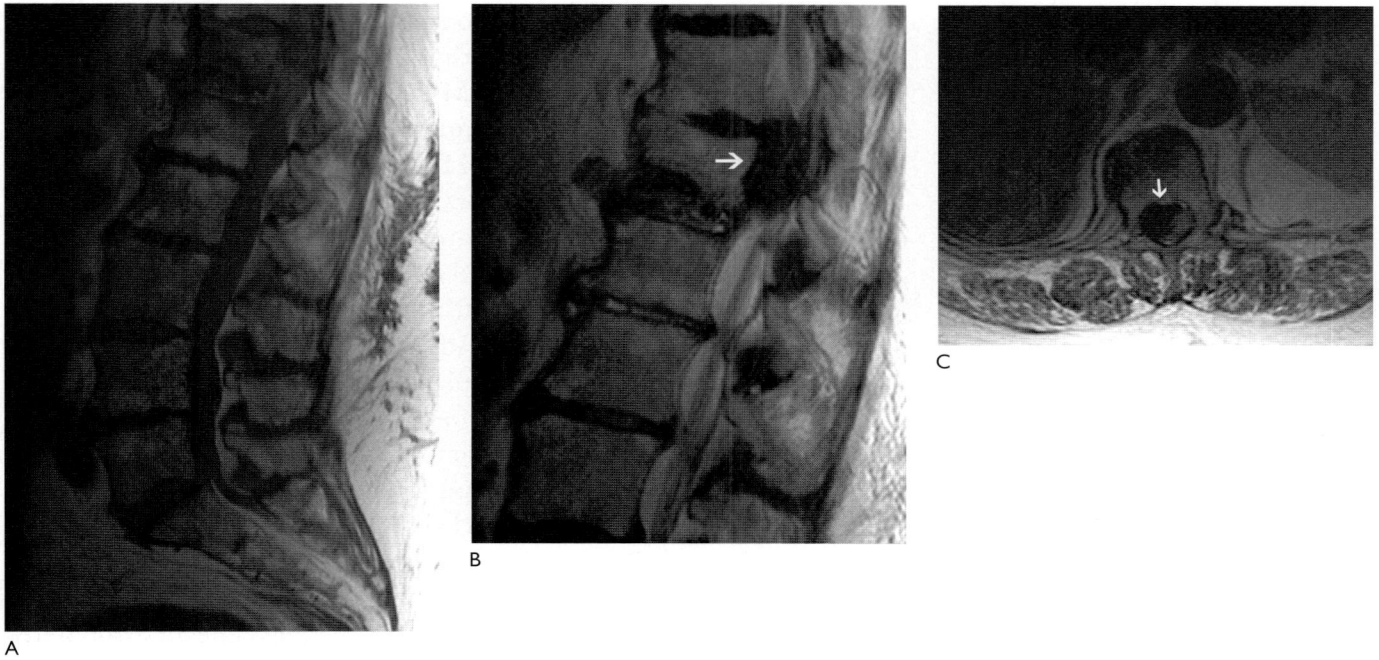

FIGURE 13-3
(A) Sagittal T1- and (B) T2WI showing a hypointense mass behind a vertebra with compression fracture attesting to the chronicity of the hematoma. (C) Axial MRI showing the hematoma occupying about two thirds of the spinal canal and compressing the thecal sac. Courtesy Dr. N. Haramati.

Type One AVM

Type one AVM occurs predominantly in the lower thoracic and upper lumbar regions of adult males in the fifth through seventh decades and represents about 60–80% of AVM diagnoses. In this condition an intradural-extramedullary fistula develops. The fistula drains into the vertebral venous outflow system. Symptoms develop secondary to increased venous pressure, which results in venous stasis within the spinal cord. These changes lead to increased intramedullary pressure and congestion. Cord edema and decreased perfusion develop into cord ischemia and, eventually, irreversible cord damage may develop.

Clinical presentation. The most common presentation of type one AVM is that of slowly evolving myelopathy. Over the course of months or years, patients develop increasing motor deficits such as paraparesis and sensory loss. Subsequently disturbances in micturition may occur as well. It is believed that the myelopathy develops secondary to sustained increased venous pressure, which results in venous engorgement and spinal cord ischemia. Physical examination reveals myelopathic findings: a combination of upper and lower motor neuron signs. At times, the symptoms are aggravated by exercise and may be accompanied by low back pain. In rare instances, when thrombosis or hemorrhaging occurs, sudden deterioration may evolve with progressive neurological loss.

Imaging studies. Plain radiographs remain normal throughout the course of the disease and are therefore not helpful. CT may detect an enlarged spinal cord. Post–contrast administration there may be enhancement of pial veins along the cord surface. It is difficult to diagnose this condition solely on CT. MRI, however, is much more sensitive than CT. On T1WI the cord appears hypointense. The most sensitive, pervasive, but nonspecific MRI finding is increased cord signal on T2WI. This finding, however, may be also observed following an infection, inflammatory conditions, demyelinating diseases, vasculitis, or cord neoplasms. The increased cord signal will disappear following embolization or resection of the fistula. The coronal venous plexus may enhance as well. Multiple flow voids may be found on the cord surface. These correspond with dilated pial veins, which are usually seen on the dorsum of the cord and are found in only half of the patients. At times, it is difficult to differentiate between flow voids and cerebrospinal fluid pulsation artifacts, thus rendering this finding less reliable. Another common finding on MRI is the associated mass effect or cord swelling. This usually appears over several cord segments and may raise the suspicion that the patient is suffering from a spinal cord tumor (Figures 13-4A and 13-4B). It is felt that the mass effect corroborates the presence of venous hypertension and cord edema. Following contrast administration multiple serpentine veins may be seen on the cord surface with occasional patchy enhancement within the cord. None of the MRI findings is pathognomonic of AVM. The combination of several findings, however, raises the suspicion for AVM, at which point an angiographic study should be ordered. This allows direct visualization of the coronal venous plexus (Figure 13-5). A reliable finding attesting to the presence of venous hypertensive myelopathy is peripheral cord hypointensity on T2WI. This finding, which has been recently described, is probably caused by sluggish blood flow containing deoxyhemoglobin within the distended capillary system.

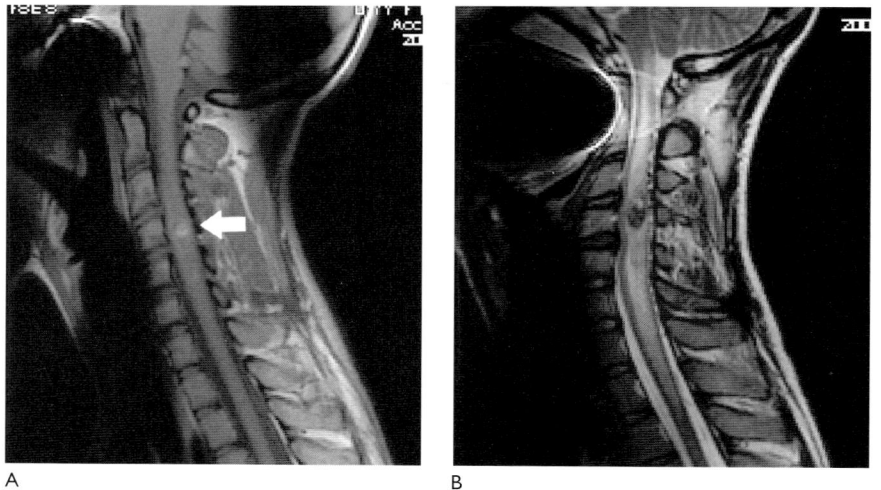

FIGURE 13-4
Sagittal MRI in a patient with a bleeding AVM. (A) T1WI shows a lesion located within the cord at the level of C4. The lesion is slightly hyperintense to the cord. The cord appears swollen at that area. (B) In T2WI the lesion appears hypointense. Note the cord swelling and the extensive hyperintense area in the cord above and below the lesion. Courtesy Dr. T Miller.

Management. Preoperatively, spinal angiography is obtained in order to precisely localize the arteriovenous fistula location. The lesion is then resected. At times endovascular interruption of the venous side of the fistula is performed with cyanoacrylic glue. Severe deficits prior to treatment usually result in worse prognosis with poor functional outcome. The duration of symptoms, however, does not have a predictive prognostic value. Lesions above T9 are far worse than those below that level.

Type Two AVM

Type two AVM is the second most common spinal AVM. The lesions in type two are intramedullary, that is, located within the spinal cord, usually in the cervical or upper thoracic regions. Direct arteriovenous communications are formed within the cord. The nidus of the AVM is compact and is commonly associated with aneurysms. The incidence of type two AVM is identical in both genders. The lesions usually appear in the third or fourth decades.

Clinical presentation. Unlike the clinical presentation in type one AVM, patients with type two AVM present with sudden, acute deterioration of neurological function due to hemorrhage within the cord substance. Axial pain with myelopathy will be the presenting symptoms. The source of the bleeding is an aneurysm that may be arterial, nidal, or venous. The blood frequently extends into the subarachnoid space.

Imaging studies. MRI is the investigation of choice in these patients. It will detect close to a 100% of cases. Flow voids, cord enlargement, and hematomyelia will be detected on T1WI. On T2WI the cord will be hyperintense. After contrast administration the nidus, cord, and dilated vessels may further enhance. Spinal angiography will show the feeding artery and the drainage pattern.

Management. Type two AVM should be embolized prior to surgical resection.

Type Three AVM

This type of AVM usually occurs in juvenile patients, is very rare, and will not be discussed here.

Type Four AVM

In the final type of AVM, perimedullary lesions, intradural-extramedullary arteriovenous communications between the anterior and the posterior spinal arteries and perimedullary veins belonging to the coronal venous plexus, develop. These lesions are usually located on the lateral or ventral aspect of the spinal cord.

Clinical presentation. Patients usually present with progressive neurological deficits involving the cauda equina or the conus. Some patients present with subarachnoid hemorrhage of a sudden onset.

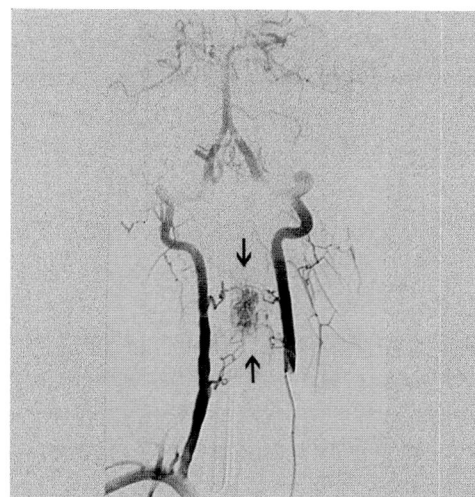

FIGURE 13-5
Angiography showing a large AVM within the upper cervical cord (arrows). Note the vessels connecting the AVM to the vertebral arteries. Courtesy Dr. T. Miller.

Imaging studies. The best diagnostic modality is MRI. It may show flow voids, cord displacement due to the ventral fistula, and cord hyperintensity on T2WI. Postcontrast studies will demonstrate multiple enhancing intradural vessels.

Management. These lesions can be embolized and operated upon.

Bibliography

Cenzato M, Versari P, Righi C, Simionato F, Casali C, Giovanelli M: Spinal dural arteriovenous fistulae: Analysis of outcome in relation to pretreatment indicators. Neurosurgery 55: 815–821, 2004.

Dommisse GF: The blood supply of the spinal cord: A critical vascular zone in spinal surgery. J Bone Joint Surg Br 56: 225–235, 1974.

Doppman JL, DiChiro G, Dwyer AJ, Frank JL, Oldfield EH: Magnetic resonance imaging of spinal arteriovenous malformations. J Neurosurg 66: 830–834, 1987.

Ferch RD, Morgan MK, Sears WR: Spinal arteriovenous malformations: A review with case illustrations. J Clin Neurosci 8: 299–304, 2001.

Gilertson JR, Miller GM, Goldman MS, Marsh WR: Spinal dural arteriovenous fistulas: MR and myelographic findings. Am J Neuroradiol 16: 2049–2057, 1995.

Gillilan LA: Veins of the spinal cord. Neurology 20: 860–868, 1970.

Groen RJM, Groenewegen HJ, Van Alphen HA, Hoogland PVJM: Morphology of the human internal vertebral plexus: A cadaver study after intravenous Araldite CY 221 injection. Anat Rec 249: 285–294, 1997.

Hassler O: Blood supply to human spinal cord. A micro angiographic study. Arch Neurol 14: 302–307, 1976.

Hughes JT, Phil D: Venous infarction of the spinal cord. Neurology 21: 794–800, 1971.

Ishizawa K, Komori T, Shimada T, Aria E, Imanaka K, Kyo S, Hirose T: Hemodynamic infarction of the spinal cord: Involvement of the gray matter plus the border-zone between the central and peripheral arteries. Spinal Cord 43: 306–310, 2005.

Ko J, Fischgrund J, Biddinger A, Herkowitz H: Risk factors for spinal epidural hematoma after spinal surgery. Clinical case series. Spine 27: 1670–1673, 2002.

Masson C, Pruvo JP, Meder JF, Cordonnier C, Touze E, De La Sayette V, Giroud M, Mas JL, Leys D: Spinal cord infarction: Clinical and magnetic resonance imaging findings and short term outcome. J Neurol Neurosurg Psychiat 75: 1431–1435, 2004.

Meder JF, Chiras J, Barth MO, N'Diaye M, Bories M: Myelographic features of the normal external spinal veins. J Neuroradiol 11: 315–325, 1984.

Muraszko KM, Oldfield EH: Vascular malformations of the spinal cord and dura. Neurosurg Clin N Am 1: 631–652, 1990.

Rodesch G, Hurth M, Alvarez H, Tadie M, Lasjaunias P: Classification of spinal cord arteriovenous shunts: Proposal for a reappraisal—The Bicetre experience with 155 consecutive patients treated between 1981–1999. Neurosurgery 51: 374–380, 2002.

Rodesch G, Hurth M, Alvarez H, Tadie M, Lasjaunias P: Spinal cord intradural arteriovenous fistulae: Anatomic, clinical, and therapeutic considerations in a series of 32 consecutive patients seen between 1981 and 2000 with emphasis on endovascular therapy. Neurosurgery 57: 973–983, 2005.

Schick U, Hassler W: Treatment and outcome of spinal dural arteriovenous fistulas. Eur Spine J 12: 350–355, 2003.

Somayaji HS, Saifuddin A, Casey AT, Briggs TW: Spinal cord infarction following therapeutic computed tomography-guided left L2 nerve root injection. Spine 30: E106–108, 2005.

Spetzler RS, Detwiler PW, Riina HA, Porter RW: Modified classification of spinal cord vascular lesions. J Neurosurg Spine 96: 145–156, 2002.

Stevens JM: Imaging of the spinal cord. J Neurol Neurosurg Psychiat 58: 403–416, 1995.

Turnbull IM: Microvasculature of the human spinal cord. J Neurosurg 35: 141–147, 1971.

Ueda Y, Kawahara N, Tomita K, Kobayashi T, Murakami H, Nambu K: Influence on spinal cord blood flow and function by interruption of bilateral segmental arteries at up to three levels: Experimental study in dogs. Spine 30: 2239–2243, 2005.

SYRINGOMYELIA

14

Syringomyelia (from *syrinx* meaning *tube* and *myelos* meaning *marrow*, referring to the spinal cord) is a condition in which a longitudinal cavity forms within the spinal cord. The syrinx, which is separated from the spinal canal, is filled with cerebrospinal fluid (CSF) and usually extends over several spinal segments. As it evolves, it may enlarge the affected cord region and compress the cord from within.

Syringomyelia can occur anywhere along the cord and is frequently found in separate locations within the cord presenting as short longitudinal cavities. When the syrinx is located in the brain stem it is called syringobulbia.

The pathophysiological mechanisms leading to the formation of syringomyelia are still poorly defined and debatable. It is believed that syrinx formation is related to abnormalities of CSF physiology. Impaired outflow of CSF at the fourth ventricle or increased CSF flow into the spinal canal due to increased intracranial venous pressure combined with hindbrain anomalies are two common theories proposed to explain the development of syringomyelia.

Syringomyelia has been classified into five categories: communicating, post-traumatic, tumor-related, arachnoiditis-related, and idiopathic.

In over 50% of syringomyelia patients Chiari malformation may be found. In these patients the syrinx is usually located in the cervical cord, with occasional extension into the thoracic cord. Syringomyelia can develop following spinal cord injury, spinal trauma, or spinal surgeries, and in patients with intramedullary tumors, adhesive arachnoiditis, spinal dysraphism, tethered cord, myelitis, or spondylosis. The pathogenesis of post-traumatic syringomyelia is multifactorial and may include hematoma formation within the cord, liquefaction, necrosis, and meylomalacia. When a syrinx is detected without any other association a complete neuroimaging evaluation of the entire neuraxis should be obtained in order to rule out a remote cord or brain stem pathology. In post-traumatic and postoperative patients the syrinx is most commonly found in the thoracic region and around the site of the original spinal injury and may extend above and below the level of injury. The interval between the original spinal trauma and the appearance of a syrinx varies from several months to many years.

CLINICAL PRESENTATION

Syringomyelia has no gender preference. It may be asymptomatic (usually centrally located) and found incidentally in patients undergoing imaging studies for spinal column pathology. At times, it presents with clinical symptoms such as gait disturbances due to spastic paraparesis or radicular pain, weakness, and dissociated sensory loss: pain and temperature sensation are affected whereas light touch, position, and vibration sense remain intact. The patient may sustain painless burns or injuries in the affected areas. Atrophy and weakness of small muscles of the hands may be found. In established spinal cord injury patients the appearance of signs and symptoms above the affected cord region or the appearance of new-onset spine pain may be due to a developing syrinx. Patients with tonsillar herniation usually present with suboccipital headache that may radiate upward toward the back of the head or downward toward the neck and shoulders. The pain typically increases with head movements, physical exertion, and valsalva maneuvers.

Scoliosis may be the first presenting symptom of syringomyelia, especially when it is accompanying a spinal tumor. In longstanding cases Charcot's arthropathy may develop.

IMAGING STUDIES

Plain radiographs are noncontributory in these patients. CT is frequently interpreted as negative as the syrinx may be small or isodense to the cord and thus may remain invisible. Occasionally, a large-diameter syrinx may be seen on CT studies. Frequently the only clue to the presence of a syrinx may be spinal cord expansion. Postcontrast CT, especially when films are obtained an hour or more after contrast administration, may demonstrate the cyst as it fills with contrast.

MRI is the study of choice. T1-weighted images (T1WI) will show a hypointense space, similar to that of the CSF, within the cord. Sagittal views help determine the extent of the syrinx. On T2-weighted images (T2WI), the signal within the cavity should correspond to that of the CSF: hyperintense (Figures 14-1A and 14-1B). Occasionally the cranial and caudal ends of the syrinx may enhance on T2WI, representing reactive gliosis. Axial cuts determine whether the syrinx is symmetrical, centrally located (relatively asymptomatic lesions), centrally located with paracentral expansion (usually associated with segmental signs), or eccentrically located (following trauma, producing combination of segmental signs and long tract signs). Contrast administration is necessary in order to rule out intramedullary tumors. The syrinx itself does not enhance (Figures 14-2 and 14-3).

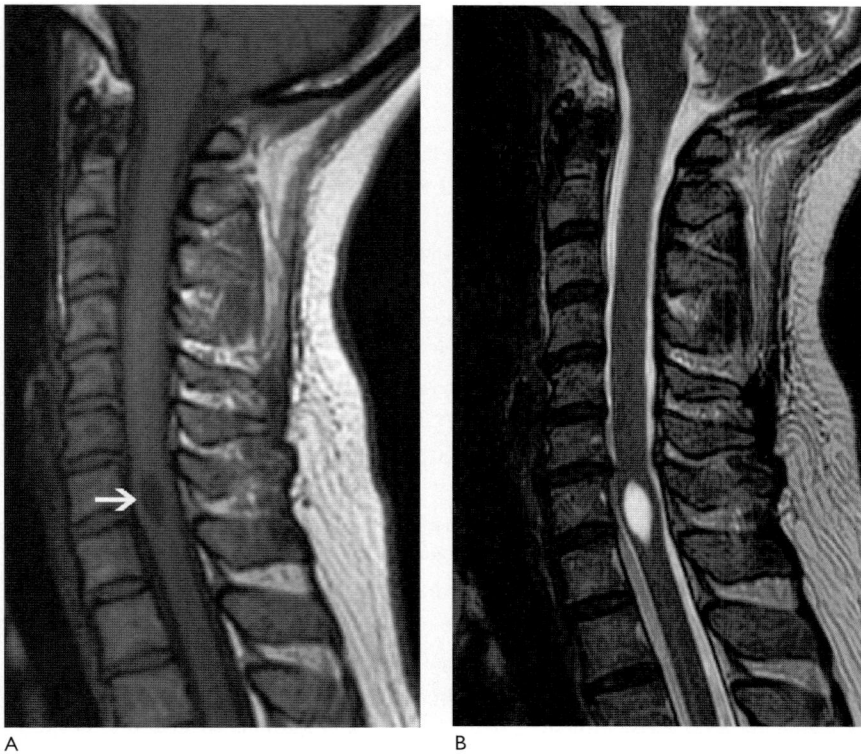

A   B

FIGURE 14-1
Sagittal MRI of a 52-year-old female who presented with unilateral severe right upper extremity pain and numbness. (A) On T1WI an oval hypointense lesion is seen within the cord (arrow) in the C7-T1 region. The cord seems slightly enlarged at that region. (B) On T2WI the lesion is well defined and hyperintense.

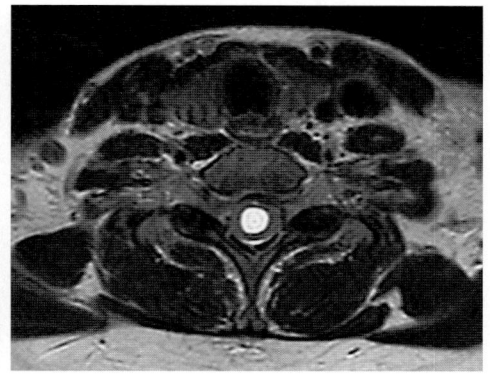

FIGURE 14-2
Axial T2WI MR of the cervical spine through the syrinx shows that it is rather large and occupies a larger portion of the right side of the cord, a fact that may explain the unilateral symptoms.

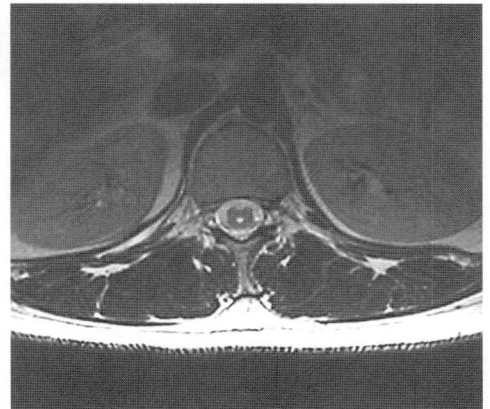

FIGURE 14-3
Axial T2WI of the lumbar spine in a 20-year-old patient with persistent low back pain. Within the distal cord/conus a hyperintense rounded syrinx was found (arrow). The lesion did not enhance with contrast and no tumor was found.

MANAGEMENT

The natural history of symptomatic syringomyelia is one of progressive neurological deterioration that may last years. Patients should be monitored and, whenever indicated, operated upon. If cerebrospinal dynamics cannot be restored, shunting procedures such as a syringoperitoneal shunt should be performed. Spontaneous resolution is exceptionally rare and is seen only when CSF obstruction has spontaneously resolved.

Bibliography

Asano M, Fujiwara K, Yonenobu K, Hiroshima K: Post-traumatic syringomyelia. Spine 21: 1446–1453, 1996.

Banerji NK, Millar JHD: Chiari malformation presenting in adult life. Brain 97: 157–168, 1974.

Batzdorf U: Primary spinal syringomyelia. J Neurosurg Spine 3: 429–435, 2005.

Carroll AM, Brackenridge P: Post-traumatic syringomyelia: A review of the cases presenting in a regional spinal injuries unit in the north east of England over a 5-year period. Spine 30: 1206–1210, 2005.

Chang HS, Joko M, Matsuo N, Kim SD, Nakagawa H: Subarachnoid pressure-dependent change in syrinx size in a patient with syringomyelia associated with adhesive arachnoiditis. J Neurosurg Spine 2: 209–214, 2005.

Chang HS, Nakagawa H: Theoretical analysis of the pathophysiology of syringomyelia associated with adhesive arachnoiditis. J Neurol Neurosurg Psychiatry 75: 754–757, 2004.

Di Lorenzo N, Cacciola F: Adult syringomyelia: Classification , pathogenesis and therapeutic approaches. J Neurosurg Sci 49: 65–72, 2005.

Gamache FW, Ducker TB: Syringomyelia: A neurological and surgical spectrum. J Spinal Disord 3: 293–298, 1990.

Heiss JD, Patronas N, DeVroom HL, Shawker T, Ennis R, Krammerer W, Eidsath A, Talbot T, Morris J, Eskioglu E, Oldfield EH: Elucidating the pathophysiology of syringomyelia. J Neurosurg 91: 553–562, 1999.

Hida K, Iwasaki Y, Imamura H, Abe H: Posttraumatic syringomyelia: Its characteristic magnetic resonance imaging findings and surgical management. Neurosurgery 35: 886–891, 1994.

Jaksche H, Schaan M, Schulz J, Boszczyk B: Posttraumatic syringomyelia: A serious complication in tetra- and paraplegia patients. Acta Neurochir Suppl 93: 165–167, 2005.

Klekamp J, Iaconetta G, Samii M: Spontaneous resolution of Chiari I malformation and syringomyelia: Case report and review of the literature. Neurosurgery 48: 664–667, 2001.

Lee BCP, Zimmerman RD, Manning JJ, Deck MD: MR imaging of syringomyelia and hydromyelia. Am J Roentgenol 144: 1149–1156, 1985.

Lee J-H, Chung C-K, Kim HJ: Decompression of the spinal subarachnoid space as a solution for syringomyelia without Chiari malformation. Spinal Cord 40: 501–506, 2002.

Lyons BM, Brown DJ, Calvert JM: The diagnosis and management of post-traumatic syringomyelia. Paraplegia 25: 340–350, 1987.

Medlock MD: Syringomyelia. Semin Spine Surg 12: 141–150, 2000.

Milhorat TH, Capocelli AL, Anzil AP, Kotzen RM, Mihorat RH: Pathological basis of spinal cord cavitation in syringomyelia. Analysis of 105 autopsy cases. J Neurosurg 85: 802–812, 1995.

Milhorat TH, Chou MW, Trinidad EM, Kula RW, Mandell M, Wolpert C: Chiari I malformation redefined: clinical and radiographic findings for 364 symptomatic patients. Neurosurgery 44: 1005–1017, 1999.

Milhorat TH, Johnson RW, Milhorat RH, Capocelli AL Jr, Pevsner PH: Clinicopathological correlations in syringomyelia using axial magnetic resonance imaging. Neurosurgery 37: 206–213, 1995.

Rossier AB, Foo D, Shillito J, Dyro FM: Posttraumatic cervical syringomyelia. Incidence, clinical presentation, electrophysiological studies, syrinx protein and results of conservative and operative treatment. Brain 108: 439–461, 1985.

Squier MV, Lher RP: Post traumatic syringomyelia. J Neurol Neurosurg Psychiatry 57: 1095–1098, 1994.

Takigami I, Miyamoto K, Kodama H, Hosoe H, Tanimoto S, Shimizu K: Foramen magnum decompression for the treatment of Arnold Chiari malformation type I with associated syringomyelia in an elderly patient. Spinal Cord 43: 249–251, 2005.

Uhlenbrock D, Henkes H, Weber W, Felber S, Kuehne D: Non-dysraphic malformations, pp. 133–141 in Uhlenbroch D: MR imaging of the spine and spinal cord. Georg Thieme Verlag, 2004.

CHRONIC ADHESIVE ARACHNOIDITIS

15

Chronic adhesive arachnoiditis (CAA) is a progressive inflammatory disorder that starts with radiculitis and gradually evolves to intrathecal scarring and granulation that encapsulate the nerve roots and lead to clumping of nerve roots to each other or to the dura. CAA tends to develop following multiple spinal surgeries, spinal infection, spinal trauma, intraspinal hemorrhage, intrathecal steroid administration, or oil-based myelograms. Up to 16% of failed back surgery patients develop CAA.

The condition affects both genders equally and typically evolves over weeks to months following the precipitating events. Initially, an inflammatory process develops in the pia-arachnoid with nerve root swelling and hyperaemia. Subsequently, collagen is deposited and the nerve roots adhere to each other and later on are completely encapsulated with dense collagen tissue. The scar tissue interferes with the neural blood supply, resulting in neural atrophy. It may also cause disturbances of cerebrospinal fluid flow, which may lead to interstitial edema and increased pressure within the cord and, eventually, syringomyelia. In late stages of the disease calcification or ossification surrounding the arachnoid may occur.

CLINICAL PRESENTATION

Most cases of CAA develop in the lumbosacral spine, mainly in the posterior region. Occasionally, the cervical or thoracic spine may be involved.

Patients present with nonspecific complaints such as severe chronic back pain that may increase with exertion. Often patients develop unilateral or bilateral chronic radicular pain. Neurological deficits such as lower extremity weakness, hypaesthesia, sphincter dysfunction, and gait abnormalities may be seen. Multiple roots in both lower extremities may be affected, leading, occasionally, to cauda equina syndrome. As the symptomatology varies from case to case, establishing the diagnosis at an early stage may be difficult, and most patients are

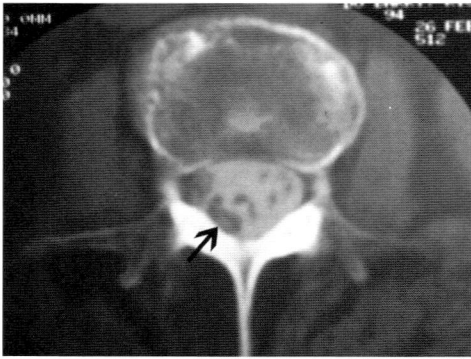

FIGURE 15-1
Axial CT-myelography in a patient with anky-losing spondylitis. Adhesive arachnoiditis is seen with nerve root clumping at the periphery of the thecal sac.

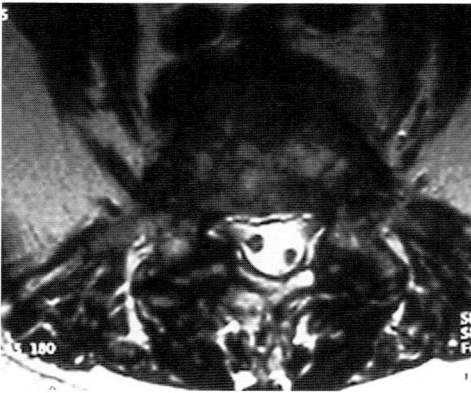

FIGURE 15-2
Axial T2WI MR of the lumbar spine showing the nerve roots clumped together in two distinct "bundles."

initially incorrectly diagnosed. The disease may be static or progressive. In the latter case, progressive neurological deficits appear resulting in severe disability.

IMAGING STUDIES

Plain radiographs are not helpful in this condition.

In the past, the CT diagnosis of CAA required the use of intrathecal water-soluble contrast agents, the so-called CT myelogram. Non-enhanced CT may detect calcifications or ossification in the shape of thin circumferential rings that surround the arachnoid. Occasionally a large calcified or ossified tubular mass may be seen (Figure 15-1).

MRI, the diagnostic modality of choice, provides conclusive evidence for the disease with high sensitivity (92%) and specificity (100%). T1-weighted images may identify clumped nerve roots within the thecal sac. T2-weighted images will show the nerve roots to be thickened due to clumping of several roots together. The clumped nerve roots may be located centrally or peripherally (Figure 15-2). In the latter situation the thecal sac may look empty. The thecal sac diameter may be decreased and occasionally deformed. Following contrast administration there may be very mild neural (cord, nerve root) enhancement.

MANAGEMENT

The management of CAA is challenging. No treatment thus far has been able to arrest or reverse the effects of CAA. The chronic pain is debilitating, and when it is combined with significant neurological deficits it results in major suffering and disability. Most patients end up frustrated due to the chronicity of pain. Multiple pain medications including narcotics are usually tried with various amount of success. Some patients benefit from spinal cord stimulation. Surgery is usually unrewarding and should be avoided if possible.

Bibliography

Chang HS, Nakagawa H: Theoretical analysis of the pathophysiology of syringomyelia associated with adhesive arachnoiditis. J Neurol Neurosurg Psychiatry 75: 754–757, 2004.

Chang KH, Choi YW, Kim OI, Han MC, Kim CW: Tuberculous arachnoiditis of the spine: Findings on myelography, CT, and MR imaging. Am J Neuroradiol 10: 1255–1262, 1989.

Delamarter RB, Ross JS, Masaryk TJ, Modic MT, Bohlman NH: Diagnosis of lumbar arachnoiditis by magnetic resonance imaging. Spine 15: 304–310, 1990.

Esses SI, Morley TP: Spinal arachnoiditis. Can J Neurol Sci 10: 2–10, 1983.

Fitt GJ, Stevens JM: Postoperative arachnoiditis diagnosed by high resolution fast spin-echo MRI of the lumbar spine. Neuroradiology 37: 139–145, 1995.

Hoffman GS: Spinal arachnoiditis. What is the clinical spectrum? I. Spine 8: 538–540, 1983.

Ido K, Urushidani H: Fibrous adhesive entrapment of lumbosacral nerve roots as a cause of sciatica. Spinal Cord 39: 269–273, 2001.

Kaufman AB, Dunsmore RH: Clinicopathological considerations in spinal meningeal calcification and ossification. Neurology 21: 1243–1248, 1971.

Kroin JS, Buvanendran A, Cochran E, Tuman KJ: Characterization of pain and pharmacologic responses in an animal model of lumbar adhesive arachnoiditis. Spine 30: 1828–1831, 2005.

Long DM: Chronic adhesive arachnoiditis: Pathogenesis, prognosis and treatment. Neurosurgery Q 2: 296–319, 1992.

Malcolm IVJ: The role of vascular damage and fibrosis in the pathogenesis of nerve root damage. Clin Orthop 279: 40–48, 1992.

Miaki K, Matsui H, Nakano M, Tsuji H: Nutritional supply to the cauda equina in lumbar adhesive arachnoiditis in rats. Eur Spine J 8: 310–316, 1999.

Nakano M, Matsui H, Miaki K, Yamagami T, Tsuji H: Postlaminectomy adhesion of the cauda equina. Changes of postoperative vascular permeability of the equina in rats. Spine 22: 1105–1114, 1997.

Rice I, Wee MYK, Thomson K: Obstetric epidurals and chronic adhesive arachnoiditis. Br J Anaesth 92: 109–120, 2004.

Ross JS, Masaryk TJ, Modic MT, Delamater R, Bohlman H, Wilbur G: MR imaging in lumbar arachnoiditis. Am J Roentgenol 149: 1025–1032, 1987.

Ross JS, Robertson JT, Frederickson RC, Petrie JL, Obuchowski N, Modic MT, deTribolet N: Association between peridural scar and recurrent radicular pain after lumbar discectomy: Magnetic resonance evaluation. Neurosurgery 38: 855–861, 1996.

Shaw MD, Russell JA, Grossart KW: The changing pattern of spinal arachnoiditis. J Neurol Neurosurg Psychiatry 41: 97–107, 1978.

Takahashi N, Konno S, Kikuchi S: A histological and functional study on cauda equina adhesion induced by multiple level laminectomy. Spine 28: 4–8, 2003.

Uhlenbrock D, Henkes H, Weber W, Felber S, Kuehne D: Inflammatory disorders of the spine and spinal canal, pp. 424–426 in Uhlenbroch D: MR imaging of the spine and spinal cord. Georg Thieme Verlag, 2004.

COCCYGODYNIA

16

The term *coccygodynia* is a descriptive name meaning pain in the coccygeal area and does not identify specific coccygeal pathology. The condition occurs most frequently in females in the third and fourth decades. It may appear following trauma, such as a fall, following childbirth, or idiopathically (with no apparent cause). Coccygodynia typically occurs in females with an elevated body mass index.

The anatomical differences between the female and male pelvis help explain the increased incidence of coccygodynia in the former group. The female coccyx is prone to trauma more than the male's due to the increased distance between the ischial tuberosities in females and the lower and more posterior coccygeal position. These anatomical differences leave the coccyx less protected and more vulnerable to trauma.

Most cases of coccygodynia are, however, idiopathic as no direct trauma to the pelvic area is recalled. Postacchini and Massorbio (1983) found an increased incidence of coccygodynia in individuals with a forward angulated coccyx or with a coccyx that is subluxed at the sacrococcygeal or intercoccygeal joint. They postulated that the first intercoccygeal joint plays an important role in the pathogenesis of idiopathic coccygodynia. Other researchers have connected coccygodynia with psychological problems, pelvic muscles spasm, chronic inflammation, coccygeal hypermobility, coccygeal hypomobility, coccygeal luxation, and coccygeal retroversion.

CLINICAL PRESENTATION

The predominant clinical symptom in coccygodynia is coccygeal pain aggravated by sitting (and sometimes by standing) and relieved in the recumbent position. The pain may be severe and exacerbated during defecation. In some patients simultaneous low back pain is reported. The physical examination reveals tenderness over the coccygeal region. Mobilization of the coccygeal bone during rectal examination elicits intense pain. The neurological examination remains normal throughout.

IMAGING STUDIES

Radiographic studies should include AP and lateral views of the pelvis. The latter should be obtained standing and sitting. Normally, the coccyx pivots only slightly anteriorly or posteriorly when the sitting posture is adopted (Figures 16-1A and 16-1B). In patients with coccygodynia increased anterior hypermobility (over 25 degrees) or posterior subluxation may be disclosed. This hypermobility may be missed if films are obtained in the standing posture only. At times, sharp angulation of the coccyx can be seen or a true subluxation of the sacrococcygeal or the first intercoccygeal joints may be observed. X-ray studies can also identify a fracture following trauma, osteoarthritic changes, tumors, or infection. Whenever doubt arises and space-occupying lesions such as cysts, tumors, or infection are suspected, CT or preferably MRI studies should be obtained.

MANAGEMENT

Conservative management of this condition is often empiric and consists of analgesic and anti-inflammatory medications. The patients are instructed to use a soft pillow or a donut-shaped pillow with a hollowed center when sitting. Manual interventions such as

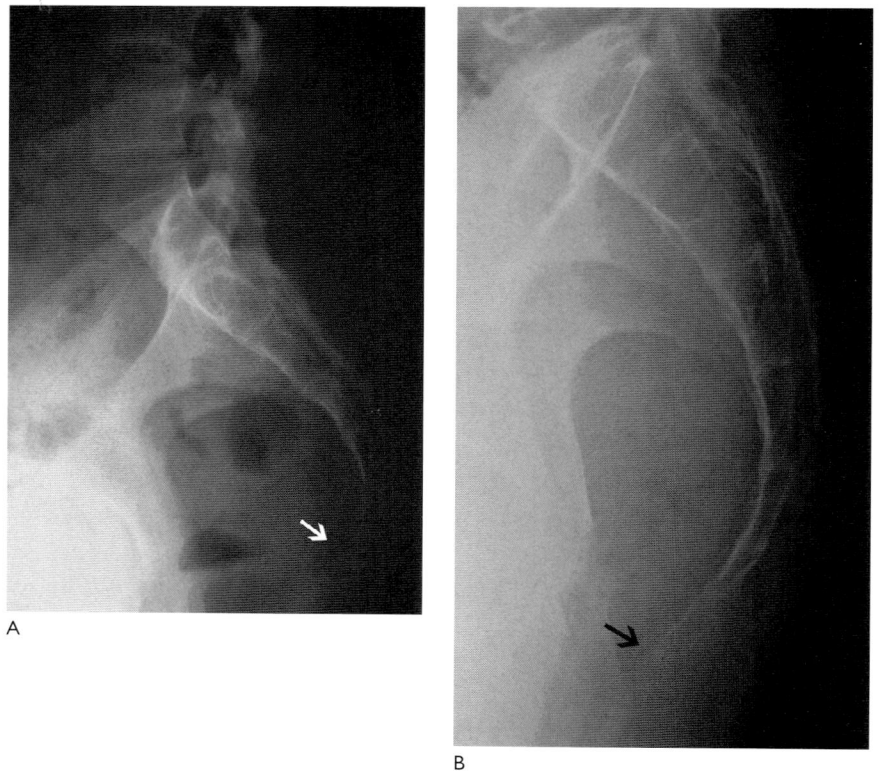

A

B

FIGURE 16-1
Lateral view of the sacrum and coccyx in individuals not suffering pain. In (A) the coccyx is facing more anteriorly than in (B).

levator ani massage, levator ani stretching, and sacrococcygeal joint mobilization may bring relief to some patients but the overall results are often frustrating.

Coccygeal manipulation in combination with a steroid injection at the sacrococcygeal junction may bring relief to a significant number of patients. These are performed under general anesthesia and can be repeated if a positive response is obtained in the first trial. Patients who fail conservative care and continue with persistent severe pain may be referred for surgery. Partial or total coccygectomy may bring relief to these patients.

Bibliography

Beinhaker NA, Ranawat CS, Marchisiello P: Coccygodynia: Surgical versus conservative treatment. Orthop Trans 1: 162, 1977.

Bernini P: Point of view. Spine 26: E484, 2001.

De Andres J, Chaves S: Coccygodynia: A proposal for an algorithm for treatment. J Pain 4: 257–266, 2003.

Dennel LV, Nathan S: Coccygeal retroversion. Spine 29: E256–E257, 2004.

Eng JB, Rymaszewski L, Jepson K: Coccygectomy. J R Coll Surg Edinb 33: 202–203, 1988.

Feldbrin Z, Singer M, Keynan O, Rzetelny V, Hendel D: Coccygectomy for intractable coccygodynia. Isr Med Assoc J 7: 160–162, 2005.

Fogel GR, Cunningham PY III, Esses SI: Coccygodynia: Evaluation and management. J Am Acad Orthop Surg 12: 49–54, 2004.

Grosso NP, Van Dam BE: Total coccygectomy for the relief of coccygodynia: A retrospective review. J Spinal Disord 8: 328–330, 1995.

Lithwick NH: Coccygodynia: Evaluation and management. J Am Acad Orthop Surg 12: 289, 2004.

Maigne JY, Chatellier G: Comparison of three manual coccydynia treatments: A pilot study. Spine 26: E479–E483, 2001.

Maigne JY, Guedj S, Straus C: Idiopathic coccygodynia: Lateral roentgenograms in the sitting position and coccygeal discography. Spine 19: 930–934, 1994.

Maigne JY, Lagauche D, Doursounian L: Instability of the coccyx in coccydynia. J Bone Joint Surg Br 82: 1038–1041, 2000.

Maigne JY, Tamalet B: Standardized radiologic protocol for the study of common coccygodynia and characteristics of the lesions observed in the sitting position: Clinical elements differentiating luxation, hypermobility and normal mobility. Spine 21: 2588–2593, 1996.

Porter KM, Kahn MA, Piggott H: Coccygodynia: A retrospective review. J Bone Joint Surg Br 63: 634–636, 1981.

Postacchini F, Massorbio M: Idiopathic coccygodynia: Analysis of 51 operative cases and a radiographic study of the normal coccyx. J Bone Joint Surg Am 65: 1116–1124, 1983.

Ramsey ML, Toohey JS, Neidre A, Stromberg LJ, Roberts DA: Coccygodynia: Treatment. Orthopaedics 26: 403–405, 2003.

Thiele GH: Coccygodynia. Dis Colon Rectum 6: 422–436, 1963.

Traycoff RB, Crayton H, Dodoson R: Sacrococcygeal pain syndromes: Diagnosis and treatment. Orthopedics 12: 1373–1377, 1989.

Wood KB, Mehbod AA: Operative treatment for coccygodynia. J Spinal Disord 17: 511–515, 2004.

Wray CC, Easom S, Hoskinson J: Coccydynia: Aetiology and treatment. J Bone Joint Surg Br 73: 335–338, 1991.

IMAGING OF THE POSTOPERATIVE DEGENERATIVE SPINE

17

Spinal surgery usually consists of one or more basic operative procedures such as decompression of the neural elements (cord, cauda equina, or nerve roots), reconstruction of the load-bearing capacity of the spine (bone grafting, cement injection, or internal fixation), and correction of spinal deformities (normalization of coronal and sagittal alignment). Many of these operative procedures are performed in concert with fusion surgery.

The most frequent spinal pathology for which surgery is performed is degenerative disc disease. Most patients with this condition do well after spinal surgery, whether it is simple disc excision or more complex fusion procedures. Some patients, however, have persistent or recurrent symptoms that necessitate re-imaging of the spine, and the diagnostic imaging of these patients will be the focus of this chapter.

The yearly increase in the number of spinal surgeries for degenerative disc disease in the United States and worldwide has resulted in a parallel rise in the number of spinal imaging studies that are performed after surgical interventions. The main goal of spinal imaging of symptomatic patients who have undergone previous spinal surgery is to correctly identify the reason for the patient's persistent, recurrent, or new pain. Such imaging studies are undertaken to determine whether or not additional surgery may help the patient.

When evaluating symptomatic patients after surgery, one has to keep in mind the classic three *W*'s related to failed back or neck surgery: *w*rong patient selection, *w*rong diagnosis, and *w*rong surgery (the latter including a wrong operated level). Mere repetition of diagnostic scans per se obviously cannot remedy poor preoperative patient selection.

A close collaboration between the managing physician and the neuroradiologist is important. Precise knowledge of the patient's symptoms (leg or arm vs. back or neck pain and the symptomatic side of radiculopathy) and what was done in surgery are all-important for the radiological evaluation. Even before performing diagnostic imaging, obtaining a detailed history on the temporal sequence of the patient's complaints after surgery may distinguish between having failed to address the patient's problem, a surgical complication, a recurrent problem, or a new pathology altogether. Indeed, the appearance of a new problem may be related to the original degenerative process and/or to the surgical procedure or, alternatively, unrelated to it altogether.

TYPES OF SPINAL PROCEDURES

This chapter will deal with postoperative imaging in patients with degenerative disc disease, the most frequent spine pathology requiring surgery.

Lumbar Spine

There are several main categories of surgical procedures for treating degenerative lumbar spine conditions:

1. Disc excision
2. Laminectomy and partial facetectomy to relieve central, lateral, subarticular, or foraminal stenosis
3. Fusion procedures: posterolateral, posterior, or interbody (Figure 17-1)
4. Disc replacement surgery (Figure 17-2)
5. Fracture reduction and stabilization, including vertebroplasty and kyphoplasty
6. Deformity correction
7. Tumor excision

There are two types of interbody fusion procedures: posterior lumbar interbody fusion (PLIF) and transforaminal lumbar interbody fusion (TLIF) (Figure 17-1). Fusion procedures are performed with autogenous bone graft or with allograft and are usually combined with spinal instrumentation (pedicle screws that are connected to rods or plates). Interbody cages are also used and may be implanted through a posterior or anterior approach.

The most frequent conditions that need to be evaluated in symptomatic patients after discectomy/laminectomy procedures are persistent or recurrent disc herniation, epidural hematoma, epidural fibrosis, spinal stenosis, instability, pars fracture, arachnoiditis, spinal infection, and dural tears. Plain X-rays and computerized tomography (CT) are the imaging procedures of choice for evaluating instability, pars fracture, and facet arthritis. The others are best evaluated nowadays by magnetic resonance imaging (MRI) with or without intravenous (IV) contrast medium.

The most frequent conditions that need to be evaluated in symptomatic patients after spinal instrumentation and fusion are residual stenosis at the operated level(s) or at an adjacent level, epidural hematoma, epidural scarring, infection, pseudoarthrosis, instability, misplaced instrumentation, failed instrumentation, and loosening of implants. Plain films and CT with or without myelography are applicable for most of these complications.

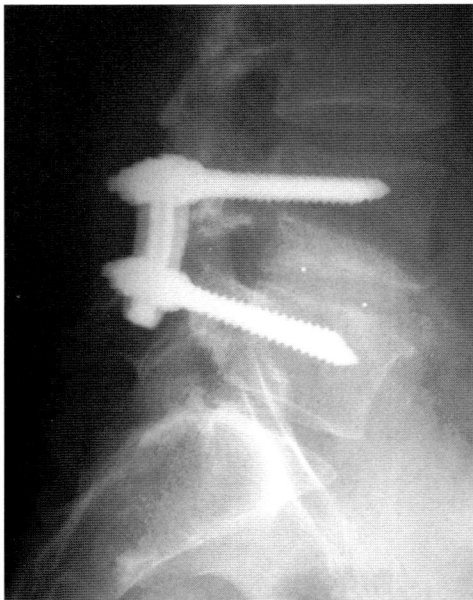

FIGURE 17-1
Transforaminal lumbar interbody fusion (TLIF). Lateral view of an instrumented fusion at L4-L5 with pedicle screws, plates, and interbody radiolucent carbon cage (with metal dotes as markers). Note the bony fusion within and around the cage.

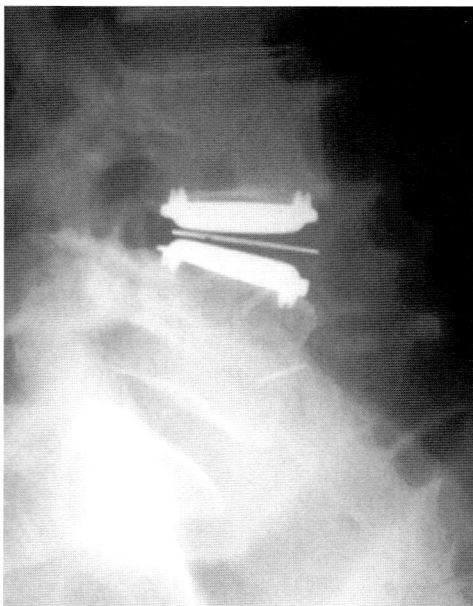

FIGURE 17-2
Lumbar disc replacement. Lateral view of disc replacement at L4-L5 with a Charite artificial disc.

Cervical Spine

The modern most common surgical approach for cervical spondylosis is the anterior one. It allows a direct approach to the cervical spine
and allows complete disc and osteophyte excision with decompression of
the spinal cord. The procedure is usually completed with fusion of the
operated segment, which is known as anterior cervical discectomy with
fusion (ACDF) (Figure 17-3A), or with disc replacement (Figure 17-3B).
An anterior cervical corpectomy may be considered if the site of epidural compression extends beyond the disc space. This approach has the
advantage of allowing a thorough decompression, including the resection
of osteophytes, and also improves fusion rates in cases where multilevel
decompression is needed, such as in patients with multilevel spondylosis
or ossification of the posterior longitudinal ligament (OPLL). Reconstruction of the spine is traditionally performed with a strut bone graft. A variety of strut-grafting techniques have been described, including a tricortical
autogenous iliac crest bone graft or a fibular strut (autologous or allograft).
The tricortical autogenous iliac crest bone graft is most often utilized for
corpectomy of one or two levels, whereas autogenous fibular grafts may be
required to reconstruct corpectomies of more than two levels. The structural stability of the cervical spine may be then supplemented with various
anterior plates or external immobilization. Vertical titanium-mesh fusion
(Harms) cages have been used to replace the resected vertebral body to
avoid low fusion rates with allograft use and donor site morbidity with
autograft harvesting (Figure 17-4). A "hybrid decompression fixation"

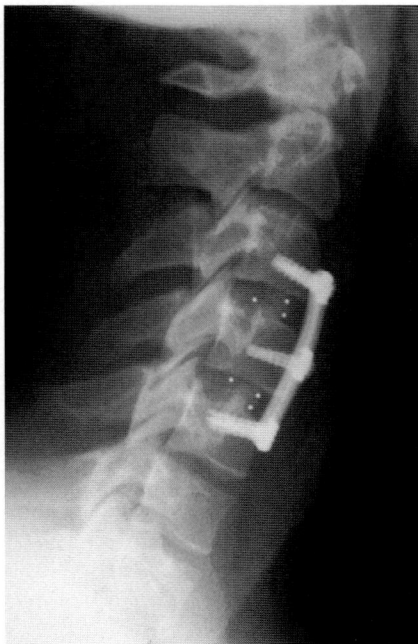

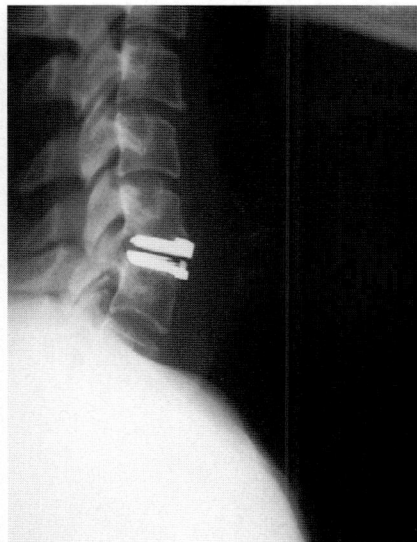

B

A

FIGURE 17-3
Anterior cervical discectomy with (A) fusion or (B) disc replacement. (A) Lateral view
of ACDF at C3-C4 and C4-C5 with interbody cages (with metal dotes as markers)
and anterior plate. (B) Lateral view of disc replacement at C5-C6 with porous coated
motion (PCM) artificial cervical disc.

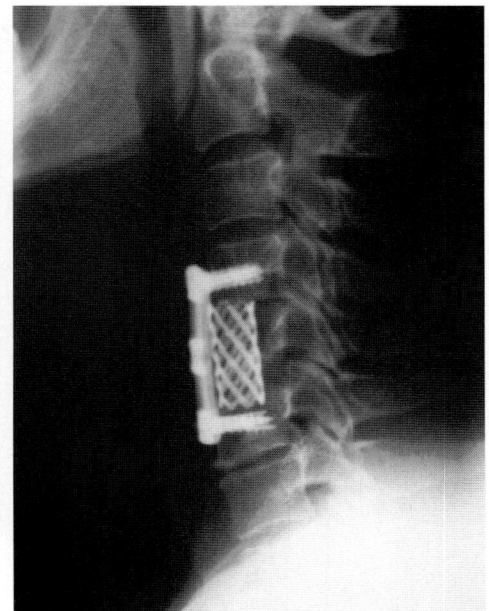

FIGURE 17-4
Anterior cervical decompression with corpectomy and adjacent discectomies. Lateral view
of the cervical spine showing a corpectomy
of C5. Reconstruction was achieved with a
Harms titanium mesh cage and anterior plate
fixing C4 to C6.

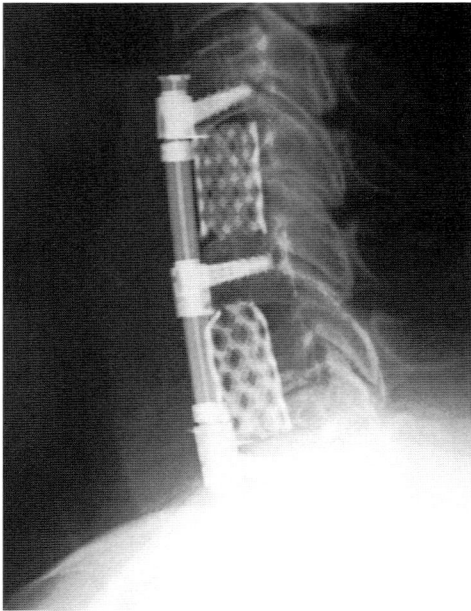

FIGURE 17-5
Anterior decompression of multilevel cervical myelopathy. Lateral X-ray of the cervical spine showing corpectomies of C4 and C6, with sparing of the middle vertebral body (C5) for instrumentation anchorage. The spine was reconstructed with Harms cages and DOC platform.

technique was recently proposed for multilevel cervical myelopathy (Figure 17-5). An alternative for the hybrid technique would be an open-door laminoplasty (Figure 17-6).

PLAIN FILMS

Plain X-rays allow the verification of laminectomy site(s) and placement of internal fixation devices (pedicle screws, hooks, plates, rods, bone cement, etc.). The placement may be graded as either appropriate and at the right level or inappropriate and/or at the wrong level. Plain X-rays may also allow evaluation of the general sagittal alignment of the spine and bone quality. They also enable the detection of breakage or loosening of the implants, pulling out of pedicle screws, and/or subsidence of intervertebral cages.

Plain films may also provide the means to evaluate bony fusion (posterior, interbody, or intertransverse fusion). The assessment of fusion quality is based on the appearance of bridging trabecular bone. It may be classified as fused (when no loss of continuity of the trabecular bone is observed), not fused (when bone continuity is interrupted), or uncertain (when bone continuity across the operated segment is questionable). There may, however, be a high false positive rate (up to 42%) if one relies solely on X-rays to diagnose solid bony fusion.

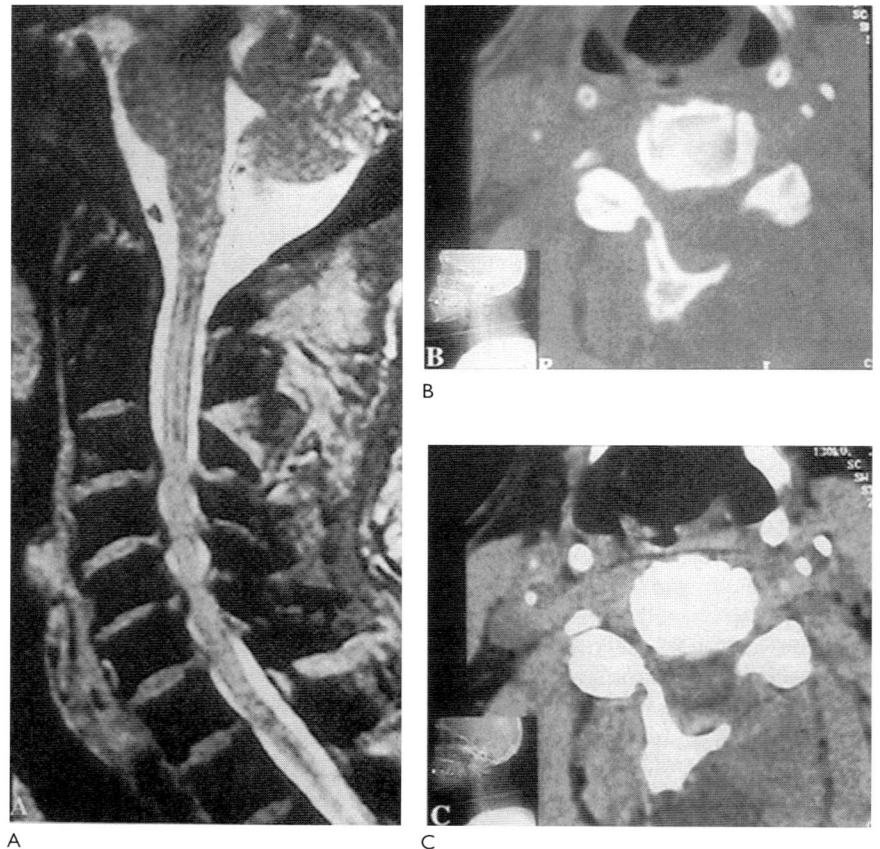

FIGURE 17-6
Open-door laminoplasty. (A) Preoperative sagittal T2WI showing cord compression at four discal levels. (B, C) Postoperative CT axial cuts showing an open-door laminoplasty.

Oblique views may sometimes be helpful in evaluating a posterolateral fusion mass. Dynamic lateral flexion-extension X-rays can further help in the assessment of solid bony union. Plain films may also detect the presence of adjacent level disc degeneration with or without subluxation, such as spondylolisthesis, retrolisthesis, or, less often, lateral subluxation (Figure 17-7). They can also corroborate whether disc space infection has evolved, mostly after intradiscal surgery (i.e., after discectomy or intervertebral fusion, usually with cages) (Figure 17-8). Although plain films have a limited value in assessing recurrent herniation or residual stenosis, they are invaluable for the appropriate postoperative assessment, and one should almost always obtain at least one postoperative X-ray, preferably in the standing position.

NUCLEAR MEDICINE IMAGING

Bone scanning detects disturbed osseous metabolism by highlighting changes in blood flow and metabolic activity of bone. Increased uptake reflects increased osteoblastic activity and/or blood flow.

Mildly increased radiotracer localization at operated levels can be detected for several years after surgery. A more pronounced radiotracer

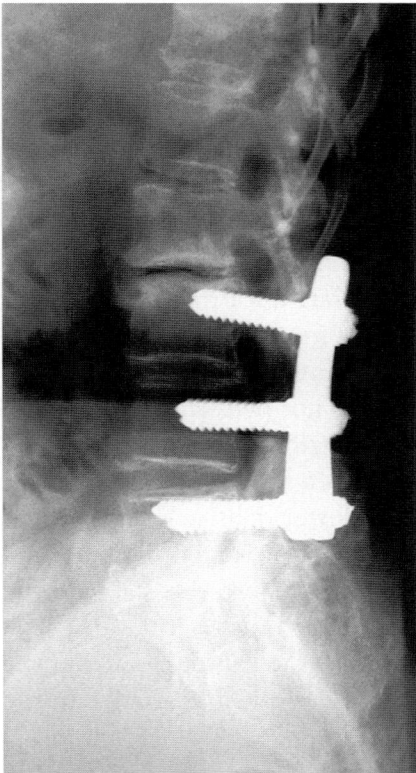

FIGURE 17-7
Adjacent level disc degeneration following lumbar fusion. Lateral view of the lumbar spine after pedicle screw fixation of the L3 through L5 segments. Note the adjacent level disc degeneration at L2-L3 with endplate sclerosis and mild spondylolisthesis.

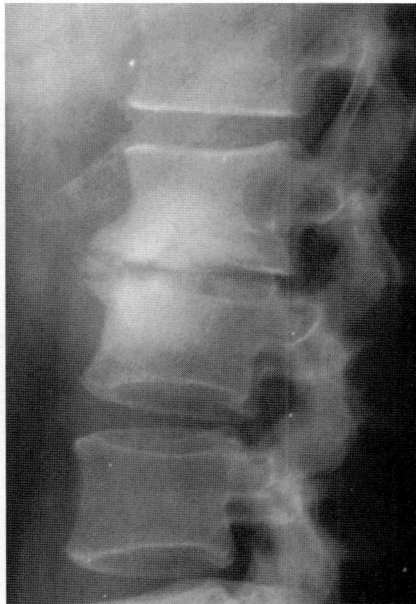

FIGURE 17-8
Disc space infection following discectomy. Lateral X-ray of the lumbar spine of a patient following L1-L2 discectomy, showing intervertebral disc space narrowing with endplate irregularities and anterior new bone formation suggesting postoperative disc space infection (see also MRI, Figure 17-17A).

uptake may indicate that a pseudoarthrosis has developed, that a surgical infection has evolved, or that a degenerative process such as adjacent level disc degeneration or the development of Modic type III changes has taken place.

In cases of pseudoarthrosis, there is continuous motion with impact loading on the bone surfaces at the non-union site, resulting in osteoblast cell activation and increased technetium-99 diphosphonate uptake at the non-union site. Pronounced uptake at the site of attempted fusion, when seen more than a year after surgery, is highly suspicious of a pseudoarthrosis. Single photon emission computed tomography (SPECT) might further delineate the site of non-union.

Combined technetium-99 and gallium-67 citrate scintigraphy is an accurate test for evaluating patients suspected as having postoperative disc space infection. Although dual-phase (i.e., blood pool and bone imaging) scintigraphy has been reported as being insensitive in detecting vertebral osteomyelitis, the sensitivity of delayed bone imaging has been reported to be excellent, ranging from 86 to 100%. The concern is that bone scan may be nonspecific in the early postoperative period due to noninfectious inflammatory reaction. Gallium imaging with SPECT analysis may be helpful in such situations. A disproportionate focal increased uptake on both the technetium and gallium scans is indicative of vertebral osteomyelitis.

COMPUTED TOMOGRAPHY (CT)

CT yields excellent images and anatomical details of the bony structures and, as such, provides important data in patients with residual central, lateral, or foraminal stenosis. Although CT is an outstanding tool in the diagnosis of lumbar disc herniations in a "virgin" spine, it is less effective in distinguishing between postoperative scarring and recurrent disc herniation. The previous laminectomy site is easily recognized on the axial CT images, when a portion of the lamina is missing. In cases of microdiscectomy where bone resection was not performed, the operative site may be recognized by the missing ligamentum flavum.

On CT, the extradural scar appears as a soft tissue lesion with a higher density than the thecal sac and a lower density than the disc. The scar appears anteriorly at the discectomy site and/or laterally and posteriorly. The dural sac is usually retracted toward the scar; and the scar does not compress the sac (as opposed to disc herniation). The scar is usually enhanced with IV contrast (see later discussion), but the accuracy of differentiating between scar and residual or recurrent disc herniation with CT is low.

Residual stenosis, especially foraminal narrowing, is one of the most frequent causes of failed back surgery syndrome and is easily detected on postoperative CT imaging (Figure 17-9).

The CT examination can reveal changes outside the spinal canal, such as atrophy of the multifidus and fat replacement of the muscle fibers.

CT with IV iodinated contrast medium may be occasionally used to demonstrate active infection of scarring. The ability of the IV con-

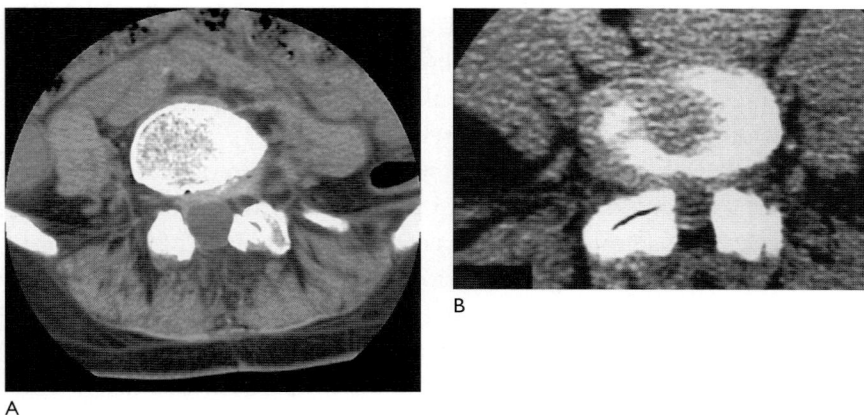

A

B

FIGURE 17-9

(A) Residual foraminal and (B) central stenosis after laminectomy. (A) Axial CT through a lumbar vertebra showing a bilateral midline laminectomy defect and residual foraminal stenosis on the left. (B) Axial CT showing residual central and foraminal stenosis after midline laminectomy. Note the severe facet arthritis.

trast to enhance scar tissue may also help to better demonstrate recurrent disc herniation; the recurrent disc occurs in an area rich in scar tissue, thus the enhanced scar will better delineate the non-enhanced recurrent disc. The differentiation between scar and recurrent disc is of utmost importance because surgery for an epidural scar is mostly unsuccessful, whereas surgery for a recurrent disc will result in significant pain relief in most patients.

CT is usually superior to plain X-rays for assessing bony fusion and pseudoarthrosis (Figures 17-10 and 17-11), pedicle screw placement, and residual stenosis at the operated level or at an adjacent level.

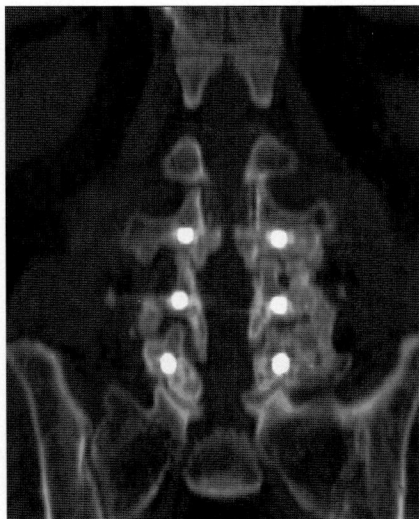

FIGURE 17-10

Pseudoarthrosis after intertransverse spondylodesis. Coronal CT reformation showing proper placement of pedicle screws at L3, L4, and L5. Note the absence of intertransverse bony fusion on the right and a pseudoarthrosis at L3-L4 on the left.

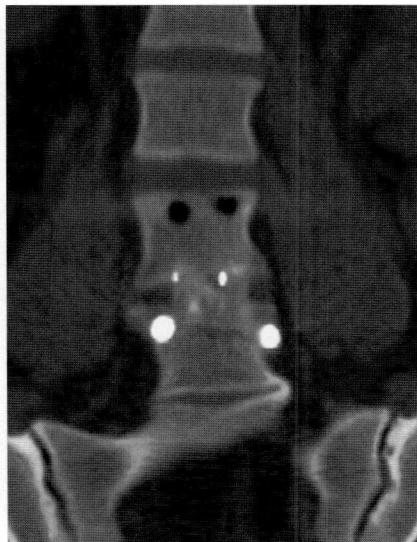

FIGURE 17-11

Solid interbody bony fusion after PLIF. Coronal CT reformation showing solid interbody bony fusion at L4-L5.

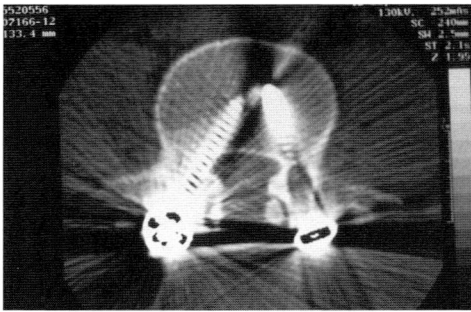

FIGURE 17-12
Misplaced pedicle screw. Axial CT cut through
a lumbar pedicular level showing bilateral pedicle screw placement. The right-side screw is
violating the lateral recess.

CT is an excellent diagnostic tool in the immediate postoperative period for evaluating pedicle screw placement, especially if the CT
cuts are done parallel to the pedicular screws and sagittal and coronal
reformations are obtained (Figures 17-10 and 17-12).

When evaluating non-union, it is important to obtain thin slices
through the intended fusion area by means of coronal and sagittal reformations. For example, plain films may show evidence of bony union,
but a CT with coronal reconstructions may indicate that a plate pseudoarthrosis has developed (Figure 17-13). The CT demonstration of
bridging bone trabeculae between the instrumented vertebrae may
indicate that the fusion is solid. On the other hand, gas in a disc within
the fusion area or lucency around pedicle screws may indicate a pseudoarthrosis. The presence of pseudoarthrosis per se is not proof for its
being the source of a patient's symptoms.

Stainless steel pedicle screws, and to a lesser extent titanium
implants, may cause artifacts on CT scans. It is better in the latter case
to evaluate the spine with bone windows or, even better, with myelography and post-myelography CT. Another advantage of CT-myelography is that it is a true dynamic examination. Although CT-myelography
can also detect arachnoiditis and pseudomeningocele, both entities are
better delineated on MRI.

Cervical Spine

There are many pitfalls with CT evaluation of the cervical spine.
The cervical cord is poorly visualized, disc pathology is not clearly
delineated, and beam hardening artifacts from the shoulders at the
cervicothoracic junction (C6 to T2) blur most of the anatomical
details. In addition, the use of metal spinal implants blurs the obtained
images even further. CT-myelography may help to better visualize the
anatomical details, especially in the cervicothoracic junction and in
the presence of metal artifacts. Cord pathology, however, will still be
missed on CT-myelography.

MAGNETIC RESONANCE IMAGING (MRI)

Although clinical imaging with conventional X-rays or CT is
reflective of tissue density, imaging with MR is much more complex.

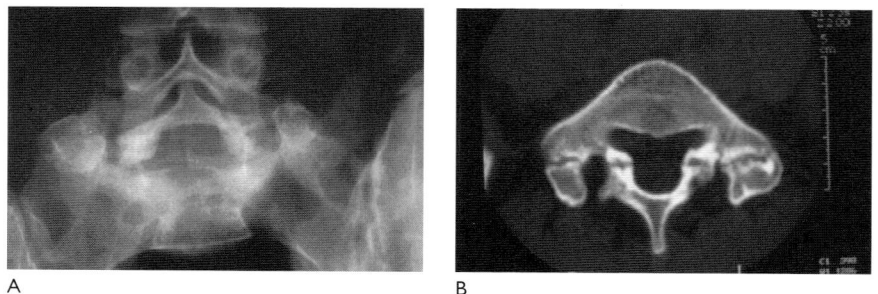

A   B

FIGURE 17-13
Plate pseudoarthrosis. (A) AP X-ray of the lumbosacral junction showing bilateral lateral bony fusion between the transverse processes of L5 and the sacral ala. (B) Axial CT
through the same area as (A), showing a plate pseudoarthrosis.

For example, the T1- and T2-weighted images (T1WI and T2WI) reflect different aspects of proton relaxation, and therefore the examined substance will appear differently in the two sequences. This becomes even more intricate as a substance on T2WI will appear differently according to the pulse sequence used for acquisition of the image. Thus, fat will appear bright on fast-spin echo (FSE), whereas it will appear darker or with an intermediate signal when acquired with conventional spin echo.

MRI is an excellent diagnostic tool for providing detailed anatomical features of soft and neural tissues and also for depicting sagittal coronal reformation by showing the spinal canal and intervertebral foraminae. In addition, because MRI is capable of revealing not only morphological alterations but also biochemical changes, it is the imaging procedure of choice for patients following spine surgery. It also has the ability to differentiate between fat, scar tissue, and disc material by using various MR sequences with or without a magnetic contrast medium such as gadolinium diethylenetriamine penta-acetic acid (Gd-DPTA).

Early Normal Postoperative Changes in the Lumbar Spine

A previous laminectomy site is identified on T1WI as a loss of the normal low signal of the cortical bone and of the high signal of the bone marrow. If the laminotomy is relatively small, the absence of ligamentum flavum may be the only sign of a laminectomy. The postoperative signal obliterates the typical paraspinal fat-muscle planes. The normal epidural pattern is replaced in the immediate postoperative period by a variable amount of heterogeneous intermediate signal on the T1WI and by a hyperintense signal on T2WI. These altered signals represent soft tissue edema. Discectomy produces an intermediate soft tissue signal anterior to the thecal sac at the site of the disc herniation. This soft tissue signal blends with the posterior disc on T1WI and may produce a mass effect on the dural tube. The amount of anterior extradural soft tissue decreases by 2–6 months after surgery. On sagittal T2WI, a tear in the anulus may be seen as a high-intensity signal, which tends to fade after a few months. To summarize, in the immediate postoperative period, an epidural soft tissue mass effect, which mimics the preoperative findings, is seen at the operative site. The soft tissue mass effect in the immediate postoperative period almost precludes the differentiation between this normal soft tissue response to surgery and a residual or recurrent disc herniation. Often, this postoperative appearance mimics the preoperative disc herniation. In some cases, this mass effect can persist, as long as one year after clinically successful discectomy.

Postoperative hematoma will ordinarily show increased signal intensity on both T1WI and T2WI. It may, however, have a variable MRI appearance according to the age of the hemorrhage. Postoperative hematoma can be confused with disc herniation on T1WI and T2WI. A better differentiation is possible with a T1-weighted gradient echo (GE) out-of-phase sequence, in which a hematoma will appear bright.

Bone marrow edema may sometimes be observed on both sides of the disc space following simple discectomy or after interbody fusion. This may be associated with intense back pain and should be distinguished from vertebral osteomyelitis. The absence of fever and normal erythrocyte sedimentation rate (ESR) and C-reactive protein (CRP) values usually rule out vertebral infection. Bone marrow edema is usually a self-limiting process.

MRI is the most useful imaging tool for distinguishing residual or recurrent disc herniation from normal postsurgical epidural scar tissue. Intravenous contrast will identify scar tissue because of its relative vascularity (compared with the avascular nature of discal material). It must be remembered that postsurgical changes and resolving hematoma or fluid collection following successful surgical intervention (discectomy or decompression) produce a mass effect on MRI, and this may preclude proper interpretation during the first six postoperative months. Nevertheless, it must be borne in mind that postoperative scarring is part of a normal process.

Although most authorities recommend the use of IV contrast (gadolinium) in the diagnosis of scar tissue, some have found that routine use of contrast material is not mandatory and obtaining FSE or FLAIR T2WI may suffice in the differentiation between scar and recurrent disc. Epidural scarring shows an intermediate signal intensity on both T1WI and T2WI and cannot be easily differentiated from disc material. Intravenously injected Gd-DPTA will enhance the fibrous tissue but not disc material. Thus, the lack of early central (as opposed to peripheral) contrast enhancement is a clear indication of recurrent disc herniation, whereas a more uniform enhancement pattern indicates epidural scarring (Figures 17-14 and 17-15). In most cases MRI

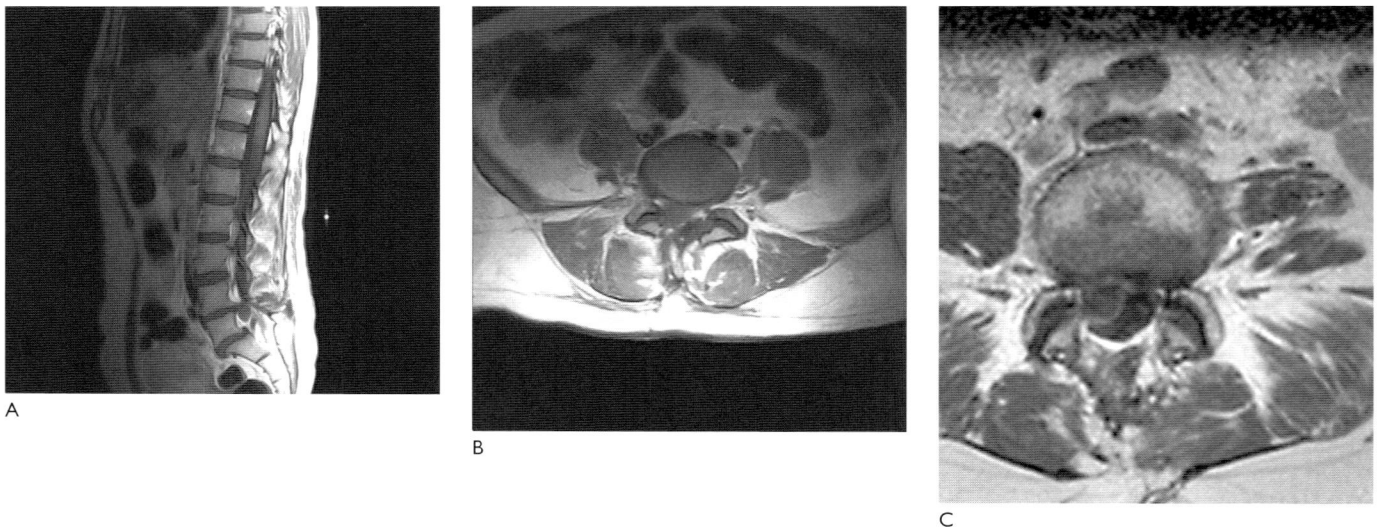

FIGURE 17-14
Recurrent disc herniation. (A) Sagittal MRI of the lumbar spine (T1 spin echo) showing a non-enhancing mass behind the L5 vertebral body that proved to be a recurrent disc herniation. (B) Axial T1WI with IV contrast showing a large right-side non-enhancing mass displacing and compressing the dural sac posteriorly and to the left. The mass was found at surgery to be a large free discal fragment. (C) Axial T1WI with IV contrast showing a rim enhancement around a right recurrent disc herniation at L4-L5.

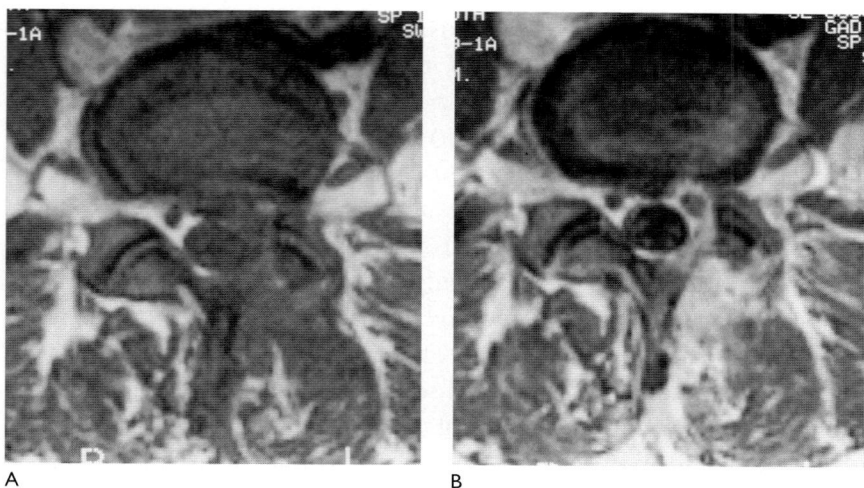

A   B

FIGURE 17-15
Postdiscectomy epidural scarring. (A) Axial T1WI without contrast showing a mass effect around the left nerve. (B) After IV injection of gadolinium, enhancing scar tissue around the left nerve root is noticed.

with IV contrast enables the physician to distinguish between scar and recurrent disc (see Table 17-1).

Occasionally, T1WI may be obtained with fat suppression in order to augment weak Gd enhancement. The enhancement of scar tissue on MRI subsides after one year. The role of epidural scar tissue in relation to patient symptoms is not clear. Scarring is usually asymptomatic, and contribution of the scar tissue to the clinical symptoms is at best controversial.

A word of caution: Gd-GDTA enhancement may also occur around a herniated disc (rim or peripheral enhancement; Figure 17-14C). In addition, the involved nerve roots may be enhanced proximally toward the conus medullaris following decompression, and this enhancement usually resolves by six months after surgery. It may happen in up to 20% of asymptomatic patients following successful disc excision. In contrast to the intrathecal spinal nerve roots, which have a visually intact blood-brain barrier and are not enhanced under normal conditions, the dorsal root ganglion may be enhanced with injected contrast material when under compression.

TABLE 17-1
Characteristics of Epidural Scarring and Recurrent Disc Herniation on MRI

	Epidural Scar	**Recurrent Disc**
Epidural location	Follows line of surgery	Opposite disc space
Mass effect	Conforms to space, retracts dura	Compresses, displaces dura
Signal intensity	Hypo- or isointense on T1WI	Hypo- or intermediate intensity on T1WI
Gadolinium	Enhances	Does not enhance centrally, may enhance peripherally

Adapted from McCulloch JA, Transfeldt EE: *Macnab's Backache*, 3rd edition, Williams and Wilkins, 1997, p. 719.

Arachnoiditis can be well visualized on MRI. There are three most common patterns typical of arachnoiditis: (1) central clumping of nerve roots (Figure 17-16), (2) adherence of the nerve roots to the dura giving an empty sac appearance, and (3) nonvisualization of roots because of an increased T1 intradural signal complicating the differentiation between CSF and neural structures.

Postoperative spondylodiscitis is characterized by the loss of the normal outline of the vertebral endplates with low signal intensity of the bone marrow on T1WI and high signal intensity on T2WI (Figure 17-17A). Contrast enhancement of the disc, the adjacent endplates, and the surrounding paravertebral soft tissue and epidural space make the diagnosis of pyogenic vertebral osteomyelitis almost certain. MRI is also useful in monitoring response to antibiotic treatment of the infection, in conjunction with ESR and CRP levels. The differential diagnosis of disc space infection is type I Modic changes in which low signal intensity appears in the disc on T2WI. In cases in which discec-

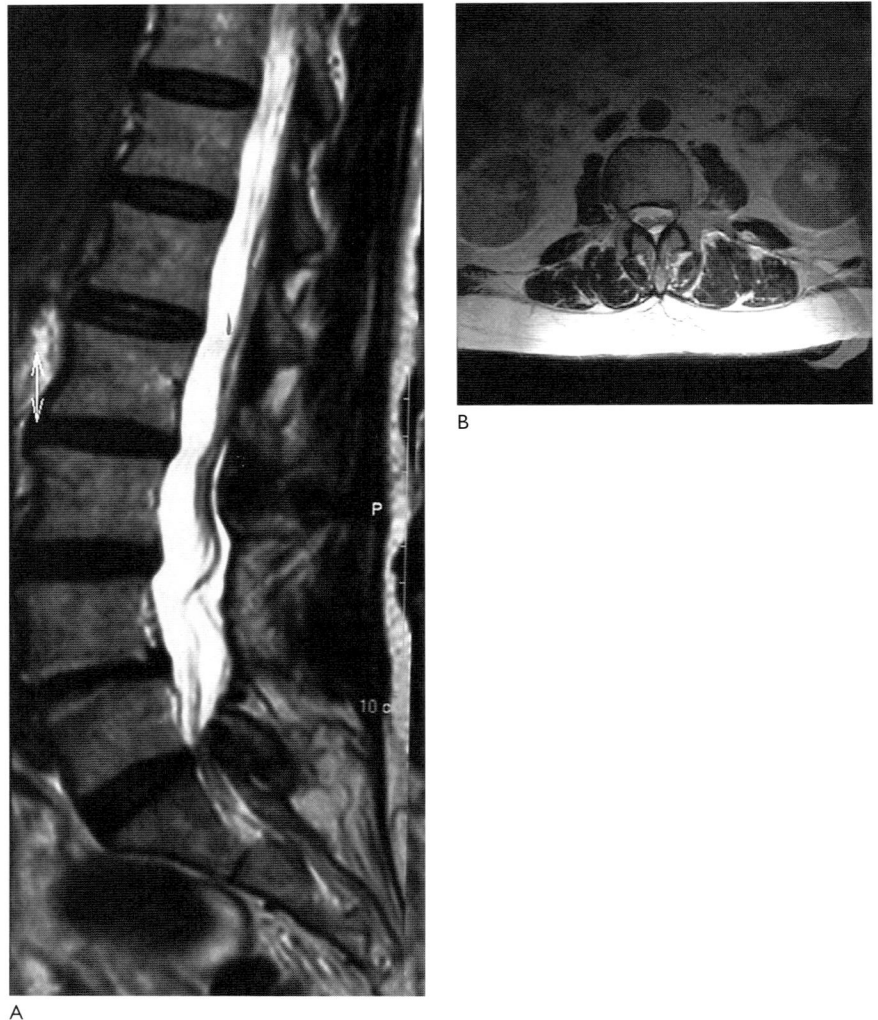

FIGURE 17-16
Arachnoiditis. (A) Sagittal T2WI showing nerve root clumping at the lower lumbar spine (following laminectomy). (B) Axial T2WI of the lumbar spine showing nerve root clumping indicating arachnoidis.

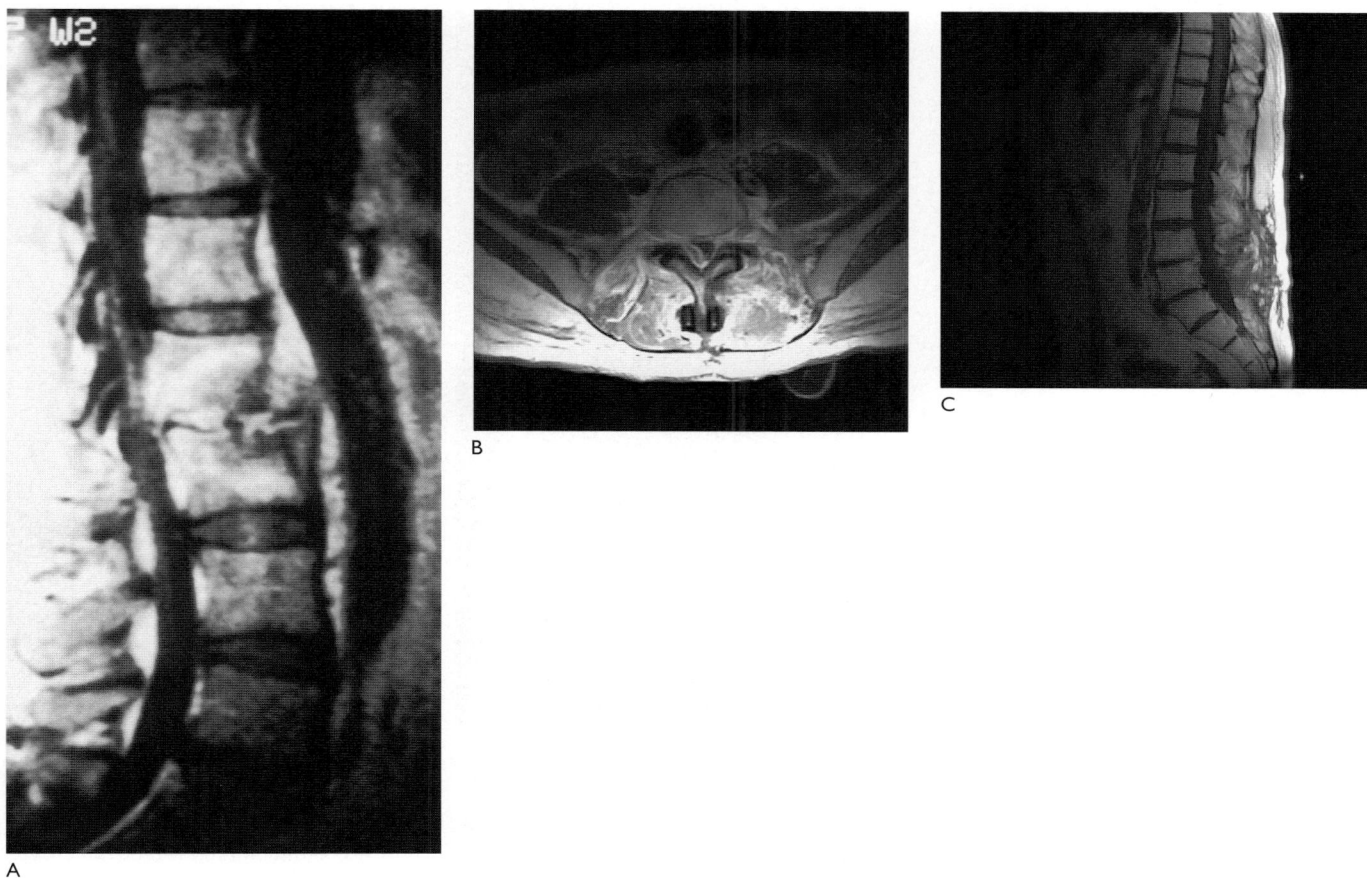

FIGURE 17-17

Postsurgical vertebral osteomyelitis and epidural abscess. (A) Sagittal T1WI showing endplate irregularities with bone edema suggesting spondylodiscitis (same patient as in Figure 17-8). (B) The best sequence for evaluating an epidural abscess is the postcontrast T1WI because the signals of an abscess and of CSF are both hyperintense, making it difficult to distinguish between them on T2WI. Following contrast administration enhancement at the periphery of the epidural abscess is noted. (C) Sagittal T1WI with IV contrast showing enhancement in both L4 and L5 vertebral bodies and a small epidural abscess at the L4-L5 disc level.

tomy was accompanied by endplate curettage, the MRI picture may mimic postoperative spondylodiscitis.

The best sequence for evaluating an epidural abscess is the contrast T1 study because the signals of an abscess and of CSF are both hyperintense on T2WI, making it difficult to distinguish between them on those images (Figures 17-17B and 17-17C). On the other hand, the two different enhancing T1 patterns contribute to the diagnosis of epidural abscesses in two ways: homogenous or heterogeneous enhancement in the granulomatous type of abscess, and the rim enhancement pattern typical of the liquefied type.

Pseudomeningoceles appear as well-circumscribed areas of abnormal fluid collection, similar to the appearance of CSF, which is located posterior to the dural sac (Figure 17-18). There are some variations in the signal intensity according to the composition of the fluid in the meningocele, including an increased signal on T1WI if the fluid is xanthochromatous. The normal posterior bulging of the thecal sac after a laminectomy should be taken into consideration in the differential diagnosis of a pseudomeningocele.

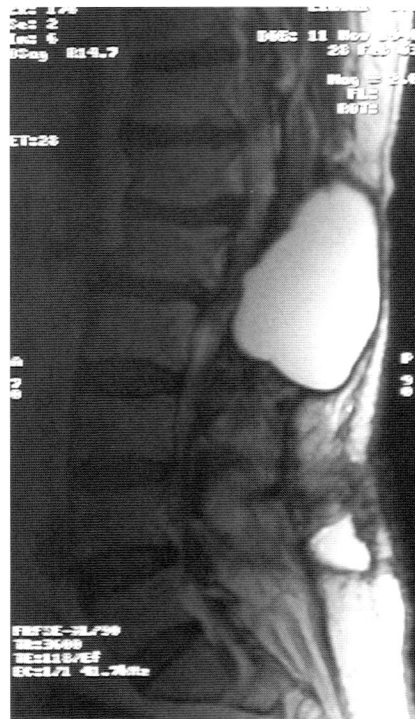

FIGURE 17-18
Postlaminectomy pseudomeningocele. Sagittal T2WI showing a hyperintense fluid collection.

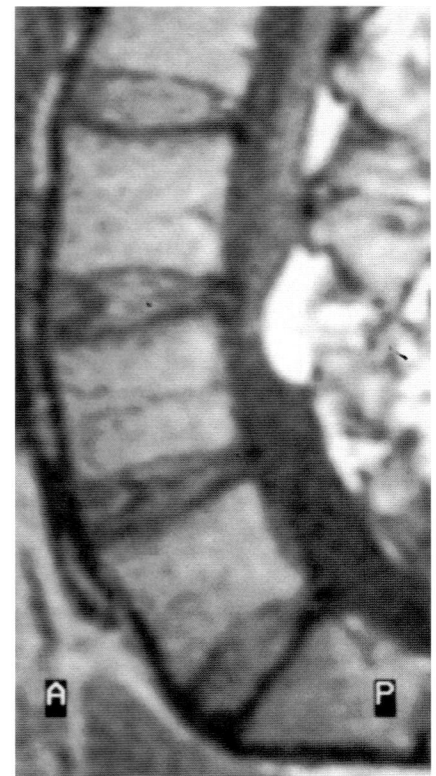

FIGURE 17-19
Postdiscectomy epidural fat graft. Sagittal T1WI of the lumbar spine showing a fat graft compressing the thecal sac.

Surgeons sometimes use autologous fat grafts to reduce postoperative epidural scarring. Occasionally, these grafts may compress the thecal sac (Figure 17-19). The characteristic appearance of fat grafts is on T1WI, in which they display as a high-signal-intensity mass.

Residual bony stenosis, in particular lateral recess stenosis, is the most frequent finding in symptomatic postsurgical patients. Bony stenosis may have a variable appearance on MRI due to the variability of the marrow content of the bone. Osteophytes or sclerotic bone will have a low signal intensity on both T1WI and T2WI. Bony spurs, on the other hand, may produce a bright signal on T1WI due to their rather fatty marrow.

MRI is also useful after fusion surgery with instrumentation. Placement of spinal implants degrades MRI quality by producing streak artifacts that may make the evaluation of the tissues adjacent to the implants challenging. Artifacts are especially prominent with stainless steel implants. In contrast, titanium implants cause minimal distortion in homogeneity, and spine-echo and FSE sequences show the least interference with metal implants. The use of drills in spine surgery, a technique that is associated with local shedding of metallic debris, may also cause artifacts on MRI.

Cervical Spine

The ability of MRI to evaluate the spinal cord is unsurpassed. On gradient echo images CSF demonstrates greater signal intensity than the cord, producing a pseudomyelographic effect. On the other hand gradient echo images tend to exaggerate the severity of bony canal stenosis. A better evaluation of the latter condition can be obtained by axial T1WI.

MRI images obtained shortly after ACDF surgery will display the graft material within the disc space or cage. The signal of the bone graft compared with that of the adjacent marrow will be varied. This varied appearance depends on the composition of the graft marrow (i.e., cellular, fatty). The endplates adjacent to the operated disc may display features of bone edema. Between 6 and 12 months following surgery, however, the MRI will usually display a bony union (i.e., a continuous marrow signal without evidence of the disc space). It will show either an isotense or a patchy increased signal on T1WI.

Gradient echo sequences are more sensitive to metal artifacts, and therefore are a poor choice for imaging the postoperative cervical spine. It is better to obtain the T2 FSE sequence, which is less susceptible to metal artifacts, thus facilitating the evaluation of residual stenosis or disc herniation (Figure 17-20). Gradient echo sequences also show artifacts within the spinal cord and so they, too, are not suitable for evaluating postoperative spinal cord pathology. Intravenous contrast adds no useful information to the evaluation of the postoperative degenerative cervical spine. Unlike the difficulty encountered in the lumbar spine, it is less problematic to distinguish between scar and recurrent disc herniation in the cervical area. Gadolinium does not cross an intact blood-brain barrier. Gadolinium concentrates in areas of inflammation and infection and in tumors, making these areas more conspicuous on T1WI.

Some shortcomings of the FSE sequence are the possibility to overlook a small hemorrhagic focus in the cord and the difficulty in differentiating between osteophytes and disc fragments. Three-dimensional imaging with a fast imaging sequence (gradient refocused echo imaging, GRE) is preferred to better delineate residual foraminal herniation.

Finally, MRI is useful in evaluating postoperative epidural hematoma (Figure 17-21), and in evaluating cord pathology, such as myelomalacia or cord atrophy.

Contraindications for Performing MRI

In addition to the classic contraindications to MRI (i.e., cardiac pacemakers, intracardiac wires, various types of artificial heart valves, intracranial aneurysm clips, ferromagnetic intraocular foreign bodies), the only absolute contraindication to MRI after surgery is an implanted epidural spinal cord stimulator.

PAIN PROVOCATION OR PAIN BLOCKADE

In addition to their application for radiological investigation, various image-controlled injection techniques are available to evaluate

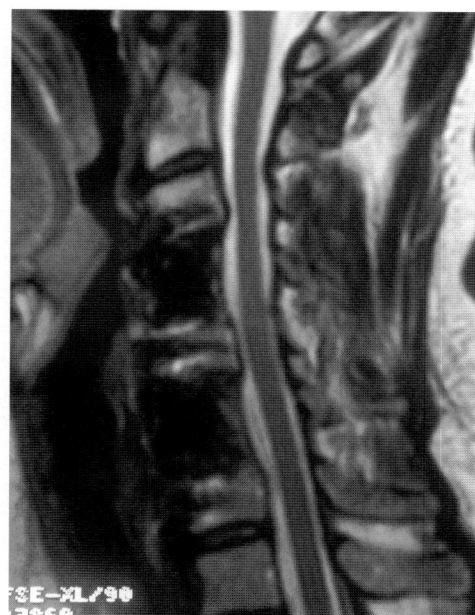

FIGURE 17-20
MRI with titanium implants. Sagittal MRI (T2 FSE) of the cervical spine after four-level decompression and fixation (corpectomy of C4 and C6, discectomies at C3-C4, C4-C5, C5-C6, and C6-C7). Despite the presence of titanium implants (mesh cages and anterior plate), cord decompression can be well visualized without interference of metal artifacts (same patient as in Figure 17-5).

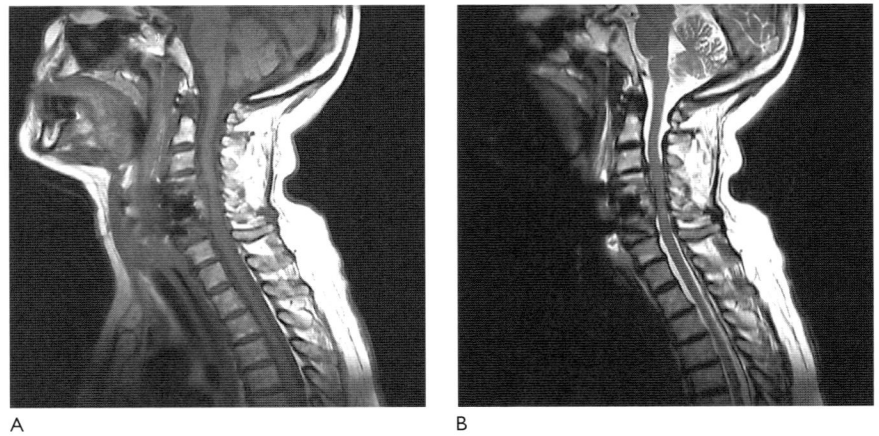

A   B

FIGURE 17-21
Epidural hematoma folowing cervical corpectomy. (A) T1 and (B) T2 FSE MRI of the cervical spine following C5 corpectomy with C4 through C6 fixation, showing a compressive epidural hematoma. Note also the high signal within the spinal cord indicating myelomalacia.

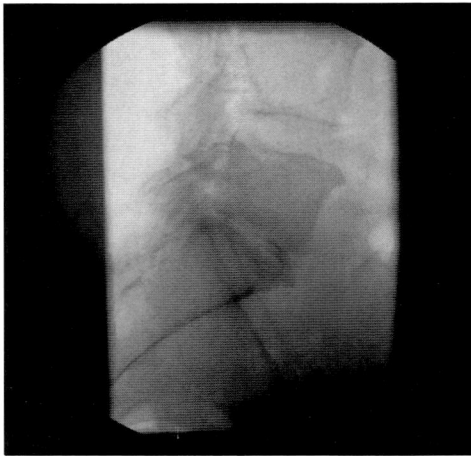

FIGURE 17-22
Lumbar discography. Lateral X-ray of the lumbar spine showing contrast dye in the L5-S1 space post discography. The patient has had a previous L5-S1 discectomy.

postoperative symptoms, such as root and facet blocks, sacroiliac joint injection, and discography (Figure 17-22). These diagnostic injections may complement the investigation of the symptomatic patient after surgery. Whereas root or facet blocks are intended to abolish the pain originating from the "blocked" anatomical structures, and thus imply that surgery on these structures will help the patient's symptoms, discography is intended to provoke the pain typically experienced by the patient. Again, performing surgery on the painful disc—be it fusion surgery, dynamic stabilization, or disc replacement—will abolish the patient's symptoms.

Selective nerve root blocks are performed to better localize the source of pain from an irritated or compressed spinal nerve root. Facet blocks or sacroiliac joint injections are used to identify the source of pain from these structures, because the radiological appearance of these joints alone is not diagnostic in localizing the pain source.

Discography must not only recreate the patient's concordant pain at a certain level, but it must also fail to reproduce the patient's symptoms at a different level. It is an interactive test that allows the patient's input when CT and MRI are equivocal in identifying the source of pain or when multilevel pathology is present. In addition to the reproduction of concordant pain, disc morphology may be evaluated by post-discography CT. Posterior annular tears will allow the contrast dye to leak into the epidural space, usually toward the side with radiculopathy, and confirm that a certain level is producing the patient's symptoms. Although some authors consider discography controversial at best, others claim a 94% clinical correlation between lumbar MRI and discography in degenerative lumbar disc disease. Similar data for cervical discography are still scarce.

Bibliography

Ashkenazi E, Smorgick Y, Rand N, Millgram MA, Mirovsky Y, Floman Y: Anterior decompression with combined corpectomies and discectomies in the management of multilevel cervical myelopathy: A hybrid decompression fixation technique. J Neurosurg Spine 3: 205–209, 2005.

Blumenthal SL, Gill K: Can lumbar spine radiographs accurately determine fusion in postoperative patients? Correlation of routine radiographs with a second surgical look at lumbar fusions. Spine 18: 1186–1189, 1993.

Boden SD, Davis DO, Dina TS, Parker CP, O'Malley S, Sunmer JL, Wiesel SW: Contrast-enhanced MR imaging performed after successful lumbar disc surgery: Prospective study. Radiology 182: 59–64, 1992.

Brantigan JW, Steffee AD, Lewis ML, Quinn LM, Persenaire JM: Lumbar interbody fusion using the Brantigan I/F cage for posterior lumbar interbody fusion and the variable pedicle screw placement system: Two year results from a Food and Drug Administration investigational device exemption clinical trial. Spine 25: 1437–1450, 2000.

Burton K, Kirkaldy-Willis WH, Yong Hing K, Heitoff KB: Causes of failure of surgery on the lumbar spine. Clin Orthop Rel Res 157: 191–199, 1981.

Coskun E, Suzer T, Topuz O, Zencir M, Pakdemirli E, Tahta K: Relationship between epidural fibrosis, pain, disability, and psychological factors after lumbar disc surgery. Eur Spine J 9: 218–223, 2000.

Davis RA: A long-term outcome of 984 surgically treated herniated lumbar discs. J Neurosurg 80: 415–421, 1994.

DePalma AF, Rothman RH: The nature of pseudoarthrosis. Clin Orthop Rel Res 59: 113–118, 1968.

Deutsch AL, Howard M, Dawson EG, et al: Lumbar spine following successful surgical discectomy. Magnetic resonance imaging features and implications. Spine 18: 1054–1060, 1993.

Dixon AK, Bannon RP: Computed tomography of the post-operative lumbar spine: The need for, and optional dose of, intravenous contrast medium. Brit J Radiol 60: 215–222, 1987.

Dreyfuss P, Schwartzer AC, Lau P, Bogduk N: Specificity of lumbar medial branch and L5 dorsal ramus blocks. A computed tomography study. Spine 22: 895–902, 1997.

Fandino J, Botana C, Viladrich A, Gomez-Bueno J: Reoperation after lumbardisc surgery. Results in 130 cases. Acta Neurochir 122: 102–104, 1993.

Findlay GF, Hall BI, Musa BS, Oliverira MD, Fear SC: A 10-year follow-up of the outcome of lumbar microdiscectomy. Spine 23: 1168–1171, 1998.

Glickstein MF, Sussman SK: Time dependent scar enhancement in magnetic resonance imaging of the postoperative lumbar spine. Skeletal Radiol 20: 333–337, 1991.

Gundry CR, Heithoff KB: Epidural hematoma of the lumbar spine: 18 surgically confirmed cases. Radiology 187: 427–431, 1993.

Hirabayashi K, Satomi K: Operative procedure and results of expansive open-door laminoplasty. Spine 13: 870–876, 1988.

Jinkins JR: Magnetic resonance imaging of benign nerve root enhancement in the unoperated and postoperative lumbosacral spine. Neuroimaging Clin N Am. 3: 525–541, 1993.

Kostuik JP: Failures after spinal fusion in Frymoyer JW, ed.: The adult spine: Principles and practice, 2nd edition. Lippincott-Raven, 1997.

Linson MA, Crowe CH: Comparison of magnetic resonance imaging and lumbar discography in the diagnosis of disc degeneration. Clin Orthop Rel Res 250: 160–163, 1990.

Maldjian C, Mesgarzadeh M, Tehranzadeh J: Diagnostic and therapeutic features of facet and sacroliac injections. Radiol Clin N Am 36: 497–508, 1998.

Mullin WJ, Heitoff KB, Gilbert TJ, Renfrew DL: Magnetic resonance evaluation of recurrent disk herniation: Is gadolinium necessary? Spine 25: 1493–1499, 2000.

Nachemson AL: Lumbar discography—where are we today. Spine 14: 555–557, 1989.

Palestro CJ, Torres MA. Radionuclide imaging in orthopedic infections. Semin Nucl Med 28: 334–345, 1997.

Post MJD, Sze G, Quencer RM, Eismont FJ, Green BA, Gahbauer H: Gadolinium-enhanced MR in spinal infection. J Comput Assist Tomogr 14: 721–729, 1990.

Ross JS: Newer sequences for spinal MRI: Smorgasbord or succotash of acronyms? Am J Neuroradiol 20: 361–373, 1999.

Ross JS, Masaryk TJ, Modic MT et al.: Lumbar spine: Postoperative assessment with surface coils MR imaging. Radiology 164: 851–860, 1987.

Ross JS, Masaryk TJ, Modic MT et al.: MR imaging of lumbar arachnoiditis. Am J Roentgenol 149: 1025–1032, 1987.

Ross JS, Masaryk TJ, Modic MT, Delamater R, Bohlman H, Wilbur G, Kaufman B: MR imaging of lumbar arachnoiditis. Am J Roentgenol 149: 1025–1032, 1987.

Ross JS, Masaryk TJ, Schrader M, Gentili A, Bohlman H, Modic MT: MR imaging of the postoperative lumbar spine: Assessment with gadopentetate dimeglumine. Am J Roentgenol 155: 867–872, 1990.

Ross JS, Masaryk TJ, Schrader M, et al.: MR imaging of the postoperative lumbar spine: assessment with gadopentate dimeglumine. Am J Neuroradiol 11: 771–776, 1990.

Ross JS, Robertson JT, Fredrickson RCA, Petrie JL, Obuchowski N, Modic MT, de Tribolet N: Association between peridural scar and recurrent radicular pain after lumbar discectomy: Magnetic resonance evaluation. Neurosurgery 38: 855–863, 1996.

Rudisch A, Kremser C, Peer S, Katherin A, Judmaier W, Daniaux H: Metallic artifacts in magnetic resonance imaging of patients with spinal fusion: A comparison of implant materials and imaging sequences. Spine 23: 692–699, 1998.

Schellhas K, Smith M, Grundy C, Pollei S: Cervical discogenic pain: Prospective correlation of MRI and discography in asymptomatic subjects and pain sufferers. Spine 21: 300–312, 1996.

Schubiger O, Valavanis A: CT differentiation between disc herniation and postoperative scar formation. The value of contrast enhancement. Neuroradiology 22: 251–254, 1980.

Schwartz AJ: Imaging of the degenerative cervical spine, in Floman Y, Onesti ST, Ashkenazi E: Degenerative disc disease of the cervical spine. Spine: State of the Art Review 14: 545–570, 2000.

Schwarzenbach O, Berlemann U, Jost B, Visarius H, Arm E, Langlotz F, Nolte LP, Ozdoba C: Accuracy of computer-assisted pedicle screw placement: An in vivo computed tomography analysis. Spine 22: 452–458, 1997.

Tehranzadeh J: Discography 2000. Radiol Clin N Am 36: 463–495, 1998.

Teplick JG, Haskin ME: Computed tomography of the postoperative lumbar spine. Am J Roentgenol 141: 865–884, 1983.

Teplick JG, Haskin ME: CT of the postoperative lumbar spine. Radiol Clin N Am 21: 395–420, 1983.

Thalgott JS, Xiongsheng C, Giuffre JM: Single stage anterior ccervical reconstruction with titanium mesh cage, local bone graft and anterior plating. Spine J 3: 294–300, 2003.

Vanderburg DF, Kelly WM: Radiographic assessment of discogenic disease of the spine. Neurosurg Clin N Am 4: 13–33, 1993.

Van Goethem JWM, Van de Kelft E, Biltjes IGGM, et al.: MR findings after successful lumbar discectomy. Neuroradiology 38: S90–S96, 1996.

Watanabe N, Ogura T, Komori K, et al.: Epidural hematoma of the lumbar spine, simulating extruded lumbar disk herniation: Clinical, discographic and enhanced magnetic resonance imaging features. Spine 22: 105–109, 1997.

Zinreich SJ, Long DM, Davis R, Quinn CB, McAfee PC, Wang H: Three dimensional CT imaging in postsurgical "failed back" syndrome. J Comput Assist Tomogr 14: 574–580, 1990.

SPINAL INJECTIONS AND MINIMALLY INVASIVE PROCEDURES

18

Fluoroscopically guided precision injections can aid both in localizing the pain-generating structures (diagnostic) and in the treatment of several painful conditions (therapeutic) of the spine. The concept of diagnostic precision injection blocks was developed with the increasing popularity of the fluoroscope and the realization that there are no diagnostic tools to precisely determine pain-generating pathology or structures. The use of fluoroscopy is absolutely necessary; it was documented that up to 30% of nonfluoroscopically (blind) simple interlaminar injections are off the target. It is inconceivable that facet joints or sacroiliac joints could be blocked reliably in a blind fashion. Using a diagnostic workup protocol and flow sheet can standardize spine pain workup and serve as a base for treatment and for reproducible research.

For therapeutic injections the precise localization of the needle tip is necessary if complications are to be avoided and smaller, more circumscribed pathologies, such as neurotomy of the medial branch of the posterior division of the spinal nerve or drainage of a facet joint synovial cyst, are to be treated.

Common diagnostic injections will be discussed first, followed by examples of therapeutic injections.

MATERIALS AND GENERAL PROCEDURE NOTES

For fluoroscopy, the following materials are required:

- A C-arm or biplane fluoroscope is necessary for proper placement of the needle.
- A fluoroscopically transparent procedure table is required. It is useful to have an adjustable table or to use an assortment of transparent bolsters and pillows to properly position the patient.
- An assortment of needles of different gages, lengths, and tip configurations facilitates a variety of procedures.
- Nonionic iodinated contrast may be injected after the initial placement of the needle tip to document its position

and to exclude intravascular placement. The amount of contrast necessary to reach the intended structures to treat will determine the optimal volume of injectate to use for the specific diagnostic injection.

- The injectate solutions should be preservative-free solutions to avoid potential seizures and arachnoiditis.
- Small particulate steroids such as triamcinolone acetonide are used for injections of the lumbar spine.
- Fine particulate steroids such as betamethasone or non-particulate steroid injectates that are usually prepared by specialized pharmacies and are not commercially available are used for injections of the cervical spine.

Sterility is another important consideration. Observation of aseptic local technique is fundamental for these procedures. It implies sterile gloves and equipment and the formation of a sterile field after aseptic preparation of the skin. Generally three Betadine passes are used as well as alcohol or Hibiclean scrub.

DIAGNOSTIC INJECTIONS

These injections are intended to selectively anesthetize (block) potential pain-generating structures, or to reproduce the patient's characteristic pain. They are particularly useful in patients with multi-level pathology and help localize the pain generator. If one can selectively "block" the pain fibers in a structure so that the characteristically usual pain of the patient disappears, or if one can selectively stimulate a structure and reproduce the same characteristically usual pain, then it is highly likely that the pain-generating structure was precisely localized and diagnosed. Usually after a block injection the patient is asked to get up from the procedure table and reproduce the preinjection pain-generating movement. A temporal "pain diagram" is given to the patient to mark the pain level every half hour for at least four hours after the block. A clear drop in the preblock pain level is considered diagnostic. This usually means a complete elimination of the pain or reduction of more than five levels on a pain visual analog scale. Because of almost 30% placebo effect for injections, it is advisable to repeat the block a second time to reproduce and confirm the block result.

Precision fluoroscopically guided injections are the main tool in the diagnostic workup of chronic low back pain of more than 12 weeks duration. Statistically the pain generator is discogenic in 40%, zygoapopheseal (Z) joint in 15–20%, and sacroiliac joint in 15% of cases. As in other medical pathologies, the best successful treatment depends on precise diagnosis of the pain-generating structure. In today's medical reality there is no other reliable diagnostic tool to determine the pain-causing anatomical structure comparable to precision diagnostic blocks.

The following most common diagnostic precision injections will be described:

- Selective spinal nerve block
- Sacroiliac joint block

- Intra-articular zygoapopheseal joint (ZJ) block
- Medial branch (MB) nerve blocks
- Discogram and disc provocation.

Selective Spinal Nerve Block

This is a commonly performed precision injection that utilizes injection of an anesthetic solution near the spinal nerve to block the pain transmission of only one spinal nerve.

Indications Selective spinal nerve blocks are indicated to precisely determine the spinal nerve mostly involved in the patient's pain picture. This information is necessary when multilevel pathology can cause nerve irritation and pain, such as in multilevel foraminal stenosis from diverse causes, or when the clinical picture is only in part radicular and there is a need to distinguish referred pain from joints or disc versus pure radicular pain from spinal nerve involvement. Better surgical outcome may be expected when the painful level and structure are identified.

Procedure The nerve block is being achieved by placing the needle tip in proximity to the spinal nerve dorsal root ganglion (DRG) or just distal to the external opening of the intervertebral foramen at the nerve sleeve level. The nerve or DRG should be blocked by no more than one-half milliliter (mL) of anesthetic so that no spillover into the epidural space should occur. This prevents blocking of multiple nerve roots, which would defeat the selectivity of the diagnostic block. Injecting nonionic contrast before the injection of the anesthetic block is useful for documentation of the needle tip position in relationship to the spinal nerve sleeve and epidural space, to exclude intravascular placement, and to determine the optimal volume of anesthetic required to cover the desired spinal nerve DRG or root. After the block, the patient is instructed to fill out a temporal pain diagram.

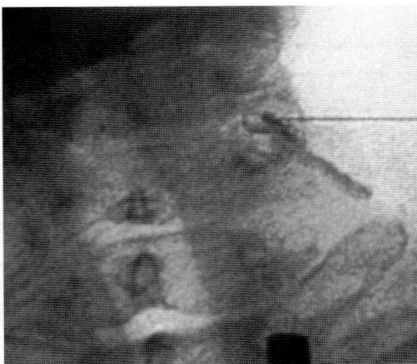

FIGURE 18-1
Cervical selective spinal nerve block, anteroposterior view.

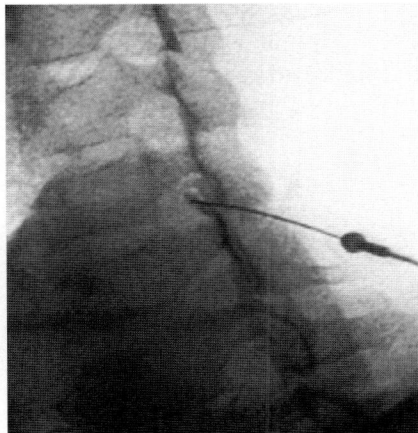

FIGURE 18-2
Cervical selective spinal nerve block, lateral view.

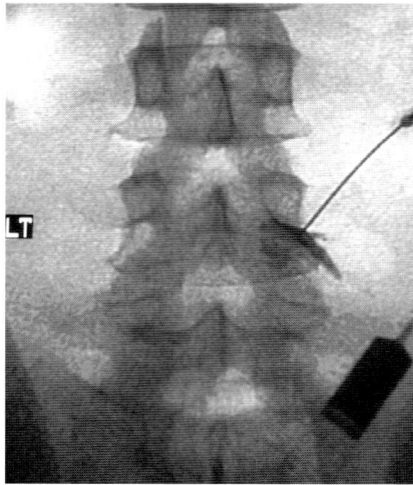

FIGURE 18-3
Lumbar selective spinal nerve block,
anteroposterior view.

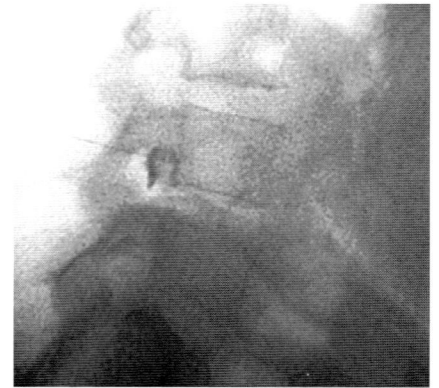

FIGURE 18-4
Lumbar selective spinal nerve block, lateral view.

A selective spinal nerve block can be done at the cervical (Figures 18-1 and 18-2), thoracic, lumbar (Figures 18-3 and 18-4), and
sacral spinal levels.

Sacroiliac Joint Block

The intra-articular injection of an anesthetic solution is utilized
to block the pain generation from this joint.

Indications   A sacroiliac joint block is used to determine the role of
this joint in the pain picture, especially in chronic low back pain workup.

Procedure   The caudal portion of the joint is accessed under fluoroscopy, and 0.5 to 1 mL of contrast material is injected to visualize an arthrogram (Figures 18-5 and 18-6). Generally 1 to 2 mL of local anesthetic is
injected, and the patient is instructed to fill out the temporal pain diagram.

Intra-articular Zygoapophyseal Joint (ZJ) Block

The intra-articular injection of an anesthetic solution is utilized
to block the pain generation from this joint.

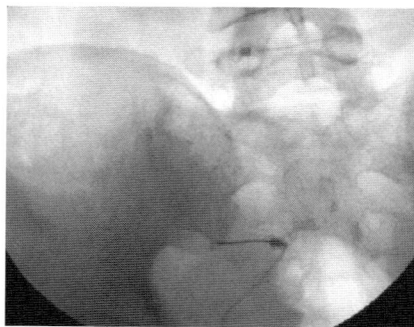

FIGURE 18-5
Sacroiliac joint block, anteroposterior
view.

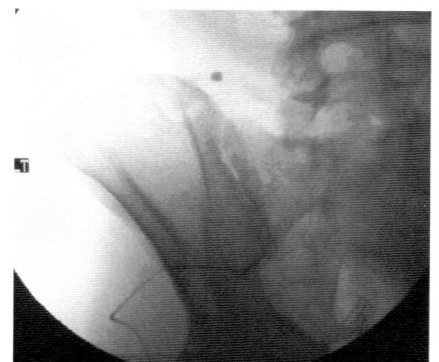

FIGURE 18-6
Sacroiliac joint block, oblique view.

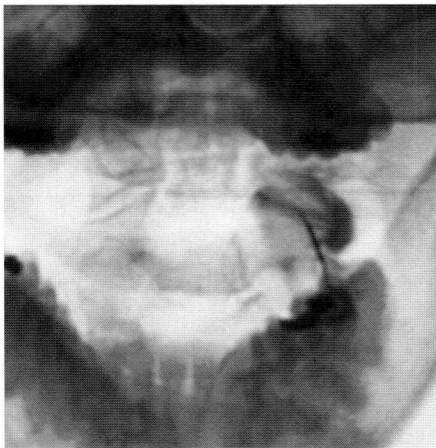

FIGURE 18-7
Cervical C1-C2 Z joint block, antero-posterior view.

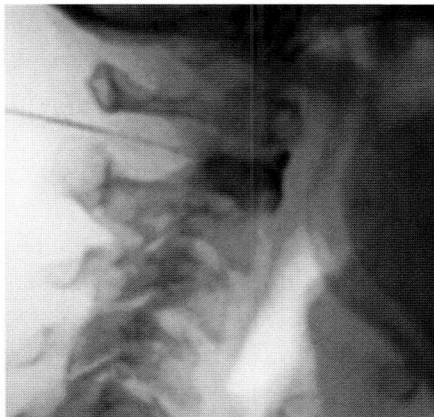

FIGURE 18-8
Cervical C1-C2 Z joint block, lateral view.

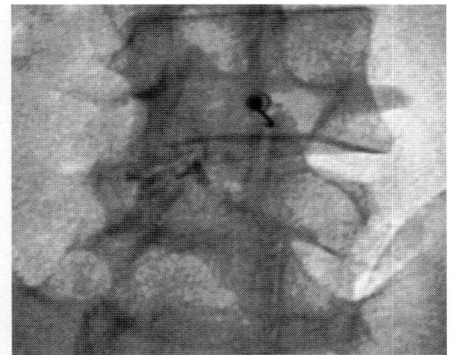

FIGURE 18-9
Lumbar Z joint block, oblique view.

Indications   The ZJ block is used in the workup of chronic low back pain or in case of concomitant radiographic picture of pathology at the spinal nerve level and of the ZJ with a nonclassic radicular-type pain distribution. At times, joint aspiration can shed light on unexpected pathology, such as crystal arthropathy.

Procedure   Under fluoroscopy the Z joint is accessed by a 25-gage needle, and 0.3 mL of contrast is injected to visualize an arthrogram. Generally 0.5 to 1 mL of local anesthetic is then injected, and the patient is instructed to fill out a temporal pain diagram.

The ZJ block can be performed at the cervical (Figures 18-7 and 18-8), thoracic, and lumbar (Figure 18-9) levels.

Medial Branch (MB) Nerve Block

An anesthetic solution injected near these nerves will block the pain transmission from the respective ZJ.

Indications   Indications for the MB nerve block are the same as for the ZJ block. The MB nerve block is used when it is technically difficult to access the Z joint. As each Z joint is innervated by two medial branch (MB) nerves; both nerves must be blocked to have an effective diagnostic block of the Z joint.

Procedure   Because of the close proximity of the MB nerves to the spinal nerves, only a small amount of anesthetic (0.25 to 0.5 mL) is to be deposited on each nerve to avoid spillover on the spinal nerve. It is important to first inject 0.1 to 0.2 mL of contrast material to make sure the needle tip is not intravascular or close to the spinal nerve.

Under fluoroscopy the needle tip is being advanced to the groove at the junction of the superior articular process (SAP) and the transverse process (TP) at the intermamillary ligament area. Block of the MB nerves can be done at the cervical and lumbar (Figures 18-10 and 18-11) levels.

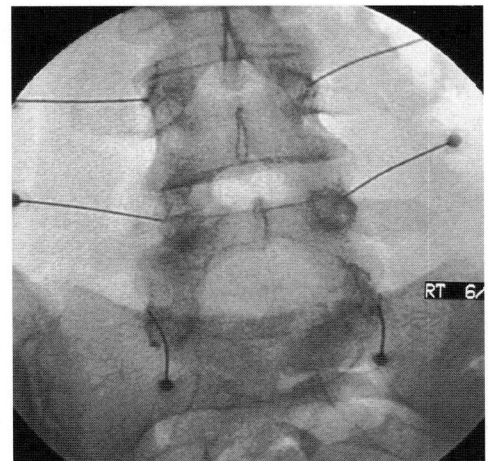

FIGURE 18-10
Medial branch nerve block, lumbar, anteroposterior view.

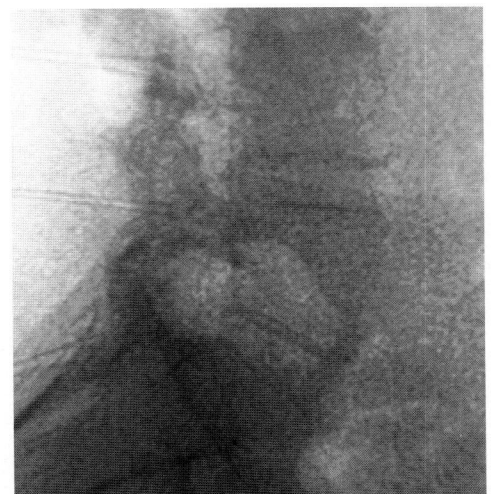

FIGURE 18-11
Medial branch nerve block, lumbar, lateral view.

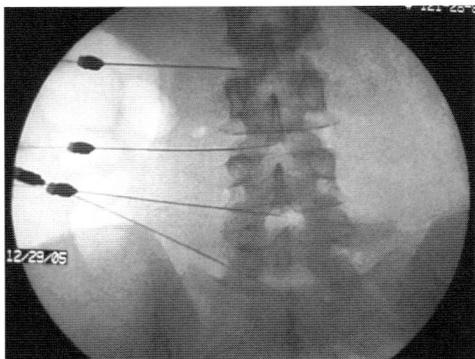

FIGURE 18-12
Needle placement for discogram, lumbar, anteroposterior view.

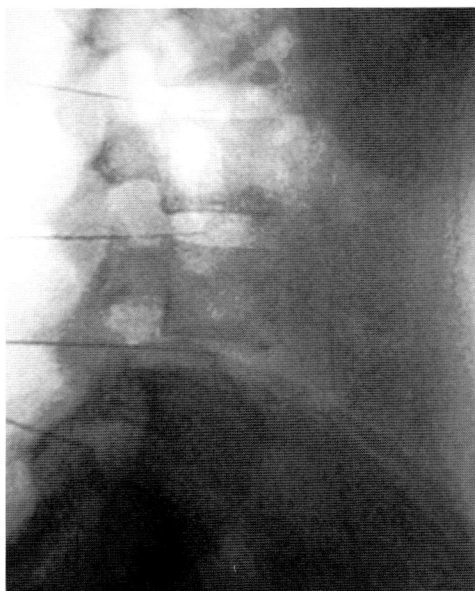

FIGURE 18-13
Needle placement for discogram, lumbar, lateral view.

Discogram and Disc Provocation

Intradiscal injection of contrast will provoke characteristic pain and will allow for a radiographic visualization of the annular tear and disc protrusion.

Indications Often, multilevel disc pathology is observed on MRI, and the determination of the painful pathologic disc is necessary for planning the appropriate treatment or surgical intervention. Discogram is necessary in the workup of chronic back pain when Z joint or SI joint pathology is also present. In case of discogenic low back pain from an internal disc disruption, the MRI might be negative and only a discogram and provocation may pinpoint the cause of the pain.

Procedure Intravenous antibiotics are administered prior to the procedure to minimize the chances of infection. A needle is introduced into the center of the disc (Figures 18-12 and 18-13). The disc is then injected with a mixture of contrast and antibiotic solution via a graded syringe connected to a pressure monitor. Recording is made of the intradiscal pressures, volume injected, and pain provocation and concordance. Important is the pressure above the opening pressure at which the concordant pain was evoked. Less than 25 pounds per square inch (psi) differential pressure indicates certainty of a sensitized disc. The pattern of the contrast material in the disc is often classified using the Dallas classification. Several consecutive discs are injected till a normal disc is identified. After the needles are removed a computerized tomography (CT) scan is being taken to better visualize tears or disruptions in the annulus.

Discogram is performed routinely in the cervical, thoracic, and lumbar (Figures 18-14 through 18-18) discs.

THERAPEUTIC INJECTIONS AND INTERVENTIONS

Fluoroscopically guided precision therapeutic injections are used to treat painful conditions of the spine. Steroid and anesthetic solu-

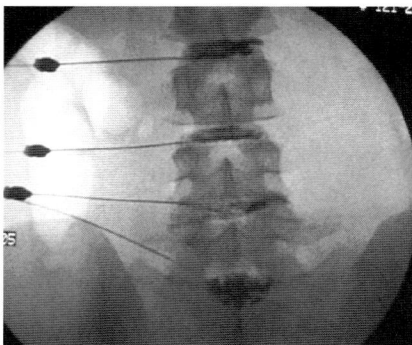

FIGURE 18-14
Discogram, lumbar, anteroposterior view.

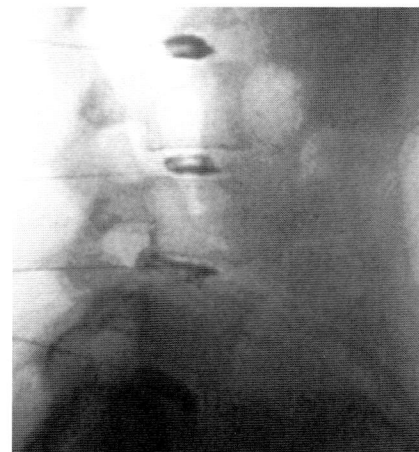

FIGURE 18-15
Discogram, lumbar, lateral view.

FIGURE 18-17
CT-discogram, lumbar, lateral view.

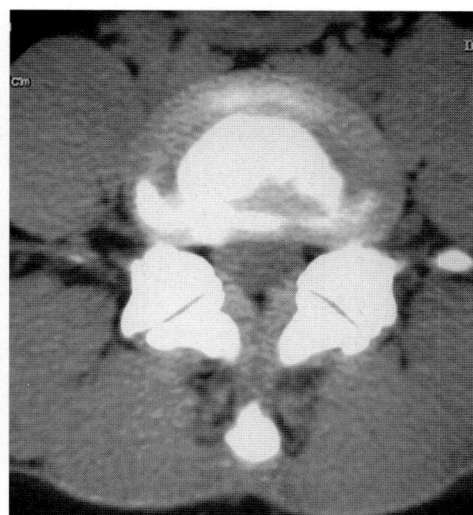

FIGURE 18-18
CT-discogram, lumbar, coronal view.

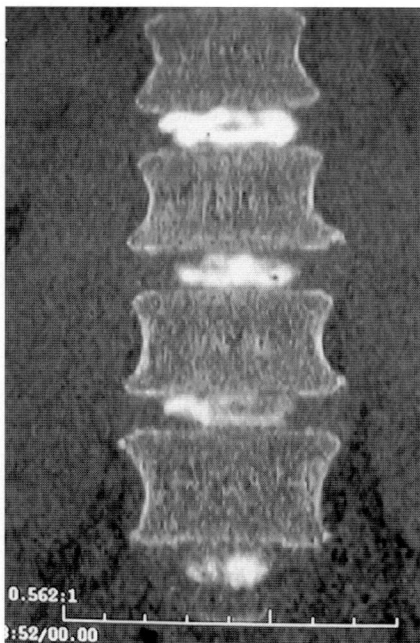

FIGURE 18-16
CT-discogram, lumbar, anteroposterior view.

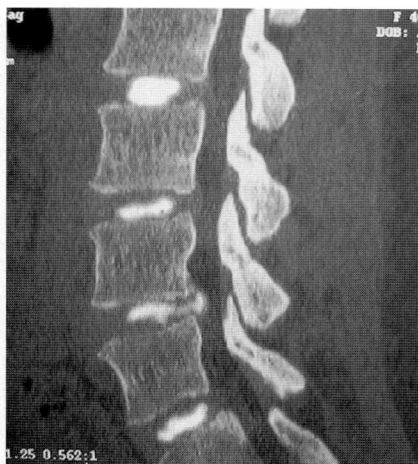

tions are used to control the pain. It is believed that it is more effective to deposit the steroids as close as possible to the pathologic processes that are thought to cause the pain.

The use of fluoroscopy allows safe deposition of steroids and anesthetic solutions in the anterior or posterior epidural space of the vertebral canal or in the epidural space of the spinal nerve sleeves.

Common fluoroscopically guided precision therapeutic injections include the following:

- Interlaminar epidural steroid injection
- Caudal epidural steroid injection
- Transforaminal epidural steroid injection
- Selective spinal nerve sleeve steroid injection
- Z joint intra-articular injection
- SI joint intra-articular injection

Fluoroscopy allows performing percutaneous interventions that require precision localization of a needle tip at the level of the targeted structure.

Common fluoroscopically guided interventions include the following:

- Radiofrequency (RF) neurotomy
- Intradiscal electrothermal therapy (IDET)
- Annuloplasty
- Lyses of adhesions
- Percutaneous disc decompression
- Spinal cord stimulation

Interlaminar Epidural Steroid Injection

Deposition of a steroid and local anesthetic solution in the dorsal epidural space via a posterior approach placing the needle between the laminas.

Indications   The main indication is deposition of steroids in the dorsal epidural space. It is usually not a technique that can deposit the steroids near the pain-generating structure, but it is the most commonly performed procedure in pain control.

Procedure   The needle is introduced into the dorsal epidural space using an interlaminar approach (Figures 18-19 through 18-23). and identifying the epidural space utilizing the loss of resistance technique. Some practitioners do not use fluoroscopy for this technique ("blind" technique) even though it has been demonstrated that the blind technique leads to up to 30% mislocalization of the needle.

Caudal Epidural Steroid Injection

Deposition of a steroid and local anesthetic solution in the epidural space via a caudal approach placing the needle through the sacral epidural space.

Indications   The main indication for caudal epidural steroid injection is for the deposition of steroids in the dorsal epidural space of the sacral and lumbar spine. The injectate usually reaches up to L3 level and not above. It is a useful technique when there is severe ste-

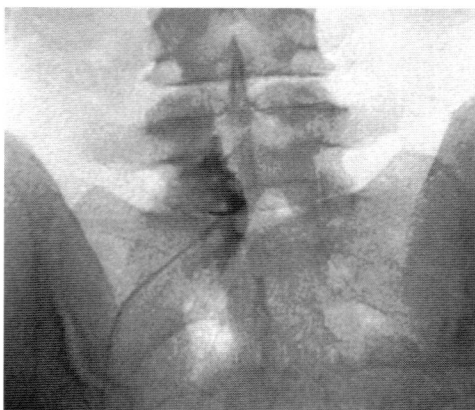

FIGURE 18-19
Interlaminar epidural injection, lumbar, anteroposterior view.

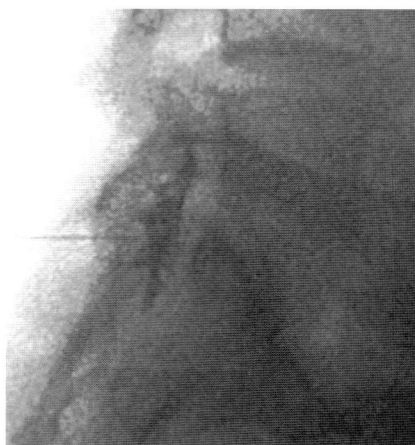

FIGURE 18-20
Interlaminar epidural injection, lumbar, lateral view.

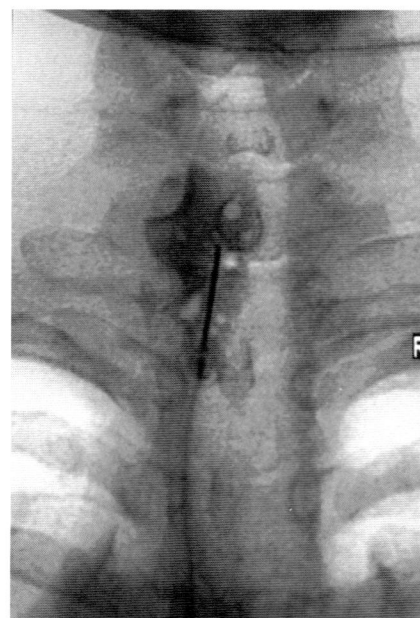

FIGURE 18-21
Interlaminar epidural injection, cervical, anteroposterior view.

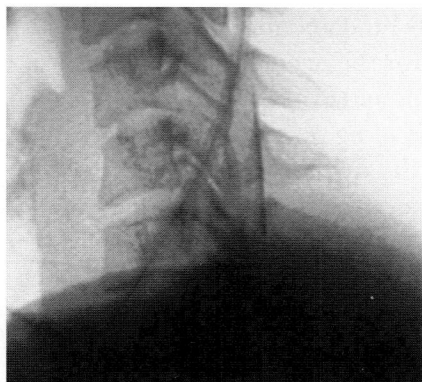

FIGURE 18-22
Interlaminar epidural injection, cervical, lateral view.

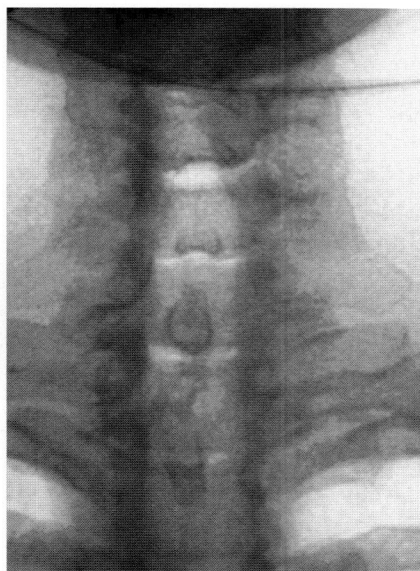

FIGURE 18-23
Interlaminal epidural injection, cervical, anteroposterior view of epidurogram.

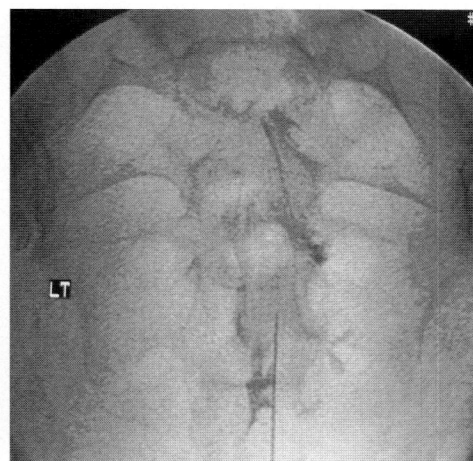

FIGURE 18-24
Caudal epidural injection, anteroposterior view.

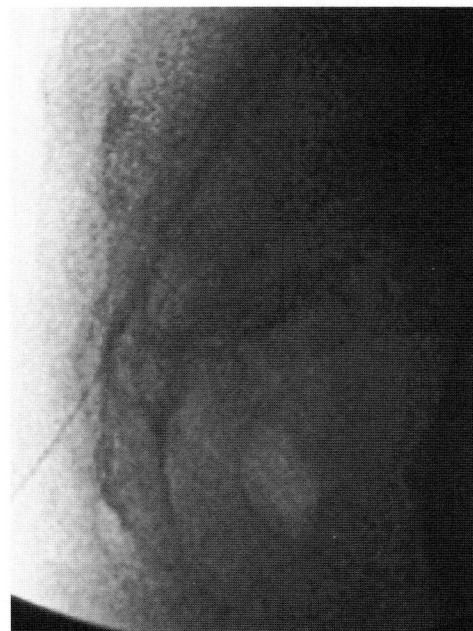

FIGURE 18-25
Caudal epidural injection, lateral view.

nosis of the lumbar spine with abundant spondylotic changes that prevent safe interlaminar or transforaminal injection of steroids. The use of fluoroscopy is helpful in this injection to document proper spread of the injectate and to exclude intravascular injection that will negate the localized effects of the steroids.

Procedure Aseptic skin preparation requires meticulous technique and extra passes with the aseptic solutions. The needle is inserted and advanced toward the notch palpated between the sacral cornucolas. The needle should penetrate the ligament covering the sacral hiatus and advanced in a cephalic direction, not above the S2 foramen where the dural sac ends (Figures 18-24 and 18-25). The needle can be directed to either side to selectively direct the injectate toward the most affected side. Larger volumes of injectate are necessary to reach the mid lumbar spine, a fact that will dilute the injectate and diminish the selectivity of the injection.

Transforaminal Epidural Steroid Injection

Deposition of a steroid and local anesthetic solution in the ventral epidural space via the intervertebral neural foramen.

Indications The main indication for transforaminal epidural steroid injection is for the deposition of steroids in the ventral epidural space. It is usually performed to treat pain caused by annulus and posterior longitudinal ligament (PLL) pathology such as tears, bulges, and herniations. The transforaminal approach was also shown to be more effective than the interlaminar epidural approach in treatment of pain of patients with spinal stenosis.

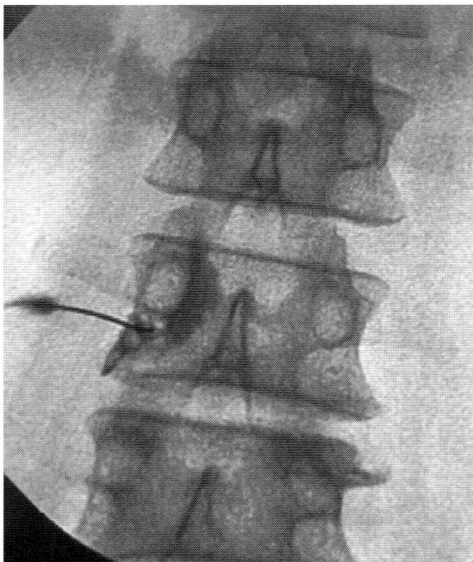

FIGURE 18-26
Transforaminal epidural injection, lumbar, anteroposterior view.

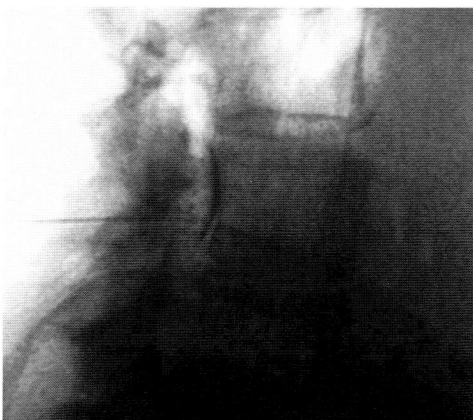

FIGURE 18-27
Transforaminal epidural injection, lumbar, lateral view.

Procedure   Use of fluoroscopy is fundamental for the proper execution of this procedure. The target for the needle tip is in close proximity to the spinal nerve and its vessels and other vital structures, such as the pleura or the spinal cord, depending on the spinal segment. In the cervical spine the target point is the midpoint of the dorsal aspect of the intervertebral foramen in a lateral view and the midfacet pillar line in an anterior-posterior view.

In the thoracic spine the target point for the location of the needle tip is the intervertebral foramen medial to the pleural lines. In the lumbar spine the target point for the location of the needle tip is the midpoint of the infrapedicle area in the so called "six o'clock position" in the "safe triangle" (Figures 18-26 and 18-27). The "safe triangle" is the area limited between the lateral border of the vertebra, the spinal nerve, and the pedicle.

Selective Spinal Nerve Sleeve Steroid Injection

Deposition of a steroid and local anesthetic solution at the spinal nerve sleeve near the intervertebral neural foramen.

Indications   The principal indication is for the deposition of steroids in the vicinity of a specific spinal nerve that is causing pain. The effect of the steroids is expected at the level of the spinal nerve and the DRG. Frequently, multiple nerves are selectively injected if they are involved in symptom generation. The common pathologies affecting the spinal nerves are herniated discs and foraminal stenosis.

Procedure   The placement of the needle is similar to the transforaminal approach, except the needle tip is placed more distally in the foramen at the level of the cervical and lumbar spine. The knowledge of the anatomical position of the spinal nerve in relation to the pedicle and the SAP is important to obtain good coverage of the specific spinal nerve. This relationship varies at different anatomical levels. In the lumbar spine the course of the spinal nerve as it exits from the intervertebral foramen is becoming less vertical and more transverse in the lower lumbar levels (see Figures 18-1 through 18-4).

Z Joint Intra-articular Injection

Deposition of a steroid and anesthetic solution into the joint.

Indications   Painful conditions originating in the Z joint such as synovitis or arthritis, and localized by a previous block, can be controlled by intra-articular injection of steroids. These injections can be repeated, but if the effect is only temporary than radiofrequency neurotomy of the medial branches may give a longer pain relief period.

Procedure   Intra-articular injections can be done at the cervical, thoracic, and lumbar levels. At times it is difficult to place the needle into the joint as it might be deformed from an arthritic process or be very curved in a transverse plane. It might be easier in these cases to place the needle in the inferior recess of the joint (see Figures 18-7 through 18-9). Use of contrast is helpful in confirming the intra-articular placement of the needle tip. Less than 1 mL of contrast is necessary to obtain a characteristic arthrogram. Volume of less than 1 mL of steroid is usually sufficient as therapeutic modality.

SI Joint Intra-articular Injection

Deposition of a steroid and anesthetic solution into the joint.

Indications Pain originating from the SI joint diagnosed by previous SI joint block is the indication for an SI joint intra-articular injection. Steroids or hyaluronidase can be injected intra-articularly to control the pain.

Procedure Use of fluoroscopy is necessary to place the needle tip in the distal centimeter of the joint line (see Figures 18-5 and 18-6). About 1 mL of contrast will demonstrate an arthrogram and confirm intra-articular placement of the needle.

RF Neurotomy

RF energy is used to coagulate the nerves involved in the pain pathway.

Indications The indications for RF neurotomy are painful conditions originating in the Z or SI joints or a spinal nerve. Neurotomy of the two medial branch nerves innervating the affected joint will reduce the pain for many months or years. RF neurotomy of a spinal nerve is done in rare cases and only after a diagnostic block has confirmed and localized the level of the painful nerve. Usually this is done at the C2 and C3 nerves. Paresthesias occur in the related dermatome. Neuritis or formation of a neuroma are possible complications.

Procedure The RF needle is placed as close as possible to the nerve to ablate. Sensory stimulation at 50 Hz followed by motor stimulation at 2 Hz is necessary to eliminate possible damage to intact spinal nerves and to confirm optimal positioning of the RF needle near the involved nerve (Figure 18-28). The needle tip is than heated to 80°C for one minute. Three or four lesions are necessary at each level to improve the chances of an effective neurotomy. Sacral medial branch neurotomy at several levels is necessary to denervate the SI joint.

Intradiscal Electrothermal Therapy (IDET)

Thermal energy is brought into the "painful" invertebral lumbar disc and applied under controlled conditions.

Indications The main indication for IDET is discogenic pain. A discogram is required to show internal disc disruption or annular tear with "bulging" of the disc or a nonextruded herniated disc.

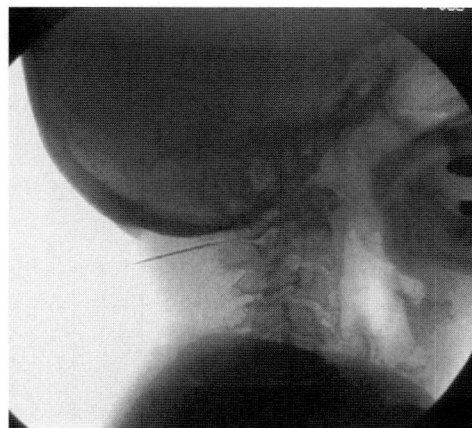

FIGURE 18-28
RF neurotomy, C2.

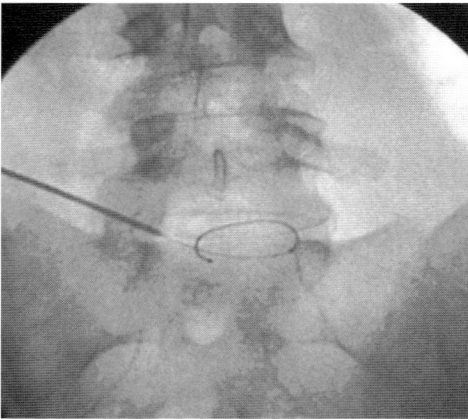

FIGURE 18-29
IDET, anteroposterior view.

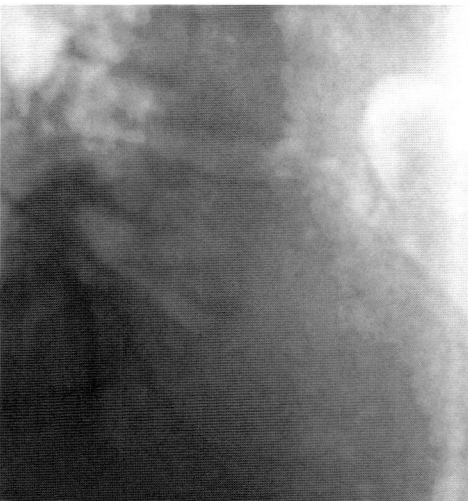

FIGURE 18-30
IDET, lateral view.

Procedure A needle is introduced into the disc and advanced to a point lateral to the center (Figures 18-29 and 18-30). A catheter is introduced through the needle and advanced. The tip reflects on the inner annular wall and is advanced to an area beyond the annular tear or bulge. Part of the catheter has a thermal element that is heated to 90°C. At times it is necessary to repeat the procedure, introducing the needle into the opposite side in order to cover the entire posterior annular part with the thermal catheter. After the procedure there is usually low back pain for about three weeks. The patient should abstain from stressing the lower back and should use a brace temporarily.

Annuloplasty

Thermal energy is brought into the "painful" lumbar disc annulus and applied under controlled conditions near the annular tear.

Indications Annuloplasty is indicated in the case of a localized annular tear.

Procedure The procedure is similar to IDET, but the thermal catheter is navigated into the annulus near the painful tear.

Lyses of Adhesions

The adhesions around spinal nerves or the epidural space are "opened" and lysed via hydraulic and mechanical force applied by a catheter tip introduced via a needle.

Indications The indications for lyses of adhesions are the presence of fibrosis and scar tissue that entrap the spinal nerve root causing radicular pain and radiculopathy. An epidurogram is necessary prior to performing lyses of adhesions in order to localize the involved area and document at least one "patent" foramen. At least one patent foramen is necessary to allow decompression of the hydraulic pressure formed inside the epidural space during the procedure. This is especially important at the cervical spine that contains the "unforgiving" cervical spinal cord.

Procedure An epidurogram is performed initially to visualize adhesions or block (Figure 18-31). A 16-gage R-K–type needle is introduced into the epidural space through the sacral hiatus or the cervical interlaminar area. A catheter with a soft spring tip (Racz catheter) is passed through the needle and advanced near the suspected pathological site. Contrast is injected to obtain an epidurogram. The presence of excluded or "cut off" nerve root sleeves or epidural filling defects is noted. Hyaluronidase followed by 10% hypertonic saline solution are injected slowly to hydraulically dissect the scar tissue and open the obstructed areas in the epidural space, especially around the spinal nerves. See Figures 18-32 and 18-33.

Postprocedural pain can persist up to three weeks.

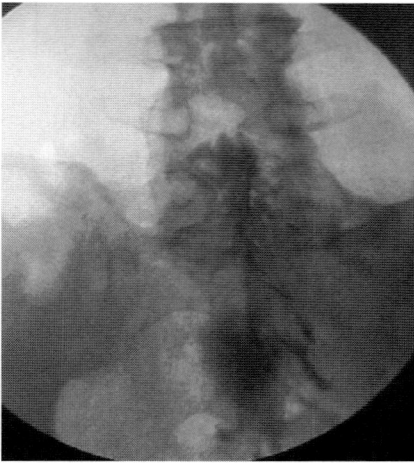

FIGURE 18-31
Epidurogram, lumbar, showing epidural
adhesions.

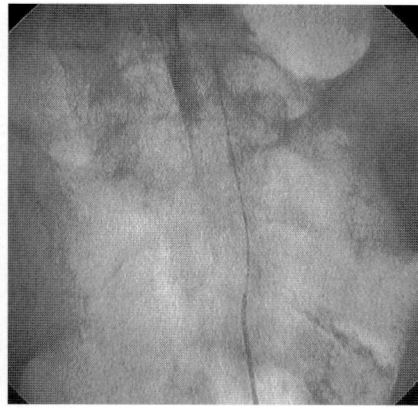

FIGURE 18-32
Racz catheter passed to blockage area.

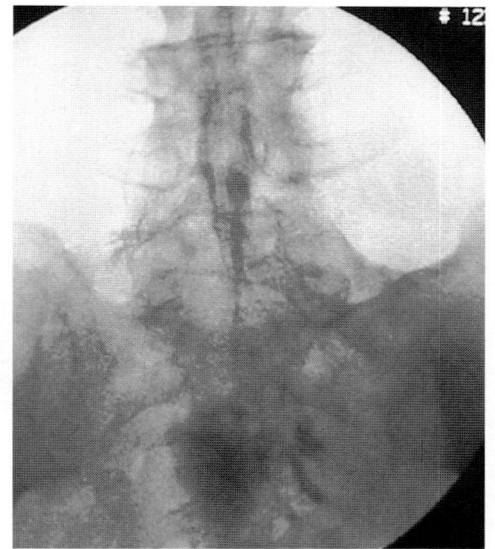

FIGURE 18-33
Epidurogram post lyses of epidural adhesions.

Percutaneous Disc Decompression

Part of the vertebral disc nucleus is removed mechanically via a needle introduced percutaneously into the disc.

Indications   The principal indication for therapeutic percutaneouds discectomy is a small, contained disc herniation with a large annular tear. A CT discogram and nerve root confirmatory block should be done prior to the procedure in order to evaluate the annular tear and to confirm the painful disc and nerve root.

Procedure   Sterility and use of antibiotics are strictly observed as in the case of performing a discogram. The disc is approached from the pathological side. A 17-gage needle trochar is introduced into the disc. A motorized augur tip cannula is passed through the trochar into the disc and advanced to the inner border of the anterolateral annulus. The motorized cannula is activated, and about 1 to 2 mL of nucleus pulposus is extracted.

Only the lumbar discs are sites for percutaneous disc decompression (Figures 18-34 and 18-35).

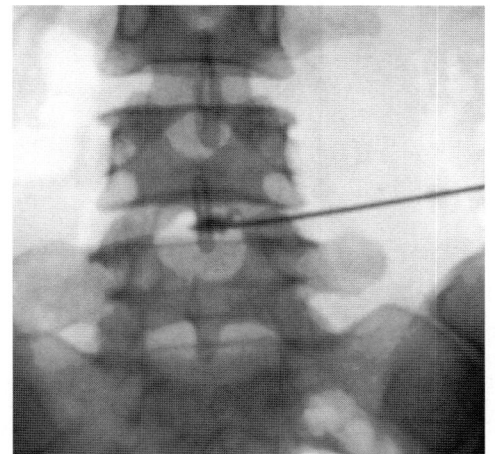

FIGURE 18-34
Percutaneous discectomy, lumbar, anteroposterior view after contrast injection.

Spinal Cord Stimulation

The posterior spinal cord columns are stimulated by a lead introduced into the epidural space resulting in block of the pain pathways.

Indications   Patients with neuropathic limb pain non controllable by medications or less invasive percutaneous procedures are candidates for spinal cord stimulation. Other indications are failed back surgery syndrome, painful arachnoiditis, and ischemic limb pain. A trial is done before the permanent implantation of the lead and stimulator. Many insurance companies request a psychiatric evaluation of the patient prior to the implant of the spinal cord stimulator.

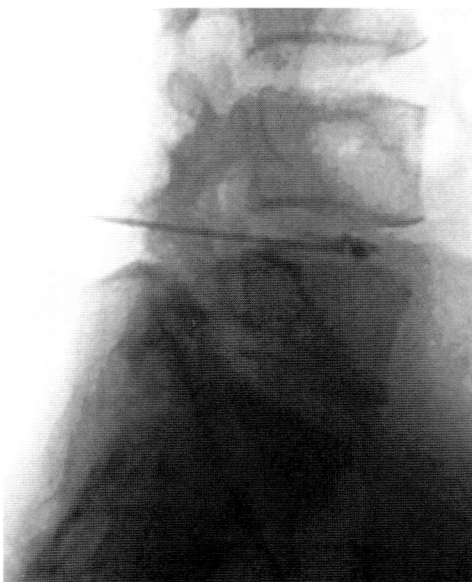

FIGURE 18-35
Percutaneous discectomy, lumbar, anteroposterior view after contrast injection.

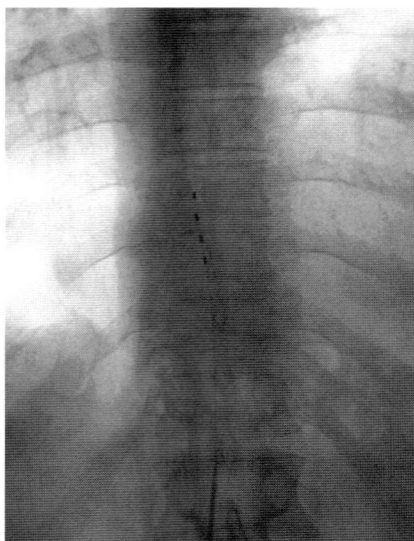

FIGURE 18-36
Percutanous lead for spinal cord stimulation of a unilateral neuropathic lower limb, anteroposterior view.

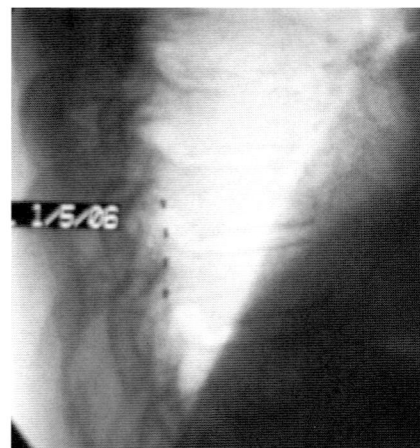

FIGURE 18-37
Percutanous lead for spinal cord stimulation of a unilateral neuropathic lower limb, lateral view.

Procedure Under local anesthesia and conscious sedation a percutaneous lead is introduced via a Touhy-type spinal needle into the epidural space and advanced to the spinal cord level corresponding to the neuropathic nerve. When the lead is in place a stimulation trial is performed and the lead is adjusted to obtain maximum pain relief. The percutaneous lead is attached to an external stimulator and the patient usually goes home for few days to try the system during his routine daily activities. About a week later the percutaneous lead is removed. After waiting at least another week the permanent system is implanted if the patient liked the pain relief obtained during the trial and there was more than 50% decrease of the pain or consumption of pain medications. See Figures 18-36 and 18-37.

Bibliography

Adams M, Bogduk N, Burton K, Dolan P: The biomechanics of back pain. Churchill Livingstone, 2004.

Bogduk N: Practice guidelines for spinal diagnostic and treatment procedures. International Spine Intervention Society, 2004.

Bogduk N, McGuirk B: Medical management of acute and chronic low back pain. An evidence-based approach. Pain Res Clin Manage 13, 2002.

Fenton D, Czervionke L: Image-guided spine intervention. Saunders, 2003.

Gauci A: Manual of RF techniques. Flivopress, 2004.

Herkowitz H, Dvorak J, Bell G, Nordin M, Grob D: The lumbar spine, 3rd edition. [Official publication of the International Society for the Study of the Lumbar Spine.] Lippincott, 2004.

Kraemer J, Koester O: MR imaging of the lumbar spine, a teaching atlas. Thieme, 2003.

McKay Best T: Fluoroscopy manual for pain management. Pain Management Innovations, 2000.

Raj P: Practical management of pain, 3rd edition. Mosby, 2000.

Raj P, Lou L, Erdine S, Staas P, Waldman S: Radiographic imaging for regional anesthesia and pain management. Churchill Livingstone, 2003.

Renfrew D: Atlas of spine injections. Saunders, 2004.

Sluijter M: Radiofrequency. Part I. Flivopress, 2001.

Sluijter M: Radiofrequency. Part II. Flivopress, 2001.

Tehranzadeh J: Interventional procedures in musculoskeletal radiology. I. Interventional techniques. Radiol Clin N Am 36 (3): 463–508.

Waldman S: Interventional pain management, 2nd edition. Saunders, 2001.

INDEX